Vegetarian Sports Nutrition

D. Enette Larson-Meyer, PhD, RD

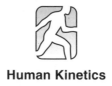

Human Kinetics

Library of Congress Cataloging-in-Publication Data

Larson-Meyer, D. Enette, 1963-
  Vegetarian sports nutrition / D. Enette Larson-Meyer.
    p. cm.
  Includes bibliographical references and index.
  ISBN-13: 978-0-7360-6361-6 (soft cover)
  ISBN-10: 0-7360-6361-7 (soft cover)
  1. Athletes--Nutrition. 2. Vegetarians--Nutrition. I. Title.
  TX361.A8L37 2007
  613.2'62024796--dc22
                                    2006013854
ISBN-10: 0-7360-6361-7
ISBN-13: 978-0-7360-6361-6

The Web addresses cited in this text were current as of June 12, 2006.

Acquisitions Editor: Martin Barnard; **Developmental Editor:** Leigh Keylock; **Assistant Editors:** Laura Koritz, Christine Horger; **Copyeditor:** Annette Pierce; **Proofreader:** Jim Burns; **Indexer:** Betty Frizzéll; **Permission Manager:** Carly Breeding; **Graphic Designer:** Robert Reuther; **Graphic Artist:** Sandra Meier; **Photo Manager:** Laura Fitch; **Cover Designer:** Keith Blomberg; **Photographer (cover):** © Skip Brown/National Geographic/Getty Images; **Art Manager:** Kelly Hendren; **Illustrator:** Figure 11.1 © Fairman Studios, LLC; all other art by Accurate Art, Inc.; **Printer:** Versa Press

Human Kinetics books are available at special discounts for bulk purchase. Special editions or book excerpts can also be created to specification. For details, contact the Special Sales Manager at Human Kinetics.

Printed in the United States of America   10   9   8   7   6   5

The paper in this book is certified under a sustainable forestry program.

Human Kinetics
Web site: www.HumanKinetics.com

United States: Human Kinetics
P.O. Box 5076
Champaign, IL 61825-5076
800-747-4457
e-mail: humank@hkusa.com

Canada: Human Kinetics
475 Devonshire Road, Unit 100
Windsor, ON N8Y 2L5
800-465-7301 (in Canada only)
e-mail: info@hkcanada.com

Europe: Human Kinetics
107 Bradford Road
Stanningley
Leeds LS28 6AT, United Kingdom
+44 (0)113 255 5665
e-mail: hk@hkeurope.com

Australia: Human Kinetics
57A Price Avenue
Lower Mitcham, South Australia 5062
08 8372 0999
e-mail: info@hkaustralia.com

New Zealand: Human Kinetics
P.O. Box 80
Torrens Park, South Australia 5062
0800 222 062
e-mail: info@hknewzealand.com

This book was written in memory of Dr. Roland L. Weinsier, MD, DrPH, a wonderful teacher, mentor, and scientist who lived an active vegetarian lifestyle.

It is dedicated to my husband, Michael, and our growing young vegetarian athletes, Lindsey, Marlena, and Ian.

And also to all the athletes, coaches, trainers, research volunteers, and training partners whom I have worked and trained with over the years. This book would not have been possible without your dedication.

Foreword. vi

Introduction. vii

1 **Gaining the Vegetarian Advantage** 1

2 **Getting Adequate Calories
From Plant Sources.** 13

3 **Finding the Right Carbohydrate Mix** 23

4 **Choosing Smart Fat Over No Fat.** 39

5 **Building Muscle Without Meat** 55

6 **Optimizing Bone Health** 65

7 **Boosting Iron Intake and Absorption.** 81

8 **Breaking Free
of Multivitamin Dependence** 95

9 **Prioritizing Eating Before,
During, and After Events.** 115

Contents

10 **Choosing Whether to Supplement** 135

11 **Reducing Muscle Cramps
and Inflammation** 151

12 **Creating a Customized Meal Plan** 171

13 **Adapting the Plan to Manage Weight** . . .189

14 **Whipping Up Quick Vegetarian
Meals and Snacks** 209

Appendix A Energy Costs of Physical Activity **227**

Appendix B Food Guidance Systems **230**

Appendix C Glycemic Index of Common Foods **232**

Appendix D Dietary Reference Intakes for Vitamins and Minerals **233**

Appendix E Metric Conversions for Common Measures **236**

Bibliography **237**

Index **257**

About the Author **263**

Foreword

With the widespread use of performance-enhancing products at all levels of sport, it is obvious the extreme measures that athletes will take in an attempt to be stronger and faster. Many athletes are constantly in search of a quick fix to optimize performance. That supposed quick fix is really just a shortcut and hardly ever works. If it does work, it likely is a temporary benefit at the expense of athletes' health.

As a competitive athlete and coach, I know there are no shortcuts. Athletes become their best—and gain better health—by getting back to the basics. More than anything else, hard work, intelligent training, adequate recovery, and good nutrition will help athletes develop to their potential. When it comes to nutrition, athletes are often overwhelmed with misinformation and marketing of fad diets and products that result in a haphazard approach of trying extreme plans that yield poor results and poor health. A plant-based diet returns athletes to the sound principles of nutrition that truly lead to optimal performance and health.

When I was introduced to a vegetarian diet in 1997, I admit it was with some reservation. Initially I was drawn to a plant-based diet not for its performance-enhancing effects but for the long-term health of my body and the planet. My reservations were sprouted by the common myths that a plant-based diet is inadequate in protein and calories, resulting in a lack of strength and endurance. Many athletes told me how they had tried a vegetarian diet only to feel depleted of energy. I questioned their results and efforts, deciding to take the initiative to learn as much as I could about sports nutrition and a plant-based diet. I focused my energies on making gradual changes. I chose not to simply eliminate animal products but to carefully learn how to replace those nutrient sources. What I found was a whole new world of foods to incorporate into my diet and exciting new lifestyle. By including a variety of whole foods, I not only avoided many of the pitfalls that others encountered, but I found myself with even more stamina as well. My performances continued to improve year after year, and I recovered from workouts and races more quickly than I had in years past.

With careful planning and a desire to explore the world of plant-based foods, all athletes can discover their bodies' potential. Dr. Larson-Meyer has done all athletes a great service by combining the current research and her wealth of experience to present *Vegetarian Sports Nutrition*. Whether you're a new or long-time vegetarian, or any type of athlete wanting to incorporate aspects of a plant-based diet into your regimen, *Vegetarian Sports Nutrition* provides the essential knowledge for optimal performance and health in a clear and concise manner. Such a comprehensive and evidence-based book has been long awaited by many athletes.

Scott Jurek
Seven-time consecutive winner and course record holder of the Western States 100-Mile Endurance Run; two-time consecutive winner and course record holder of the Badwater Ultramarathon

Introduction

Everyone is an athlete. The only
difference is that some of us are
in training, and some are not.

George Sheehan

Vegetarian athletes are a dedicated bunch! We head out for early-morning workouts while the rest of the world is still asleep, and we monitor our intake of animal products. Eating well is as important to us as keeping our bodies fit and healthy. Although most of us strive to eat a balanced plant-based diet, things do not always go as planned. Eating is sometimes haphazard and unbalanced, and we find, as we should, that this can take its toll on training, performance, and health.

This book is dedicated to active vegetarians and vegetarian athletes in all sports and of all ages and abilities—from the casual and recreational athlete to the world-class competitor—as well as to semivegetarian athletes contemplating a shift to a more vegetarian diet. Its purpose is to help athletes gain or maintain optimal nutrition for peak performance and health. The advice is based on the latest scientific knowledge combined with practical experience from my nearly 20 years as a sport dietitian, scientist, and vegetarian recreational runner and cyclist.

Specifically, this book is designed to help you optimize your training, performance, and health through better food choices. The book reviews the latest information on fueling athletic performance and offers suggestions on how you—as a busy vegetarian athlete—can easily meet your energy, carbohydrate, protein, fat, fluid, and vitamin and mineral needs. It contains sections that allow you to assess your current diet and tailor food intake according to training and wellness goals. The book also discusses many topics that periodically trouble athletes, including questions about vitamin and mineral supplements and ergogenic aids, the need for a translation of the latest nutrition lingo (including omega-3s, the carbohydrate-to-protein ratio, and the glycemic index), and the struggles associated with losing weight, gaining muscle, or remaining injury free. In addition, the last chapter focuses on vegetarian athletes who live in and cook in the real world (and a real kitchen). In a nutshell, the book provides vegetarian athletes with the tools for making consistent food choices to optimize training, peak performance, and good health.

Keep the training and the faith!

1

Gaining the Vegetarian Advantage

I met my husband on a hilly century ride—a 100-mile (160 km) bicycle ride—in the mining country just north of Phoenix. After riding with him and his buddy for a few miles, he asked me—out of the blue—if I was vegetarian. I was taken aback at first and was almost offended. I nearly snapped back, "Do I look like a vegetarian?" He skirted the question at first, explaining that he, as a physician, had been reading some of Dean Ornish's work and that he was very interested in the health aspects of vegetarian diets. He then told me that he had never known a vegetarian and finally replied, "Yes, you do look like someone who is healthy and might be vegetarian."

The rest is history. I ended up dropping him somewhere around the 70-mile (112 km) mark and—after our first date at a vegetarian restaurant—he gave up flesh foods and now kicks my butt in most athletic endeavors. I still wonder to this day, however, if it was just a lucky guess or if I somehow looked like I had the vegetarian advantage.

Scientific evidence collected over the last 10 to 20 years (since the mid-1980s or so) has noticeably changed our understanding of the role of vegetarian diets in human health and disease prevention. Vegetarian diets appear to be advantageous over omnivorous, or meat-containing, diets for promoting health and longevity, suggesting that indeed there may be a vegetarian advantage. Although our knowledge is far from complete regarding the benefits of vegetarian eating on the health and performance of athletes, it is clear that athletes at all levels can experience the vegetarian advantage.

The topic of vegetarian sports nutrition is becoming increasingly popular. It appears, for instance, that more and more athletes and active people are adopting vegetarian diets. Many more are probably interested but may not know how or if a vegetarian diet is compatible with peak performance. Although we don't know exactly how many athletes are vegetarian, we do know that many well-known (and even not-so-well-known) athletes are vegetarian, including six-time Ironman triathlon champion Dave Scott (vegan), vegan ultramarathoner and seven-time winner of the Western States Endurance Run Scott Jurek, French Olympic figure skater Surya Bonaly, Heisman Trophy–winning football player Desmond Howard, basketball center Robert Parish, powerlifter Bill Manetti, and tennis champions Martina Navratilova and Billie Jean King (see www.veggie.org).

We also have an idea that the percentage of athletes who are vegetarian is likely to be similar to that reported for the general population. The most recent estimates suggest that 2.8 percent of American adults[18] and 4 percent of Canadian adults[2] report following a vegetarian diet. The numbers are even higher when people who are "mostly vegetarian" but eat fish or poultry on occasion are included. For example, according to estimates from the Vegetarian Resource Group,[18] an additional 1.2 percent of American adults occasionally consumes fish but does not eat poultry or red meat. Furthermore, an estimated 30 to 40 percent of the U.S. population report having an interest in meatless food products, meaning that they are likely to fall in the semivegetarian category. Many may even be contemplating vegetarianism.

This chapter introduces the concept of vegetarian eating, reviews the potential benefits of vegetarian diets on health and performance, and offers tips—for those not yet vegetarian—on making the first steps toward gaining the vegetarian advantage. For both veteran vegetarians and those who are new, this chapter is also intended to help strengthen your belief in vegetarian practices whether they can be documented scientifically or simply felt intuitively (or even spiritually). The ensuing chapters are intended to help you understand and overcome the potential nutritional challenges and further your progress in gaining the vegetarian advantage. This advantage will help you feel and perform your best in your chosen sport or activity—whether it be running, cycling, swimming, soccer, tennis, golf, Olympic lifting, dancing, walking, or netball. *Is* there a vegetarian advantage? I truly believe there is.

Types of Vegetarian Athletes

The motivations for following vegetarian diets are numerous—in both athletes and nonathletes—and include health, ecological, religious, spiritual, economical, ethical, and other reasons. The most common reasons, however, are health benefits, animal rights, and spiritual beliefs. Environmental concerns, nevertheless, are becoming increasingly widespread as more and more people recognize that raising meat uses more land and resources than planting crops does. Not surprisingly, these different rationales for vegetarianism mean that vegetarians are not the same in their beliefs or their food choices. Although attempts have been made to categorize vegetarians into groups based on food choices (see box 1.1), I find that these categories don't always fit and unnecessarily label people, mainly because vegetarianism encompasses a spectrum of eating philosophies and practices that aren't easily categorized. For example, two lacto–ovo vegetarian runners may have different philosophies about dairy products. One may consume several servings of dairy products per day, and the other may consume dairy only when it is found as an ingredient in prepared foods or offered as a dish of ice cream. Similarly, some vegans may be extremely strict, eliminating all commercially prepared foods that are processed with or contain animal derivatives (e.g., commercial bread or granulated sugar), and another will simply avoid foods of obvious animal origin and show up to practice in leather athletic shoes. All are vegetarian and all have unique needs that are independent of their vegetarian classification.

Although categorizing can serve its purposes—for example, in the food labeling of vegan products—I think it is more important that athletes understand how their individual philosophies and food preferences potentially influence their nutrient intake. That said, I also think it is important to include occasional fish and poultry eaters and semivegetarians in the ranks of vegetarian athletes. I hope this will not rankle purists. In my experience training with and professionally counseling

---

Box
1.1

Types of Vegetarians

The four major groups, according to the Vegetarian Resource Group:
 - ➤ Lacto–ovo vegetarian: Does not eat meat, fish, or fowl; eats dairy and egg products
 - ➤ Ovo vegetarian: Does not eat meat, fish, fowl, or dairy; eats eggs
 - ➤ Lacto vegetarian: Does not eat meat, fish, fowl, or eggs; eats dairy products
 - ➤ Vegan: Does not eat any animal products, including meat, fish, fowl, eggs, dairy, and honey; most vegans also do not use animal products such as silk, leather, and wool

In addition, the following categories can be considered vegetarian:

 - ➤ Macrobiotic vegetarian: Avoids most animal-derived foods and emphasizes unprocessed organic foods
 - ➤ Pesco vegetarian: Does not eat red meat or fowl; eats dairy and egg products and fish occasionally
 - ➤ Pollo vegetarian: Does not eat red meat or fish; eats dairy and egg products and fowl occasionally
 - ➤ Semivegetarian: Tries to limit meat intake

Reprinted courtesy of The Vegetarian Resource Group.
www.vrg.org

fellow vegetarian athletes, I have found that many do occasionally choose to eat fish or poultry when they are attending social events or feeling somewhat insecure about their nutrition. One study of vegetarians living in Vancouver, British Columbia, documented similar findings, noting that 57 percent admitted to occasional intake of fish and 18 percent admitted to occasional intake of chicken.[4] On the other hand, many vegetarian athletes want to move toward more strict practices. According to the study of the Vancouver vegetarians, 62 percent, including four of six vegans, reported that their diets had become more restrictive over time, and 53 percent planned additional changes, most frequently a reduction in the use of dairy products.[4]

The Vegetarian Advantage

Many have felt the vegetarian advantage. I felt it the semester I gave up meat immediately after my first anatomy lab as a college junior (when I realized perhaps for the first time what meat really was). I gained nearly 7 pounds (3.2 kg) that semester as I frantically ate peanut butter and cheese and sprinkled sunflower seeds on everything to ensure that I got enough protein (the protein myth is discussed further in chapter 5). Despite the weight gain, I felt better than I ever had. I noticed an improvement in my general well-being after changing to a vegetarian diet, as did most of the female athletes in an Israeli study.[19]

Daniel, as described in the Bible, also felt it. Daniel (after being determined to be handsome, intelligent, and well trained enough to serve in the royal court) made up his mind not to let himself become ritually unclean by eating the food and drinking the wine of the royal court. He went to the guard who was placed in charge of him and his three friends and said, "Test us for 10 days. Give us vegetables to eat and water to drink. Then compare us with the young men who are eating the food of the royal court, and base your decision on how we look." Ten days later, Daniel and his friends "looked healthier and stronger than all those who had been eating the royal food" and were then allowed to "eat vegetables instead of what the king provided" (Daniel 1:8-16, Good News Bible). The feeling noted by Daniel perhaps summarizes why many major religions, except Christianity in general, emphasize vegetarian practices for spiritual reasons, healing, or meditation.

Historical records also tell us that many of the athletes of the ancient Olympics may have also felt the vegetarian advantage. Despite the fact that the most widely quoted account of an athlete of antiquity is that of the legendary wrestler, Milo of Croton, who reportedly ate a gargantuan amount of meat, the diet of most ancient-Olympic athletes was most likely vegetarian.[17] Their diets, like that of most Greeks and Romans of the time, consisted mostly of cereals, fruits, vegetables, legumes, and wine diluted with water. When meat was consumed, it consisted mostly of goat (in Greece) and pig (in Rome) flesh.[41] In fact, the earliest Greek athlete whose special diet was recorded was Charmis of Sparta, whose training diet is said to have consisted of dried figs.[20]

What Science Says

Unfortunately, we can't measure the full aspect of the vegetarian advantage and prove, for example, that switching to a vegetarian diet will promote a greater sense of well-being or improve health in its full definition. This definition—derived from the Old English word for *hale*—includes being whole and hearty and of sound mind, body [and spirit] and having the capacity to live, work, and interact joyfully with [nature] and other human beings.[8] We can, however, look at the scientific evidence supporting the advantage of the vegetarian diet compared to the typical Western diet on both physical health (from the perspective of disease risk) and performance. Admittedly, the evidence is much stronger for health advantages than for performance advantages, which should be motivating by itself, but there are also interesting indications that plant-based diets may aid in training and exercise recovery.

Potential Health Benefits

Research has shown time and time again that vegetarians living in affluent countries enjoy remarkably good health, exemplified by less obesity, high blood pressure, heart disease, diabetes, dementia, and many cancers.[1, 5] Vegetarians also appear to live longer and healthier lives.[13] The reasons for these positive health effects, however, are difficult to pinpoint and may be related to the absence of meat, the greater variety and amount of plant foods, or other lifestyle practices associated with vegetarianism. Undeniably, current evidence suggests that all three may be involved in the vegetarian advantage.[46] Numerous studies have found that meat intake is associated with increased risk for a variety of chronic diseases including heart disease,[13, 42] diabetes,[42] and some cancers.[13, 16] In contrast, an abundant consumption of fruits and vegetables,[7, 39, 44] legumes, unrefined grains,[14, 23, 24, 30, 39] and nuts[14, 22, 40] is

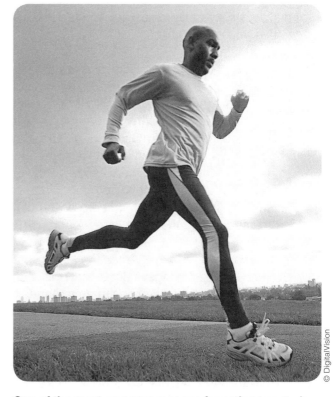

© DigitalVision

One of the most common reasons for eating vegetarian, especially among athletes, is general health benefits.

consistently associated with a lower risk for many chronic degenerative diseases and, in some cases, even with increased longevity. In addition, meat-containing diets are probably not as safe as vegetarian diets because of the recent risk of mad cow disease and elevated mercury levels in certain fish, among other things.

The beneficial effects of plant foods in the prevention of chronic diseases are, however, on their own merit, more definite than the detrimental effects of meat. In fact, large-scale studies among vegetarians and nonvegetarian populations have observed many more correlations between the protective effect of plant foods than the hazardous effects of animal foods.[13] In support of this thinking, recently published findings from the Oxford Vegetarian Study and the Health Food Shoppers Study being conducted throughout England and Wales, found that vegetarians shared similarly lower mortality rates with health-conscious omnivores who regularly shopped at health food stores.[3]

Factoring out the lifestyle factors is a bit more difficult because vegetarians as a group tend to be more physically active, less obese, more health conscious, and perhaps less stressed than their meat-eating counterparts. They also are less likely to smoke. This presents a challenge for researchers assessing the relationships between diet and disease risk, because studies must adjust research data to account for these and other differences between vegetarians and nonvegetarians. Although all major epidemiological studies attempt to statistically control for such confounding factors, study results are still often criticized because it is not possible to fully adjust for all lifestyle differences between vegetarian and nonvegetarian populations.

Fortunately, much data is available from the Adventist Health Study, a long-term study conducted by researchers at Loma Linda University, exploring the links between diet, lifestyle, and disease among Seventh-Day Adventists in the United States and Canada. What is particularly noteworthy about the Adventist Health Study is that it can compare the health risks of vegetarians (who make up 40 percent of the Adventist population), occasional meat eaters, and nonvegetarians in a population with a generally similar lifestyle. Adventists, for example, attend religious services regularly and are health conscious. They do not smoke or drink alcoholic beverages and most avoid coffee and tea. Hence, findings for the study provide more powerful (or should we say less murky) evidence supporting the benefits of vegetarian diets because the lifestyles of the vegetarians and meat eaters tend to be quite similar.

The findings from the Adventist Health Study are summarized in table 1.1. Collectively, the findings indicate that both increased plant foods and decreased animal flesh offer positive health advantages. Quite interestingly, the Adventists think it is no coincidence that the results independently emphasize the protective qualities of seeds such as nuts, beans, whole grains, and fruits because in the first chapter of the Bible, it reads that God said, "I have provided all kinds of grain and all kinds of fruit for you to eat but for all the wild animals and all the birds I have provided leafy plants for food" (Genesis 1:29, Good News Bible).

TABLE 1.1   Findings From the Adventist Health Study Conducted in Seventh-Day Adventists (SDA) in the United States and Canada

Cancer	A vegetarian diet is associated with a lower risk for prostate and colon cancers but not necessarily for cancers of the lung, breast, uterus, or stomach. Specifically, nonvegetarians have a 54% greater risk for prostate cancer and 88% greater risk for colon cancer. Frequent beef consumption increases risk for bladder cancer Legume consumption reduces risk for colon and pancreatic cancers. Higher consumption of all fruit (and dried fruit) lowers risk of lung, prostate, and pancreatic cancers.
Dementia	Meat consumption increases the risk for dementia. People who eat meat are more than twice as likely to develop dementia. People who have eaten meat for many years are more than three times as likely to develop signs of dementia.
Diabetes	Vegetarian diets appear to lower risk for type 2 diabetes. Self-reported diabetes among SDAs is less than half that reported by the general population. Among SDAs, vegetarians have lower risk of diabetes mellitus than semivegetarians and nonvegetarians.
Heart disease	Following a vegetarian, vegan, or fish-containing diet reduces the risk of heart disease. Vegetarian men have a 37% reduced risk of developing ischemic heart disease compared with nonvegetarians. Mortality from ischemic heart disease is 20% lower in occasional meat eaters, 34% lower in people who eat fish (but not meat), 34% lower in lacto–ovo vegetarians, and 26% lower in vegans compared to regular meat eaters. Beef consumption increases heart disease risk in men but not necessarily in women. Men who eat beef three or more times a week are more than twice as likely to have fatal ischemic heart disease than are vegetarians. Eating nuts and whole grains provides a protective effect against fatal and nonfatal ischemic heart disease in both men and women. People who eat nuts five or more times a week have approximately half the risk of those who eat nuts less than once a week. People who consume mainly whole-wheat bread have 59% lower risk for nonfatal coronary heart disease, and 89% lower risk for fatal heart disease compared to those who mainly consume white bread.
Hypertension	Following a vegetarian diet lowers the risk for hypertension. SDA semivegetarians are 50% more likely to have hypertension than SDA vegetarians.
Arthritis	Following a vegetarian diet lowers risk for arthritis. SDA vegetarians are at a lower risk of arthritis than nonvegetarians are.

Combined data from five prospective studies that included the Adventist Health Study[13, 15, 26, 42]

Potential Performance Benefits

Much less is known about whether a vegetarian diet offers training or sport performance advantages. Although a handful of studies in the early 1900s investigated the value of a vegetarian diet as a means of increasing physical capacity, most of these studies were not scientifically rigorous—at least based on today's standards.[33] In a few cases, the studies may have produced the answers the investigator or athlete desired, which of course was that a vegetarian diet is superior to a flesh-containing diet.

One of these studies, conducted by a professor of political economy at Yale University, consisted of a series of endurance tests made on 49 people the professor classified as flesh-eating athletes, flesh-abstaining (vegetarian) athletes, and sedentary flesh abstainers (vegetarians).[12] The endurance tasks involved holding the arms horizontally, performing deep knee bending, and doing leg raises (lying on the back) for as long as possible. The investigators found that vegetarian athletes had considerably more endurance than the flesh-eating athletes and that many of the untrained vegetarians were also able to outendure the flesh-eating athletes. In a similar type of experiment, a Belgian researcher determined that vegetarian students had greater endurance of the forearm than meat-eating students.[6] Forearm endurance was determined by measuring the maximum number of times the students could lift a weight on a pulley by squeezing a handle. The vegetarians performed an average of 69 reps, and the meat eaters performed 38.

The early research may have been provoked by reports that vegetarian athletes living in Europe and America were outperforming their meat-eating rivals and setting records in cycling, distance footraces, swimming, tennis, and the marathon[33] (see table 1.2). The United States' Will Brown, for example, who in the late 1890s switched to a vegetarian diet for health reasons, thrashed all records for the 3,218-kilometer (2,000-mile) bicycle race. About 20 years later in 1912, a runner named Kolehmainen became one of the first men to run a marathon (26.2 miles [42 km]) in less than 2 hours, 30 minutes.[33]

Why the vegetarians seemed to demonstrate superior endurance performance is certainly intriguing but, as the early investigators themselves noted, it may have been partially explained by grit and partially explained by the motivation of the vegetarians to outdo their meat-eating rivals,[12] probably something understood by many vegetarian athletes. Another reason for the increased endurance of the

TABLE 1.2 Early Feats of Vegetarian Athletes

Year	Athletic feat
1896	James Parsley led the London Vegetarian Cycling Club to victory over two nonvegetarian clubs. A week later he won the most prestigious hill-climbing race in England, breaking the hill-climbing record by nearly a minute. Other members of the club also performed remarkably.
1890s	Will Brown thrashed all records for the 3,218-km (2,000-mile) bicycle race, and Margarita Gast established a women's record for the 1,609-km (1,000-mile) race.
1893	The first two competitors to racewalk the 599 kilometers (372 miles) from Berlin to Vienna were vegetarians.
1890s (late)	Eleven of the first 14 finishers in the 100-km (62-mile) foot race across Germany were vegetarian.
1912	Kolehmainen was one of the first men to complete the marathon in less than 2 hours, 30 minutes.
Early 1900s	The West Ham Vegetarian Society fielded an undefeated tug-of-war team.

Data from D.C. Nieman, 1999, "Physical fitness and vegetarian diets: is there a relation?," *Am J Clin Nutr.* 70: 570S-575S.

vegetarians—which was not yet understood in the early 1900s—was that the carbohydrate content of the vegetarian diet was most likely much higher than that of the meat eaters.[33] Higher carbohydrate intake would give the vegetarians an endurance advantage over their opponents.

In recent years, however, the advantage in endurance performance noted in the early vegetarians has not been evident. Better-controlled comparisons have found that vegetarian men and women have aerobic or anaerobic capacities that are similar to their equally trained meat-eating counterparts[19] and also perform similarly when challenged to a 1,000-kilometer (621-mile) endurance run.[11] Short-term intervention studies that have placed omnivorous athletes on a vegetarian diet have not found this to benefit (or hinder) performance. In one investigation, the strength and endurance performance of eight male omnivorous athletes was found to be unaltered when they were randomly assigned to a lacto–ovo vegetarian diet for six weeks compared to their performance on a meat-rich diet for six weeks.[36, 38]

Indeed, even though science lacks proof that a vegetarian diet offers short-term advantage to athletic performance, this should not dissuade you from starting or sticking to a vegetarian plan. Most of the studies have been conducted only in the short term and focused simply on the completion of an exercise task under the controlled conditions of a laboratory. As athletes, we know that peak performance on the field or during a race draws on many things and often takes years of training (and eating) to achieve. Hence, to truly prove a benefit to athletic performance, scientists would have to somehow clone a group of athletes and compare how they performed over a lifetime as a vegetarian and as a meat eater. Alternately, scientists could follow closely matched vegetarian and meat-eating athletes to determine which group was more likely to perform better over the long run, and like in the Adventist Health Studies, adjust for known confounding variables such as training, motivation, injury, and overall nutrition. Despite the elusiveness of this concept, however, we can focus on the potential benefits of a vegetarian diet on recovery and, as mentioned earlier, its role in keeping us healthy as we train.

Potential Benefits During Recovery

Plant-based diets are abundant in antioxidant vitamins and many plant chemicals—called phytochemicals[43]—that may protect against more than just cancer and heart disease. Many of these compounds are able to sequester reactive by-products—called free radicals—that are produced in muscle during strenuous exercise. These reactive by-products are thought to promote exercise-induced injury to muscle proteins and contribute to muscle fatigue[35] and soreness. Although the body has a complex defense mechanism that aids in eliminating free radicals, dietary antioxidants interact cooperatively with this system to help control and sequester free radicals.

Studies have noted convincingly that vegetarians have higher circulating concentrations of the antioxidant vitamins (vitamin C, vitamin E, and beta-carotene)[29, 37] and possibly also higher levels of other beneficial phytochemicals. To this end, studies have also found—quite excitingly—that vegetarians experience less damage from free radicals to DNA (our body's genetic material) in the blood[27] and less lipid peroxidation, or damage by free radicals to lipid-containing structures.[28] Although studies have not yet addressed whether a vegetarian diet protects against free-radical damage in muscle (as it does in blood), several studies have found that supplementation with certain antioxidants reduces damage to the lipid components in the muscle cell.[10, 25, 35, 45] A recent study also found that consuming a drink containing black grape, raspberry, and red currant concentrates reduced exercise-induced oxidative stress and possibly also muscle damage.[31]

Hence, high levels of dietary antioxidant vitamins or phytochemicals may perhaps protect the muscles against free-radical damage or assist in reducing inflammation. Studies from my days as a postdoctoral student at the University of Alabama at Birmingham supported this thinking. We became interested in the exercise-overstress response in muscle, which is a phenomenon endurance athletes experience after an intense effort.[32] During exercise overstress, the muscle becomes damaged and is temporarily unable to produce high levels of energy using oxidative processes until recovery, which takes several weeks to several months depending on the severity of the initial performance effort. While attempting to recreate this overstress response, we measured many athletes before and after a marathon race or a bout of strenuous jumping in the laboratory and found that we were able to induce overstress only in the nonvegetarian subjects. The vegetarians were somehow protected, which we hypothesized was due to the high levels of antioxidants in their diets.

Do Only Purists Gain the Advantage?

Perhaps a final lingering question is whether athletes have to be purists to gain the vegetarian advantage. I think not. Although there are areas where an exclusively plant-based diet appears to produce a health advantage over dairy-containing diets, there are also cases—as will be reviewed in this book—in which consuming dairy or small amounts of other animal foods, such as fish, may make it easier to meet daily nutrient requirements without supplements. This does not imply, however, that animal foods are needed in any way, shape, or form for the diet to be nutritionally adequate. It does mean, though, that athletes who choose to eat a little fish or chicken now and again are probably just as likely to reap the major advantages of vegetarianism as a purist. The important thing is simply that you eat a diet containing ample cereals, grains, fruits, vegetables, and legumes—and limit the consumption of animal foods to fit your health and personal philosophy.

To add a little humor to this discussion, I know for certain that there are times when many vegetarian athletes have had to decide whether to pick the pepperoni off the pizza. I remember returning from my first double-century bicycle race (320 km) and finding that what I was most craving—hot vegetable soup—was made with floating specks of beef. I also remember my racing partners eating hot chili after a rainy March 10K, which prompted me to drive for miles in search of a vegetarian bowl, which I never found. Most notably, I remember asking the race director of a local bike ride to order vegetarian pizza, only to find that the

Box
1.2

Steps for an Easy Transition
to a Vegetarian Diet

1. Take stock of your current diet.

> Make a list of the foods and meals that you normally eat.

> Identify the foods and meals that are vegetarian, and build from these as a foundation. Examples include spaghetti with marinara sauce, bean burritos, or cheese sandwiches.

> Plan to eat a vegetarian meal several times a week using foods you know and enjoy.

2. Add more vegetarian meals by revising favorite recipes that are meat based.

For example, chili can be made using beans, textured vegetable protein (TVP), or tofu in place of ground beef. The beef in spaghetti sauce can be replaced with TVP or sauteed vegetables.

3. Expand your options by finding new recipes in cookbooks and trying different products from the store.

Many vegetarian meals can be made without a recipe and without much time in the kitchen. Try seasoned-rice mixes, spaghetti with sauce from a jar, vegetable chow mein, burritos with canned refried beans, and vegetarian baked beans with rice. Try various brands of vegetarian burgers and meatless hot dogs.

4. Make a list of vegetarian meals that you can eat away from home.

Inventory your options at the cafeteria, nearby restaurants, and convenience stores. Look for vegetarian soups, salads, pasta salads, pasta primavera, vegetable pizza, and baked potatoes. Chinese, Thai, Indian, and Middle Eastern restaurants offer numerous vegetarian entrees. Choices from a convenience store may include a bean burrito or a microwavable frozen entree.

Plan vegetarian meals to go using leftovers from a home-cooked or restaurant meal. Other ideas for portable vegetarian meals include bean or vegetable soup in a thermos, peanut butter and banana sandwiches, bean dip with pita bread or crackers, and cheese with bread and fruit.

5. Eliminate meat at breakfast.

Try some of the meat analogues that look and taste like bacon or sausage to make the change easier.

(continued)

(continued)

---

6. Take stock of your menu once again.

Do your meals include . . .

a variety of grains, legumes and soy products, vegetables, and fruits?

some fresh fruits and vegetables daily? (Aim for at least 5 servings per day.)

primarily whole grains with little processing? (Aim for 6 to 11 servings per day.)

---

faster guys had devoured it, leaving only pepperoni, before I crossed the finish line. Although many of us swear we would never eat meat-contaminated pizza, others would in this or similar situations pick those pieces of pepperoni off that pizza (however, they might dab the pizza with a napkin to remove any remaining highly saturated pepperoni fat). Yes, the world would be much better for vegetarian athletes if race directors just ordered vegetarian for everyone, but in the real world, our decision to occasionally eat meat-contaminated pizza does not make us less-healthy vegetarians. Indeed, some flexibility may help us fit in better with our nonvegetarian teammates, as long as we draw the line when they are headed to Bubba's Pork House for breakfast.

Going and Staying Meatless

Although many readers have been vegetarian for some time, others may be new to vegetarian eating or contemplating going meatless. If you are not yet experiencing the benefits of a vegetarian diet and are ready to move in this direction, the information presented in box 1.2 may be helpful for making an easy and gradual transition. The slow transition—which is generally recommended by dietitians—provides a comfortable progression that allows you time to find new ways to meet nutrient needs without meat. The goal is to make changes that you can live with and that are nutritionally sound. The alternative is the become-vegetarian-overnight approach that I used years ago. Although this approach works for some, it often does not give athletes enough time to educate themselves on vegetarian food choices and patterns. Box 1.2 may also be helpful if you choose the abrupt transition; however, you will have to be diligent in assessing your daily diet and finding ways to satisfy your nutrient needs. If you don't, you may experience a decline in your health and performance related to poor eating, not to the vegetarian diet. Remember that to gain the vegetarian advantage you have to eat soundly.

The remaining chapters of this book should be helpful whether you are a new, transitioning, or veteran vegetarian. They are designed to help you gain the vegetarian advantage, avoid common (and even not so common) dietary pitfalls and fine-tune your diet so that you can feel and train your best. Only then can you perform optimally.

2

Getting Adequate Calories From Plant Sources

A category III (cat III) cyclist came to see me after being coaxed by a local veteran rider. The veteran rider informed me, during a group training ride, that he thought the kid had a lot of potential but that he did not seem to eat well. "The kid" was in his early 20s and had been training hard in hopes of advancing to cat I status. But "I just feel off," he told me during our first session. "Some days I feel OK, but I don't seem to have power in higher gears," he added. With prompting, he described a food intake pattern that seemed sporadic. He also reported that eating often made him feel "bogged down."

To get a better idea of his food and fluid intakes, I asked him to record his training and racing in a log for the following two weeks and to jot down in detail what he ate and drank and when. I also had him stop by his physician's office to have his iron status checked along with a few other things. His blood work came back normal, but the logs were revealing. He had been riding relatively hard six days a week. His rides ranged from easy 35 to 40 milers (56-64 km) followed by several short sprints to grueling hilly 65 milers (105 km) at top pace. I estimated that his energy expenditure on training days ranged from 3,500 to 5,000 calories per day. His reported intake ranged from 1,700 to 2,600 calories per day, with a good portion of that energy coming from a sport beverage taken during training. The only day he came close to meeting his energy needs was on his rest day, when he reported eating slightly more than 3,600 calories.

Although methods for recording food intake often underestimate actual energy (calorie) intake, I had no doubt the "kid" was not getting enough calories to support his intense training efforts. Food made him feel bogged down because he ate only two meals a day and attempted to consume large post-training meals that were not easy to digest, e.g. four pieces of vegetarian lasagna or two large *fast-food bean burritos. He also was not drinking enough during his rides, which contributed to post-training nausea that inhibited his desire to eat (but that is another story). The trick was to teach him the importance of meeting energy needs and help him develop a plan that spread meals and snacks throughout the day.*

Meeting energy needs is the first—yet often neglected—nutritional priority for all athletes. However, discussions about meeting energy needs are usually not a priority unless the athlete needs to lose weight, gain weight, or is vegetarian. Although I sometimes find the latter amusing, I usually find it frustrating. During my years of practice, I have found that certain athletes—vegetarian or not—have trouble meeting energy needs. Typically, the athletes who struggle to meet energy needs require excessively high amounts of energy and make food choices that are bulky or too high in fiber. Many also have hectic schedules that do not allow enough time to eat. A vegetarian diet low in energy-dense foods can contribute to the problem. Therefore, this chapter focuses on enhancing your understanding of your own energy needs, why neglecting these needs over the long run may be a recipe for disaster, and how you, as a vegetarian, can meet these needs.

Energy, Calories, and Joules

In the United States, the term calorie and energy are often used interchangeably. Elsewhere, the joule is used in place of the calorie. Calories and joules are simply terms used to quantify "energy" (see box 2.1). Skipping the hard-core thermodynamics lecture, the body releases the energy stored within the chemical bonds of certain foodstuff and temporarily trap it within the chemical bonds of special molecules called adenosine triphosphate (ATP) and creatine phosphate (PCr). The energy stored within ATP and PCr is ultimately used to fuel muscle activity, producing heat energy. The overall process is similar to using wood to fuel a fire and ultimately producing heat, except that instead of using the energy immediately, the body temporarily stores food energy as ATP. Thus, the body is able to break down the energy stored within the chemical bonds of carbohydrate, protein, fat, and alcohol in food and provide 4, 4, 9, and 7 calories per gram respectively. Vitamins and other organic matter do not provide energy to the body because their chemical bonds cannot be broken down and used as fuel. That said, a calorie and a joule are both simply units of energy.

Energy Needs of Vegetarian Athletes

Daily energy needs vary considerably among individual athletes and depend on many factors. These factors include your body size, body composition, sex, training regimen, and nontraining activity patterns. If you are a teenage or young adult athlete and are still growing, this energy need is also factored into the

Box
2.1

Calories and Joules

The calorie we refer to when we discuss the energy content of food is really a big calorie, or a kilocalorie (kcal). A kilocalorie is the amount of heat required to raise one liter of water 1 degree centigrade from 14.5 to 15.5 degrees Celsius. The joule is the international unit of work or energy. It is the work done by a force equal to one Newton acting over a distance of one meter. The kilocalorie is equivalent to 4.1868 kilojoules.

equation.

Over the last 10 to 15 years researchers have learned a lot about the energy needs of athletes, thanks to the development of a technique called doubly labeled water.[8] This technique has allowed scientists to measure—outside the laboratory—free-living energy expenditure in athletes as they carry out their habitual training. Using this technique, the energy needs of athletes have been shown to vary from approximately 2,600 calories per day in female swimmers[8] to nearly 8,500 calories per day[7] in male cyclists participating in the Tour de France bicycle race. In comparison, the energy expenditure of elite female runners has been estimated to average approximately 2,800 calories per day,[8] and that of elite lightweight female rowers averages to just less than 4,000 calories per day.[10] The energy needs of a male ultramarathoner who ran around the coast of Australia averaged 6,320 calories per day.[9] The energy expenditures of less-competitive, less-active, or smaller athletes, however, are likely to be less than these examples, but certainly much greater than 2,000 calories for women and 2,500 calories for men used as reference intakes on food labels in the United States.

Vegetarianism does not necessarily affect energy needs. Nonetheless, one group of researchers found that the energy needs at rest (termed resting energy expenditure, or REE) were approximately 11 percent higher in a group of 17 young vegan and lacto vegetarian men compared to a group of 40 nonvegetarian men of similar age and aerobic fitness.[23] Although the researchers were not sure why the vegetarians had a slightly higher REE, they speculated that it was the result of the habitual high carbohydrate composition of a vegetarian diet.[23] Other researchers have hypothesized that long-term consumption of high-carbohydrate diets may somehow stimulate the sympathetic nervous system, which is a known stimulator of REE.

Estimating Your Energy Needs

Having a little knowledge of how much energy you need daily to function in your everyday activities as well as train in your given sport should help you meet your energy needs and consume a healthy, well-balanced training diet. Unfortunately, the doubly labeled water technique for measuring energy expenditure is not

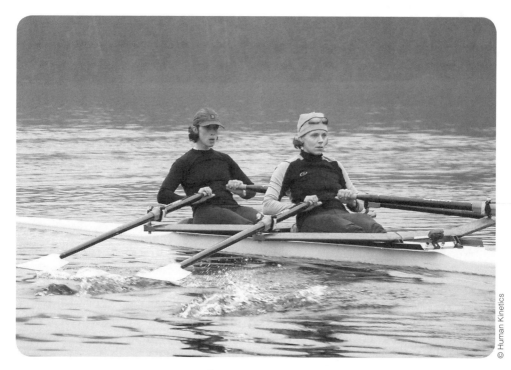

© Human Kinetics

Female rowers have different energy needs than male cyclists, but whatever your sport and body type, you can meet your needs on a vegetarian diet.

available to most athletes, unless you are lucky enough to live near a university or research institution that studies the energy needs of active people. Nevertheless, daily energy expenditure (DEE) can be approximated in several different ways. Before we begin, however, let's look at the components that make up DEE and define your daily energy needs.

In adults, the daily energy requirements are made up of various components, including the energy needed to maintain normal body functions, digest food, perform training and nontraining activities, and handle the aftermath of exercise. Specifically, resting energy expenditure, or REE, is the energy required to maintain normal body functions such as breathing, heart beating, and brain function. The thermic effect of food (TEF) refers to the energy required to digest and metabolize food. Although somewhat self-explanatory, the energy expenditure during training, or TEE, represents the energy expended during scheduled training, practice, and competition sessions that are specifically related to the athlete's sport, whereas the energy expenditure during nontraining activities, or NTEE, is the amount of energy needed to perform all physical activities that are not related to training. These activities include those associated with food preparation, health and hygiene, work, and leisure. Finally, the temporary increase in REE that occurs after a bout of exercise, termed the excess postexercise oxygen consumption, or EPOC, is partially caused by the increase in body temperature, circulation, and ventilation, which remains elevated for a time after exercise, as well as the additional energy required to remove lactate and resynthesize ATP and PCr.

Just how much these components contribute to your daily energy expenditure depend on your activity level. In nonathletes, REE typically makes up about 65 percent of DEE, but it may contribute less than 50 percent of the total needs in athletes who are training heavily. Similarly, the contribution of TEE and NTEE varies with each athlete and depends somewhat on the athlete's nontraining occupation. For example, the NTEE of an athlete whose occupation requires little physical activity (e.g., student, bank associate, secretary) will make up a much smaller part of his or her DEE than the NTEE of an athlete whose occupation requires more physical activity throughout the day (e.g., construction worker, waitress, mail carrier delivering mail on foot). An athlete's TEF and EPOC typically comprise much less of his or her DEE than the other components and, in fact, are often ignored in most methods of prediction because they are typically within the margin of error associated with the estimate. Nonetheless, research has suggested that an estimated 6 to 10 percent of the total energy consumed (or 60 to 100 calories following the consumption of a 1,000-calorie meal) is required to digest and metabolize food and an additional 100 to 200 calories may be needed after particularly long and vigorous training sessions as a result of EPOC.[1]

Although most of the components of energy expenditure need to be measured in a laboratory, a variety of prediction equations derived from laboratory data can be used to estimate DEE or the various components of TEE. Athletes can either directly estimate DEE or estimate DEE from the sum of its components. The easiest method is to directly estimate DEE by multiplying your body weight in kilograms by an activity factor that best describes your physical activity patterns (see box 2.2). By the direct method, your physical activity pattern lumps your training and nontraining activity levels into one package. For active and athletic people, the activity factors are classified as moderate, heavy, or exceptional. *Moderate* describes the activity level of a fitness enthusiast who works out for 30 minutes, three or four times a week. *Exceptional* describes the activity level of an athlete who trains for one to two hours, six days a week. The activity level of ultraendurance athletes or Ironman triathletes is not categorized in this quick method. Nevertheless, this method can at least give you a ballpark idea of your energy needs.

The second method for estimating your daily energy needs is to estimate each of the major components of DEE, and then add them together. Although somewhat cumbersome, estimating DEE from its components accommodates more variation in activity patterns and is the method I have used for years to help educate athletes about their energy needs (see table 2.1). I have found that working through the calculations with athletes helps them realize why energy needs are so high—or why they are not as high as they think—and how changes in their training during the preseason or off-season should influence their energy intake. The activity also helps athletes realize how their activities of daily living, including sitting at a desk or with their feet propped up watching television, influence their daily energy needs.

Box
2.2

Quick Calculation
for Estimating Daily Energy Needs

Obtain weight in kilograms (weight in pounds divided by 2.2). Estimate daily energy expenditure (DEE) by multiplying body weight in kilograms by the appropriate energy expenditure factor below (kcal/kg/day).

Category	Energy expenditure (kcal/kg/day)
MODERATE ACTIVITY	
Men	41
Women	37
HEAVY ACTIVITY	
Men	50
Women	44
EXCEPTIONAL ACTIVITY	
Men	58
Women	51

Adapted, by permission, from M. Manore and J. Thompson, 2000, *Sport nutrition for health and performance* (Champaign, IL: Human Kinetics), 473.

Dangers of Inadequate Energy Intake

To perform optimally and maintain good health, all athletes need to strive for what scientists call a neutral energy balance. A neutral energy balance is simply a condition in which the sum of energy consumed from food, fluids, and supplements equals the energy expended during rest, daily living, and sport-related activity. Although some athletes may need to tilt the energy balance to gain or lose body mass, which is discussed in chapter 13, it is important for athletes to maintain this energy balance, particularly during the season and during times of high-volume aerobic or strength training.

Sufficient energy consumption is important for maximizing the effect of training, promoting adequate tissue repair, maintaining or promoting lean body mass, and meeting your overall nutrient needs. Many athletes do not realize that training, hard racing, and competition are catabolic (i.e., wasting) events, and that the nonexercise, or recovery, period is when anabolic events such as tissue repair, remolding, and growth occur. Inadequate energy intake during the recovery period can result in loss of or failure to gain skeletal muscle and bone mass and can increase the risk of injury, illness, and fatigue. It may also lead to lower circulating concentrations of male and female hormones, particularly testosterone and estrogen, and result in menstrual cycle dysfunction in female athletes (see box 2.3). Information concerning testosterone will be discussed in chapter 13.

TABLE 2.1   Calculation of Daily Energy Needs

Energy expenditure component	Formula	**Example:** Female college soccer player who practices for 90 min and lifts weights for 30 min. Weight = 66 kg; body fat = 21% (lean body weight = 52 kg)	**Example:** Male cyclist who works as a musician and averages 150 miles (241 km) per week (average of 25 miles/day at 20 mph for 75 min). Weight = 86 kg; body fat = 16% (lean body weight = 72.2 kg)
Resting energy expenditure (REE)*	REE = 500 + (22 × fat-free mass in kg)	500 + (22 × 52) = 500 + 1,144 = 1,644 kcal	500 + (22 × 72.2) = 500 + 1,588 = 2,088 kcal
Energy expenditure during nontraining physical activities (NTEE)	Light activity (student, bank associate, secretary) = 0.3 × REE Moderate activity (sales clerk, fast-food worker, electrician, surgeon) = 0.5 × REE Heavy activity (construction worker, waitress, mail carrier delivering mail on foot) = 0.7 × REE	Assume light occupational activity (student): 0.3 × 1,644 kcal = 493 kcal	Assume moderate occupational activity (stands, moves, loads, and unloads equipment regularly, some sitting): 0.5 × 2,088 kcal = 1,044 kcal
Energy expenditure during training (TEE)	Refer to physical activities charts (found in many nutrition or exercise physiology texts)	A 64-kg athlete uses ~7.2 kcal/min for soccer practice and 6.1 kcal/min for weight training: 8.1 kcal/min × 90 min = 648 kcal; 6.1 kcal/min × 30 min = 183 kcal	An 86-kg male uses ~18.4 kcal/min when cycling at a steady 20 mph pace (hills and wind ignored): 18.4 × 75 min = 1,380 kcal
Total daily energy expenditure (DEE)	DEE = REE + NTEE + TEE	1,644 + 493 + 648 + 183 = 2,968 kcal/day	2,088 + 1,044 + 1,380 = 4,512 kcal/day

*The Cunningham equation for estimating REE[5] has been shown to more closely estimate the actual REE of endurance-trained men and women[22] than other available equations. Calculation of total daily energy expenditure ignores any increases in REE that may be the result of following a vegetarian diet (which may raise REE by approximately 11%), the thermic effect of food (which may increase DEE by 6-10% of energy intake), and excess postexercise oxygen consumption (which may add an additional 100-200 kcal/day) on days the training is vigorous. If you do not know your percentage of body fat, use a range of 5%-15% for a man and 17%-25% for a woman. Values for energy expenditure are for energy needs above resting and were estimated using values from appendix A.

Getting Adequate Calories From Plant Sources

Most athletes naturally consume enough calories while eating a vegetarian diet. You train, you are starving, you eat. End of the story. For some athletes, however, it is not this easy and may even pose a constant struggle. You work out, you are not in the least bit hungry, you grab a granola bar or banana, you rush to class or work, and suddenly—an hour later—you are ravenous. But, you have no food. Or, you exercise, you eat, you get full, you rush to work, and suddenly a few hours later you are hungry, and again, there's no food.

Box
2.3

Female-Athlete Triad:
Considerations for Vegetarian Athletes

Female athletes—including vegetarian athletes—who are driven to excel in their sport may be at risk for developing the disorders of the female-athlete triad. These are amenorrhea (lack of regularly occurring menstrual cycles), disordered eating, and low bone density.

Amenorrhea. Amenorrhea may be experienced by any active woman, although it is more common in athletes participating in distance running, gymnastics, and ballet. The mechanism responsible for disrupting normal menstrual function is not well understood, but accumulating scientific evidence suggests that the disruption may be caused by low energy intake or a constant energy drain. Several studies predominately involving endurance runners found that amenorrheic athletes report reduced intake of total energy,[12, 18] protein,[12, 18] and fat[6, 12] and higher intakes of fiber[6, 13] than their normally menstruating teammates. Although there is some indication that menstrual-cycle disturbances may be higher in vegetarians[2] and vegetarian athletes,[3, 12] these findings are not consistently reported[2, 21] and can be explained by study-design issues.[2] For example, studies commonly define vegetarians as people who eat small quantities of meat and not necessarily a vegetarian diet[3, 12]. Studies may also attract a biased sample of vegetarians (i.e., those with menstrual-cycle disturbances may be more likely to volunteer for a study on menstrual-cycle disturbances [2]).

Disordered eating. Disordered eating is common among female athletes who perceive that they can succeed by achieving or maintaining an unrealistically low body weight through excessive energy restriction or excess exercise or both. Several studies have noted that disordered eating behaviors tend to be more prevalent among vegetarians.[11, 19, 20] Most experts believe this is because vegetarianism is seen as a socially acceptable way to reduce energy and fat intake and *not* because being vegetarian causes eating disorders.

Low bone density and osteoporosis. Low circulating estrogen levels associated with loss of monthly cycles combined with reduced energy and nutrient intakes can predispose athletes to reduced bone density, premature osteoporosis, and increased risk of stress fractures or other overuse injuries.

Evaluation and treatment. Loss of the menstrual cycle is unhealthy and is not a normal part of training. Athletes experiencing amenorrhea should see their personal or team physician for a thorough evaluation. In many cases, reproductive function can be restored by increasing energy intake.

You can remedy this situation with a little knowledge and some planning. First, if you have not already done so, estimate your energy needs using one of the methods outlined in box 2.2 or table 2.1 and divide your requirements by three to estimate how much you would need to eat if you ate only three meals a day. If you were the female soccer player in the example in table 2.1, you would have to eat approximately 989 calories at each meal. If you were the male cyclist in the example, you would have to eat about 1,504 calories at each meal. Is this even possible? Probably not on a healthy, high-carbohydrate diet! In working with athletes over the years I have found that most with high energy needs or hectic schedules or both do better if they "graze," or strive to eat six to eight small meals or snacks throughout the day.

Next take your estimated daily energy requirement and subtract either 750 calories (if your daily needs are fewer than 4,000 calories) or 1,500 calories (if they are more than 4,000 calories). Now divide the remainder by three. The 750 or 1,500 calories was subtracted to account for three 250- or 500-calorie snacks. Again, if you were the female soccer player, you would need to eat approximately 740 calories at each of three meals and consume three 250-calorie snacks (see box 2.4 for snacks that contain approximately 250 calories). If you were the male cyclist, you would need to eat approximately 1,004 calories at each of three meals and consume three 500-calorie between-meal snacks. There is no magic to the 250- or 500-calorie snack, however. You can play around with this to help determine a pattern that works for you. Athletes with early-morning or midafternoon training sessions might also try a plan consisting of four meals plus a snack, which allows an extra meal before or after the workout.

Second, assess your food supply. Do you have food on hand when you are hungry? If not, make it a priority to stock your pantry, desk drawer, gym bag, and car with healthy nonperishable snacks, such as dried fruit, nuts, crackers, and granola bars. If you have regular access to a refrigerator or freezer, stock it also. In working with college athletes, I noticed that most—even the vegetarians—failed to eat enough fruit. I suggested they go to the grocery store once a week and buy a combination of 21 different pieces of fruit, three pieces for each day of the week. Each piece has approximately 100 calories and is full of vitamins, some minerals, and many antioxidants. You can also keep a bag of trail mix handy, or make your own by mixing different types of nuts and dried fruit.

Third, if you eat regularly but feel you get full prematurely, assess your food choices. If your diet consists of mostly whole, unprocessed foods and your energy needs are high, you may need to select breads, cereals, and grains that are more refined about a third to half of the time, and also substitute fruit juice for some of your servings of fruits and vegetables. Although fiber is important, it is common for vegetarian athletes to consume two to three times more than the daily recommended intake of 20 to 38 grams. Diets with excess fiber are not harmful but are bulkier than more-refined diets and may prohibit the intake of high volumes of food and energy. Cyclists, for example, participating in a laboratory-simulated Tour de France had difficulty meeting their daily energy needs of 8,000 to 10,000 calories

Grazing Foods That Provide Approximately 250 Calories

Granola bar

Two large or four small pieces of fruit

One large apple or banana with 1 1/2 tablespoons (24 g) of peanut butter

1/2 ounce (14 g) of nuts mixed with 1/2 ounce (14 g) of dried fruit (approximately 1/4 cup [37 g] mixture)

1 1/2 ounce (42 g) of raisins or other dried fruit

One peanut butter and jelly sandwich

2 ounces (57 g) of pretzels (regular or whole wheat)

One large bagel plus 1 tablespoon (15 g) of nut butter

1 cup (245 g) of nonfat yogurt, sweetened and with fruit

1 slice of soy cheese and 1 ounce (28 g) of regular or whole-grain crackers

Two 2 1/2-inch (6.3 cm) oatmeal or raisin cookies and 1 cup (236 ml) of soymilk

8 ounces (236 ml) of Sustacal, Ensure, Boost, or other liquid supplement beverage (Note: Boost has slightly fewer calories)

One healthy smoothie (recipe in table 14.4 contains approximately 300 calories depending on ingredients selected)

Use the food label and the information available at the USDA Nutrient Data Laboratory Web site (www.ars.usda.gov/main/site_main.htm?modecode=12354500) to estimate the energy content of your favorite snack foods.

when they selected whole-grain and high-fiber foods.[4] Some scientists also question whether diets too high in fiber interfere with mineral absorption and the normal metabolism of various steroid hormones, including estrogen and testosterone.

Finally, if you are new to vegetarianism, are striving to improve your eating pattern, or are simply overwhelmed, chapter 12 provides guidelines for customizing a meal plan to meet your energy and nutrient needs. The next three chapters offer information on fine-tuning your energy intake to ensure a balance between carbohydrate, fat, and protein fuel—which ultimately influences your performance and even your health. Read on!

3

Finding the Right Carbohydrate Mix

A freshman on the women's soccer team came to see me a week after the first Friday–Sunday match of the season. She had been one of the coach's top recruits with a good scoring record playing on the boys' (not girls') team in high school. Given her history, she was thrown into college play early in the season alongside her more-experienced junior and senior teammates. "Ever since Friday it has been an effort to run," she told me. She went on to explain that all week she had been experiencing tiredness and fatigue that was isolated to her quads and was particularly noticeable after climbing stairs or running during practice. She denied any association with muscle soreness or tenderness and then added, "I don't know what is wrong. I felt great during preseason." I inquired further and confirmed my suspicion that the coach had kept her on the field for most of the match on both Friday and Sunday. I took a detailed diet history and was not surprised to find that her carbohydrate intake over the last few weeks had been low. Overall she made good food choices and had eaten adequately during preseason (as I had also observed during my close interaction with the team), but she had somewhat unconsciously cut back on her carbohydrate intake, particularly fruit, after classes had started. I estimated that she needed at least 411 to 462 grams of carbohydrate per day (8 to 9 g/kg body weight) to support her prolonged practice and game times, but over the last week she appeared to be averaging only approximately 340 (6.6 g/kg body weight). I suspected that she was experiencing a classic bout of glycogen depletion, initiated by the weekend matches, that she had not been able to remedy during the week. I sent her home with a prescription to eat a high-carbohydrate meal that night and gave her ideas for keeping her carbohydrate intake within the recommended range during the season. I never saw her in my office again but the word from her coach was that she was feeling and playing well.

As an athlete, carbohydrate should make up the bulk of your diet. Carbohydrate—in the right mix—is needed to properly fuel your muscles and brain and to optimize your training, performance, and health. Getting the right amount of carbohydrate fuel from a vegetarian diet is easy because it is naturally carbohydrate packed, and it can also provide the right mix at the right time. That said, however, vegetarian athletes are not immune from bad training days, most noted by fatigue, reduced precision, and no power, or "dead" muscles. Bad training days may occur regularly if you don't understand the importance of carbohydrate fuel or know how much is required during each stage of your training. They may occur because you are not yet armed with the adequate carbohydrate know-how, even if you are already on a vegetarian diet. Thus, this chapter reviews how to make sure you get enough carbohydrate fuel for each stage of training and in the right mix.

Why Athletes Need Carbohydrate

In chapter 2, we briefly discussed how your body gets energy from foodstuff and that it is the energy released from within the chemical bonds of carbohydrate, fat, and even protein that allows you to live. Although carbohydrate, fat, and, to a lesser extent, protein are used to fuel physical effort, carbohydrate is the only fuel that can sustain the moderate- to high-level effort that is required in most sports and athletic endeavors. Carbohydrate is also the preferred fuel for the brain and central nervous system and the only fuel these systems can use without weeks of adaptation that allows the brain to use products of fat metabolism, called ketones or ketone bodies.

As most athletes know, carbohydrate can be stored in skeletal muscle and liver in a starchlike form called glycogen. The body's glycogen stores, however, are limited. Glycogen can become depleted during continuous steady-state exercise lasting at least 60 minutes and during intense intermittent activities that include stop-and-go running, intense court play, and brisk hiking on difficult terrain. In fact, glycogen levels are likely to be depleted at the end of an intense soccer or basketball game in team members who play the majority of the game.

Research has shown time and time again that muscle and whole-body fatigue develop at about the same time that glycogen stores become low. The reasons are relatively simple. First, active muscles that have been exhausted of their carbohydrate stores are forced to rely primarily on fat for fuel. Fat cannot be "burned" as rapidly or efficiently as carbohydrate, so you are forced to slow your pace and eventually stop exercising. Second, the liver—exhausted of its carbohydrate stores—is now unable to serve as a bank for blood sugar and must struggle to maintain blood sugar concentrations by converting protein (amino acid) sources to blood sugar. This process, termed *gluconeogenesis,* which means new-sugar formation, is slow and typically cannot keep pace with the rate at which the exercising muscle takes up sugar. The result is often low blood sugar, which is characteristically accompanied by lightheadedness, lethargy, and overall fatigue. Although the body's enzymes—machinery for making blood sugar from amino acids—are typically regulated through training, athletes at any level can experience low blood sugar. Most likely you have experienced this feeling yourself—at least once—which in some athletic circles is called *hitting the wall.*

Carbohydrate for Optimal Performance

Diets high in carbohydrate are important in most sports because they maintain glycogen stores in muscles and the liver. Extensive research conducted in this area has found that high-carbohydrate diets decrease the risk of fatigue during both continuous and highly intense intermittent exercise. Overall, diets rich in carbohydrate increase your capacity to exercise longer before exhaustion and also maintain your sprinting ability at the end of exercise. For endurance athletes, this means you will be able to maintain a faster pace for longer and better preserve your sprinting potential at the end of a long training run or race. For athletes involved in stop-and-go sports such as soccer, football, rugby, volleyball, basketball, tennis, and hockey, it means you will be able to play or practice longer before feeling fatigued and also maintain your ability to sprint, jump, bat, slam, or tackle at the end of a game. Very few studies have attempted to show the benefit of high-carbohydrate diets on performance during stop-and-go team sports. However, a study conducted at the Karolinska Institute in Stockholm, Sweden, found that male soccer players performed approximately 33 percent more high-intensity exercise movements, which were assessed by special movement-analysis equipment, during a 90-minute soccer game with four players to a side when they consumed a high- compared to a low-carbohydrate diet.[2]

Also of interest to athletes is the fact that carbohydrate can main-

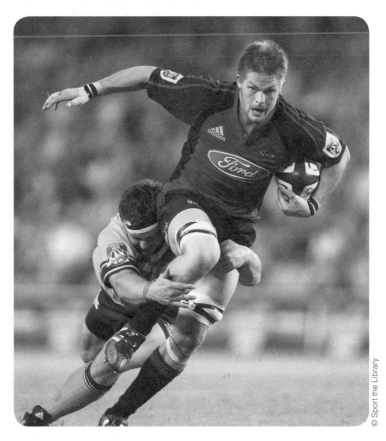

© Sport the Library

A vegetarian diet rich in a variety of carbohydrate sources can help prevent fatigue toward the end of a game.

tain an optimal bioenergetic state, the balance between creatine phosphate (PCr) and its breakdown products, in exercising muscles longer than fat can. This could ultimately affect regeneration of ATP for the ATP–PCr system, which is the energy system used primarily for power and speed activities that last less than 10 seconds, such as sprinting, jumping, serving, spiking, blocking, tackling, digging, and batting.

In a study conducted early in my career, my colleagues and I had active men and women follow a vegetarian diet that was either rich in carbohydrate (7.5 g carbohydrate/kg body weight) or low in carbohydrate (1.5 g carbohydrate/kg body weight) for five days.[6] Both diets met the subjects' energy requirements and were randomly assigned based on a coin toss. The subjects exercised their quadriceps muscles on a device similar to a knee-extension machine, and the exercise got progressively more difficult every two minutes. While they were exercising, we measured the bioenergetic state of their muscle using a magnetic resonance imaging (MRI) machine. This technique, called magnetic resonance spectroscopy allowed us to study muscle metabolism without taking a muscle biopsy. The participants were able to exercise an average of 5 minutes, 40 seconds when they followed the carbohydrate-rich diet and an average of 5 minutes, 10 seconds when they followed the carbohydrate-poor diet. Most notably, we found that the PCr concentrations in the working muscles were preserved for longer on the carbohydrate-rich diet. Had this been an athletic competition, the high-carbohydrate diet may have allowed the competitors to get in an extra jump, punch, jab, or dig. Who knows how it would have helped in double overtime?

Determining Carbohydrate Needs

Optimal carbohydrate intake depends on several factors, including your body size and the type of sport you participate in and its duration and intensity. Determining exactly how much you need involves trial and error, but it should fall between the recommended ranges for athletes and active people of 6 to 10 grams of carbohydrate per kilogram of body mass daily.[8] Focusing on a certain percentage of calories from carbohydrate is no longer recommended because percentage recommendations are not easy to understand and may be misleading (as will be reviewed in chapter 4).

Under the umbrella of these recommendations, it is suggested that athletes with higher training demands strive for the upper range of 8 to 10 grams per kilogram of body mass per day (4-4.5 g/lb), and those with lower energy needs, which includes less-active and smaller female athletes, aim for the lower range of 6 to 7 grams of carbohydrate per kilogram of body mass (2.7-3.2 g/lb). Although every athlete and training situation is different, you should aim for the upper range if you are a recreational or elite distance athlete or college or professional athlete in your preseason or competitive season. In contrast, you should strive for the lower range if you are a fitness enthusiast or athlete who is participating at a level that demands less-intense physical training. This typically describes golfers; table tennis players; baseball, softball and cricket players; weightlifters; aerobic dance participants; and most athletes during the off-season. Furthermore, if you are a male athlete with a low percentage of body fat you should strive for slightly more carbohydrate than if you are a female or less-lean athlete. But again, there is an art to using this recommendation because some athletes simply burn more carbohydrate and thus have higher demands (even when they are off the court) than other athletes have. Refer to table 3.1 to estimate your daily carbohydrate requirements.

TABLE 3.1 Estimating Daily Carbohydrate Needs

Enter your body mass (weight) in kilograms (weight in pounds divided by 2.2).	_____ kg *(line a)*
Enter estimated range of carbohydrate needed to support your current level of training and performance (see text). • 6-7 g carbohydrate/kg body mass • 7-8 g carbohydrate/kg body mass • 8-9 g carbohydrate/kg body mass • 9-10 g carbohydrate/kg body mass	_____ to _____ g/kg *(line b$_1$) (line b$_2$)*
Multiply line a by line b$_1$ to get your estimated lower range.	_____ g carbohydrate/day
Multiply line a by line b$_2$ to get your estimated upper range.	_____ g carbohydrate/day
You may need to meet or exceed your estimated upper range on the day before or after, or both, a particularly vigorous or long training session or competition.	

From *Vegetarian Sports Nutrition* by D. Enette Larson-Meyer, 2007, Champaign, IL: Human Kinetics.

Research suggests that consuming more than 10 grams of carbohydrate per kilogram of body weight daily is not associated with a performance advantage and may interfere with your ability to consume adequate protein and essential fatty acids (as we will discuss in subsequent chapters). That said, however, male athletes participating in adventure racing and ultraendurance events, including the Tour de France, are known to consume more than 12 grams of carbohydrate per kilogram of body weight during competition and sometimes also training.

Estimating Carbohydrate Intake

Every athlete should count carbohydrates at least once. This exercise helps you determine if you are meeting your estimated needs and forces even vegetarians to learn a little more about which foods are the richest sources of carbohydrate. Knowing carbohydrate sources is also useful in assuring that you consume adequate carbohydrate before, during, and after exercise, which is discussed in chapter 9.

To give carbohydrate counting a try, simply pick a day that is representative of your intake and keep a running tally of the carbohydrate-containing foods and beverages you eat and drink. All foods except cheese, oils, and meat contain countable amounts of carbohydrate. Remember to include sport drinks and supplements consumed during your workout. The carbohydrate content of selected vegetarian foods are listed in table 3.2. Serving sizes are listed according to the recommendations in the new food guide pyramid (see appendix B or www.mypyramid.gov). This information, along with the food label (which in the United States and other countries lists the carbohydrate content of most foods in grams per serving), should give you an idea of whether your intake is in the ballpark of your recommendations. An example of a carbohydrate-counting log is shown in table 3.3.

TABLE 3.2   Approximate Carbohydrate Content of Various Foods and Beverages

Food	Portion	Carbohydrate (g)
GRAIN EQUIVALENTS		
Bagel	Mini bagel	15
Bagel	Large (3-4 oz)	45-60
Biscuit	Small (2-inch diameter)	15
Bread, sliced	1 slice	15
Cornbread	1 (2-inch cube)	15
Crackers, whole wheat	5 crackers	15
Crackers, rounds or squares	6-8 crackers	15-20
English muffin (or bun)	1/2 or 1 side	15
Muffin	Small (2 1/2-inch diameter)	15-20
Oatmeal	1/2 cup (1 packet of instant)	15
Pancake	4 1/2-5 inch	15
Pasta	1/2 cup cooked (1 oz dry)	15-20
Popcorn	3 cups, popped	15
Ready-to-eat cereal	1/3-1 cup (varies)	15-20
Rice	1/2 cup cooked	15-20
Tortilla, corn or flour	5-6 inch	15
VEGETABLES		
Broccoli	1 cup cooked	5-10
Greens (collards, mustard, turnip, kale, spinach)	1 cup cooked	5-10
Salad greens (lettuce, spinach, and so on)	2 cups raw	5-10
Carrots, winter squash, pumpkin	1 cup	15
Sweet potato	1 cup	30
Beans, peas, lentils	1 cup	30-45
Food	**Portion**	**Carbohydrate (g)**

VEGETABLES *(continued)*		
Corn	1 cup	30
Potato, baked or mashed	1 medium or 1 cup	30
Other vegetables (cucumber, asparagus, green beans, mushrooms, onions, tomatoes)	1 cup raw or cooked	5-10
FRUITS		
Fruit, all	1 cup	15
Orange, peach, pear	Medium	15
Apple, banana	Large	30
Fruit, dried	1/3-1/2 cup	60
Fruit juice, lemonade	1 cup	30-45
MILK AND YOGURT		
Milk, plain yogurt	1 cup	12
Yogurt, sweetened and flavored	1 cup	40-45
SPORT AND DISCRETIONARY FOODS		
Fluid-replacement beverage	1 cup	15-19
Soda	12 oz	40-45
Sport bar	1 bar	40-60
Sport bar, high protein	1 bar	2-30
Sugar	1 Tbsp	15
Jelly, jam, honey, preserves	1 Tbsp	15

Developed based on My Pyramid Plan equivalents for Grains, Vegetables, Fruits, Milk and Discretionary Calorie; Carbohydrate content approximated according to the Dietetic Exchange List for Meal Planning, 2003, and selected food label.

Once you have tallied your daily needs, compare it to your estimated needs (table 3.1). If you are meeting your needs and are feeling strong, congratulations! If you are falling short, try to add carbohydrate foods for a week or two and see how you feel. If you notice no difference, your diet may be just fine. The volleyball player whose carbohydrate log is presented in table 3.3 was asked to add a few more servings of carbohydrate at dinner after we determined that her log accurately reported what she ate and her portion sizes. Finally, if you are falling short and feeling tired, fatigued, or dead-legged, by all means start counting daily until eating a higher-carbohydrate diet becomes second nature.

Carbohydrate counting is also particularly helpful when you are bumping up the volume or intensity of your training, or are entering an intense competitive season. For best results, counting carbohydrate during these times should be combined with the use of a training log or performance feedback from a coach or training partner. You may, for example, note that low carbohydrate intake on a particular day was followed by poor running, lightheadedness, or excessive moodiness during a training session. Occasional carbohydrate counting may also be useful

TABLE 3.3 Sample Log for Counting Carbohydrate

1 1/2 cups cornflakes (3/4 cup = 1 oz serving)	44
1 cup 1% milk	12
12 oz (1 1/2 cups) orange juice	45
White bread, 2 slices	30
Peanut butter	—
1 can (~2 cups) fruit cocktail in light syrup	60
1 large handful (~1 cup) grapes	30
Jelly beans (~2 oz)	54
1/3 cup granola	15
1/4 cup almonds	—
2 cups vegetarian chili (contains ~1 cup beans and 1 cup onion, green peppers, and tomato sauce combined)	30-45 5
~2 oz cheddar cheese	—
15 saltine crackers	30
Total	**355-370**

Reported daily carbohydrate intake for a 141-lb (64 kg) female volleyball player involved in off-season training. Her carbohydrate goal range was 384-448 g of carbohydrate/day (6-7 g carbohydrate/kg body mass). Note: Carbohydrate counting is most accurate if portion sizes are accurately measured and food labels are used to supplement the information presented in table 3.2. Refer to appendix E for guidance on converting English units to metric.

to athletes prone to weight gain because consuming excessive calories—even in the form of carbohydrate—can result in weight gain.

A recent study illustrates how the carbohydrate level of your diet might affect your training and mood, which, in addition to your teammates or training partner, may even be detected by your significant other, children, or coworkers. Researchers at the University of Birmingham in the United Kingdom asked seven trained male runners to perform two 11-day training periods in which training was intensified over the last 7 days of the 11-day session.[1] During one period, the runners consumed a moderate-carbohydrate diet (providing 5.4 g carbohydrate/kg/day). During the other period, they consumed a high-carbohydrate diet (providing 8.5 g carbohydrate/kg/day). The order of the diets was randomly assigned. The researchers found that although some aspects of the athletes' mood and performance were negatively affected by the intensified training, the high-carbohydrate diet better maintained the athletes' mood and endurance performance (measured during a 16-kilometer [10-mile] outdoor race) over the course of the 11-day training period. They concluded that a carbohydrate diet may be particularly important during periods of intensified training to reduce the symptoms of overreaching. *Overreaching* is the preferred term for what was once called overtraining.

Components of the Carbohydrate Mix

Finding the right carbohydrate mix is a bit more difficult than ensuring that you are getting enough carbohydrate. This is because the right mix is likely to be different from person to person and to vary somewhat across your training and competitive year. To help you find the right mix, this next section reviews the various components of the mix along with the definitions of simple, complex, and high glycemic–index and low glycemic–index carbohydrate. It is more important to incorporate a variety of whole and slightly processed grains, colorful fruits and vegetables, and, to a certain extent, sport products into your mix than to focus on only complex carbohydrate or foods with a low glycemic index (GI). Table 3.6 on page 37 can help you determine if you should alter your carbohydrate mix to improve your health and performance.

Important Considerations

Your daily choices of the foods presented in table 3.2—including grains, fruits and vegetables, milk, sport products, and desserts—are what make up your carbohydrate mix. Balancing these carbohydrate-containing foods in your diet is necessary to ensure that you consume adequate nutrients and obtain a variety of disease-preventing and possibly recovery-enhancing phytochemicals. Achieving this mix requires that you understand the other food categories, or food groups, which we address again in chapter 12. For now, however, let's think carbohydrate.

Grains vs. Fruits vs. Vegetables vs. Dairy

If you look at the various food guidance models available in the United States and other countries, including MyPyramid and the food plate (see appendix B), the consensus is that the bulk of your carbohydrate should come from grains supplemented with carbohydrate from vegetables, fruits, milk, and if desired, other discretionary foods. The recommendation for a 2,400- to 3,000-calorie diet is for 8 to 10 servings. The grains are a staple because, in addition to carbohydrate, they also provide some protein, B vitamins, and iron and (if not overly processed) are a more satiating source of carbohydrate than most fruits and vegetables. Whole grains, in addition, provide fiber, zinc, and selenium.

Fruits, on the other hand, provide fiber, potassium, folate, and vitamin C. Dark-green and orange-red fruits also provide carotenoids, some of which may be converted to vitamin A. Although they provide about the same amount of carbohydrate per cup, fruits are higher in natural sugar and water and are typically lower in complex carbohydrate. This may make them appealing after a workout but less likely to satisfy an hour or so after consumption. It is not understood why fruits tend to be less satiating than grains, but it may be related to their negligible protein content. Do not limit fruits because of their high sugar content. However, the sugars in many fruits—including cherries, plums, peaches, and apples—is absorbed slowly, yielding a rather low glycemic index (described later in this chapter). As is often incorrectly stated, fruits do not cause spikes and subsequent falls in blood sugar.

In contrast to grains and fruits, vegetables come in starchy and nonstarchy varieties. Starchy vegetables—including root vegetables and legumes—are carbohydrate packed (a half cup [90 g] cooked contains 15 grams of carbohydrate), whereas nonstarchy vegetables—such as asparagus, broccoli, cauliflower, snap peas, and leafy greens—contain little carbohydrate (a half cup [90 g] contains 5 grams or less of carbohydrate). Like fruit, vegetables are a source of fiber, potassium, folate, vitamin C, and carotenoids but also contain protein, iron, calcium, and other minerals. Although all vegetables are "good for you," vegetarian athletes may need to alter the mix of these vegetables according to their training regimens. For example, when energy needs are high, eating a large helping of nonstarchy vegetables can literally fill you up, at least temporarily, before you are able to consume an adequate supply of carbohydrate. When you are red-shirted or unable to compete for a prolonged period, however, eating this same serving of nonstarchy vegetables may help you feel full and prevent unwanted weight gain.

Finally, some dairy products, particularly milk and yogurt, are also sources of carbohydrate (12 grams per cup [236 ml]) as well as protein and calcium. Nearly 100 percent of the carbohydrate in milk is in the form of lactose (or milk sugar), which many adults cannot easily digest. The lactose content of yogurt is also high but is much lower than that of milk and apparently decreases daily (even as it sits in the refrigerator) because its natural bacteria breaks down lactose to glucose and galactose. Glucose, sucrose, and even high-fructose corn syrup provide additional carbohydrate in fruit-containing and flavored yogurt. It is not necessary to include carbohydrate from dairy in your mix, but it does provide additional carbohydrate for vegetarian athletes who are able to digest lactose. Athletes who experience abdominal discomfort, bloating, or gas after consuming milk or yogurt may be lactose intolerant and may want to cut back on or eliminate these foods from their diets (see chapter 6 for information on getting adequate calcium without consuming dairy products). Lactose-intolerant adults who want to continue consuming dairy products can buy low-lactose versions or take tablets that contain the enzyme lactase, which aids in the digestion of milk sugar.

Although most food guidance systems were not designed with athletes in mind, the recommendation to obtain the bulk of carbohydrate from grains is appropriate for athletes. My own eating habits follow this trend. I have found over the years that if I don't eat enough rice and grains over the course of several days, I don't feel satisfied and end up with uncontrollable cravings for grain products. The summer I participated in RAGBRAI (Register's Annual Great Bike Ride Across Iowa), I spent the week eating mostly fresh fruit, pastries, and cheese pizza because vegetarian options were hard to come by. About five days into the weeklong ride, I was craving bread so much that I stopped at a small store, bought a loaf and devoured nearly the whole thing. That said, however, I have also encountered a few vegetarian athletes who feel the food pyramid model is too heavy on the grains. These athletes claim they do fine eating mostly fruits, vegetables, legumes, and nuts, and fewer grains.

Color

Several national nutrition campaigns in the United States, including MyPyramid and the national 5 A Day for Better Health program (a partnership between the National Cancer Institute, the Produce for Better Health Foundation, the Centers for Disease Control and Prevention, and many state and local agencies), are taking the message of increasing consumption of fruits and vegetables one step further. The new emphasis is to "eat your colors." Why? Because colorful fruits and vegetables provide the range of vitamins, minerals, and phytochemicals the body needs to maintain good health. The message from MyPyramid is to include dark-green vegetables, orange vegetables, legumes, starchy vegetables, and other vegetables in your diet regularly. The message from the 5 A Day groups is to "Get 5 A Day the Color Way" (see www.5aday.com/index.php) and ensure "There is a Rainbow on [your] plate" (see www.5aday.com/html/kids/kids_home.php). The spectrum of colors is explained in table 3.4 and consists of five groups: blue or purple, green, white, yellow or orange, and red. As athletes, striving to eat a variety of colorful phytochemical-rich fruits and vegetables may not only lower

TABLE 3.4 Fruit and Vegetable Color Guide

Color	Sources of	Found in
Green	Lutein and zeaxanthin	Greens (turnip, collard, and mustard), kale, spinach, lettuce, broccoli, green peas, kiwi, honeydew melon
	Indoles	Broccoli, cabbage, brussels sprouts, bok choy, arugula, Swiss chard, turnips, rutabaga, watercress, cauliflower, kale
	Vitamin K	Swiss chard, kale, brussels sprouts, spinach, turnip greens, watercress, endive, lettuce, mustard greens, cabbage
	Potassium	Leafy greens, broccoli
Yellow and orange	Beta-carotene and vitamin A	Carrots, sweet potatoes, pumpkin, butternut squash, cantaloupe, mangoes, apricots, peaches
	Bioflavonoids and vitamin C	Oranges, grapefruit, lemons, tangerines, clementines, peaches, papaya, apricots, nectarines, pears, pineapple, yellow raisins, yellow peppers
	Potassium	Bananas, oranges, grapefruit, lemons, pineapple, apricots
Red	Vitamin C	Cranberries, pink grapefruit, raspberries, strawberries, watermelon, red cabbage, red pepper, radishes, tomatoes
	Anthocyanins	Raspberries, cherries, strawberries, cranberries, beets, apples, red cabbage, red onions, kidney beans, red beans
Blue and purple	Anthocyanins and vitamin C	Blueberries, blackberries, purple grapes, black currants, elderberries
	Phenolics	Prunes, raisins, plums, eggplant
White	Allium and allicin	Garlic, onions, leeks, scallions, chives

From http://www.5daday.gov/color/.

your risk of some chronic diseases, such as cancer and heart disease, but may also optimize your ability to recover from strenuous exercise.

Whole vs. Processed

During a meeting of the American College of Sports Medicine many years ago, I attended a session that focused on the nutritional needs of male athletes training for and competing in distance stage bicycle races such as the Tour de France. During this session, it was emphasized that focusing on whole grains was not a good idea for these athletes because the low energy density of whole compared to processed grains and other whole foods made it more difficult for these athletes to meet their extreme energy and carbohydrate needs. The point hit home. I had trouble with the same thing several years earlier (although I was not training for the Tour). At the time I had been a vegetarian for about a year and estimate that I was "burning" more than 3,000 calories a day cross-training and riding 100 to 150 miles a week. I was making spaghetti with whole-wheat pasta, eating brown rice, baking bran muffins, and eating lots of fruit, and I could not eat enough food. My stomach got full, but I still felt hungry—yes, I thought this was physiologically impossible. The solution for both the elite cyclists and me was the same—relax on the whole foods. The right mix for an athlete is one that includes some whole grains and some less-processed versions. Even the 2005 Dietary Guidelines for Americans and MyPyramid suggest that we aim for half of our grains to be whole grains.

Sport Products and Desserts

Okay, we all know modern athletes do not live by bread alone. What about other carbohydrate sources like lemonade, sport drinks, sport bars and gels, recovery drinks, and, heavens yes, frozen yogurt, dairy-free frozen dessert (such as Tofutti), and grandma's homemade cherry pie? These are "added sugar" foods and beverages in which sugar or syrups have been added during processing or preparation. On MyPyramid, they are considered luxuries and make up your discretionary calories. Although they are allowed in a healthy diet, MyPyramid suggests that you limit foods that provide discretionary calories. This limit is approximately 265 to 360 calories for an active female consuming 2,000 to 2,400 calories per day and 360 to 510 calories for an active male consuming 2,400 to 3,000 calories per day.

Given these guidelines, let's first address sport products. Although, I am a firm believer in whole foods, I find—as I suspect many athletes do—that some products (including sport drinks and gels and honey packets) can be a convenient necessity. When I competed in my first 100-mile (160 km) bike ride back in the late 1980s, I ate at least six bananas during the ride. I started the ride with two wedged in my sport bra (I was new to the sport and did not yet have a jersey with pockets), and as much as I like bananas, was pretty sick of them for weeks after the ride. I became a thankful fan when the first sport gel arrived on the market. Although there are no hard-and-fast rules for athletes concerning the use of supplemental sport foods, my rule is to eat meals and snacks made with real foods and use sport foods as supplements if needed during longer training sessions or competitions. If you followed the recommendation from MyPyramid and consume 2,400 to 3,000 calories per day, you could consume 90 to 120 grams of carbohydrate as supplements—if you ate no dessert—which is enough to supplement 90 to 120 minutes of training. This sounds fairly reasonable to me.

Now let's get to dessert. When I am training hard, I am a fan of desserts. In working with athletes over the years I have found that a daily dessert treat is usually appropriate as long as the athletes don't get carried away. Believe me, I have seen resident athletes at the U.S. Olympic Training Center in Colorado Springs attack the poor chef as he emerged from the kitchen with a plate of warm cookies. For vegetarian athletes, a few cookies, a piece of pumpkin cake, or dish of pudding, frozen yogurt, or Tofutti will add extra calories, and if the choices are right, even some nutrition. My rule on dessert is to have homemade if at all possible—that way you can sneak in some whole grains, nuts, and good oils—and to choose ones that are low in saturated fat and contain fruits or vegetables. I suppose dark chocolate is OK too. Examples of appetizing fruit desserts include frozen yogurt with bananas or berries, fruit cobbler, baked apples, pumpkin muffins, rhubarb bread, and dark-chocolate zucchini cake. Together, dessert and your sport supplements should—as the pyramid suggests—make up only a small portion (10 to 20 percent) of your calories.

Not-So-Important Considerations

If you had even a little background in vegetarian or sports nutrition before reading this book, you may be wondering why I have so far neglected to discuss simple and complex carbohydrate and the glycemic index, which is a method of classifying carbohydrate sources based on their functionality or how quickly they appear in the bloodstream after consumption. This is because I feel strongly, based on the research and my experience, that it is more beneficial to be concerned about eating a variety of wholesome foods—which include fruit and fruit juice—rather than to be concerned about whether a carbohydrate is simple or complex or elicits a certain glycemic response.

Complex vs. Simple Carbohydrate

There are several reasons that vegetarian athletes should not be overly concerned—as many still are—about the amount of simple (sugars) compared to complex (starchy) carbohydrate they consume in their diet (see table 3.5). The first is that simple carbohydrate, including fruit, fruit juice, and milk are not necessarily less healthful than more complex carbohydrate, which includes whole-wheat bread, potatoes, and cereal. Rather, it is that these foods should be consumed in the right mix, limiting the more-processed versions because these foods tend to be lower in nutrients, phytochemicals, and fiber. Second, from a performance standpoint, there is no evidence that complex carbohydrate or simple carbohydrate is more advantageous for athletes during training. In fact, researchers found that diets either high in complex carbohydrate or high in simple carbohydrate are equally effective at improving endurance (compared to a low-carbohydrate diet)[3]

TABLE 3.5   **Classification of Carbohydrate Sources**

Type	Example
Simple: Monosaccharides (one sugar unit)	Glucose or blood sugar Fructose or fruit sugar Galactose
Simple: Disaccharides (two sugar units)	Sucrose or table sugar (glucose + fructose) Lactose or milk sugar (glucose + fructose) Maltose (glucose + glucose)
Complex: Polysaccharides (many sugar units)	Maltodextrin (short straight chain) Amylose starch (straight chain of glucose) Amylopectin starch (branched chain of glucose) Polycose (commercial product of glucose units)

and in restoring glycogen in the 24-hour period after exercise.[4] The only possible benefit to a diet higher in more-complex carbohydrate was that it tended to result in slightly higher muscle glycogen stores over a 48-hour period when the athletes rested and did not train.[4]

Low Glycemic vs. High Glycemic Index

There are also several reasons that vegetarian athletes should not be overly concerned about the glycemic index (GI) of the foods that make up their carbohydrate mix. The first is that the GI, which is a measure of how quickly the carbohydrate in an individual food appears in the bloodstream after consuming a standard 50- or 100-gram portion, is extremely controversial. Although low glycemic–index diets are popular and recommended by some health professionals for weight loss[7] and improved overall health,[5] the evidence from scientific studies is not consistent or compelling. Furthermore, because the GI is measured in individual foods, its application to mixed meals and the overall diet has been criticized. Indeed, the GI of a food, such as a banana, can change quickly with ripening, cutting, or smearing with a little nut butter. With respect to its benefit to athletes, a food's GI is likely to be an important consideration only during exercise or in the preexercise and postexercise meal (as will be discussed in chapter 9), but no research suggests that athletes—particularly vegetarian athletes—will be faster, leaner, or healthier if they consume a low glycemic–index training diet.

Carbohydrate Wrap-Up

As discussed in this chapter, evaluating your carbohydrate mix is somewhat involved because it includes honestly assessing many aspects of your current eating. Some of these aspects are important for performance only, and others influence just health. Although the information in table 3.6 is helpful, keep in mind

TABLE 3.6 Are You Getting the Right Carbohydrate Mix?

Evaluation question	Suggestion for change
Do you find it a struggle to maintain your weight?	**No.** No reason to change
	Yes. I struggle to keep weight on. Replace some of your whole-grain and whole foods with more-processed versions. Eat regular pasta, white bread, and fruit and vegetable juices in place of whole-grain and whole-fruit versions.
	Yes. I am a few pounds overweight. Eat more whole-grain and whole foods. Substitute regular pasta, breakfast cereal, and fruit juice with whole-wheat pasta, cooked grains such as oatmeal and barley, and whole fruit. This will increase the fiber content of your diet and may also reduce hunger by making you feel more full or satisfied.
Do you eat a variety of carbohydrate sources from the grain, vegetable, and fruit groups?	**No.** Assess what you lack and add these to your diet. The guidelines presented in MyPyramid or the food plate model are a great place to start.
	Yes. Good job.
Do you eat a selection of colorful fruits and vegetables?	**No.** Incorporate more of the fruits and vegetables listed in table 3.4. This will help you reduce your risk of cancer and other chronic diseases and may improve your ability to recover from strenuous exercise.
	Yes. Keep up the good work. You have taken a step to reduce your risk of cancer and other chronic diseases and may even be improving your ability to recover after strenuous exercise.
Do you use sport supplements?	**No.** There is no reason to use these items. However, fluid-replacement beverages and carbohydrate bars and gels are convenient products that help athletes in heavy training meet their carbohydrate needs.
	Yes. Fluid-replacement beverages and carbohydrate bars and gels are convenient products that help athletes in heavy training meet their carbohydrate needs. These items, however, should not replace real food. Cut back on their use if they make up more than 20% of your total calories or have become your regular lunch or dinner.
Have you been trying to follow a diet that has a low glycemic index or that avoids sugar?	**No.** Because these factors don't seem to matter in the big picture, you are right on target.
	Yes. Focus instead on getting a variety of grains, whole grains, fruits and vegetables, and legumes. Glycemic index and sugar don't seem to matter in the big picture. Even if you have diabetes or prediabetes, the total carbohydrate content of the food and its nutrient content are more important. Remember also that sugar is found naturally in many foods including fruit and milk.
Do you eat sweets or dessert regularly?	**No.** Great. But allow yourself to splurge if you want to every once in a while.
	Yes. Enjoy yourself. Strive, however, for choices that are low in saturated fat and trans fat and provide nutrients. Good choices include frozen yogurt (or tofu) topped with fruit, fruit cobbler, baked apples, and whole-wheat versions of banana or pumpkin breads and oatmeal chocolate chip cookies with pecans.

that the right mix might change as you progress through your yearly season. For example, it is probably prudent to routinely emphasize eating variety and color, but you could find that you need to change your discretionary calories or amount of whole vs. processed foods or starchy vs. nonstarchy vegetables according to your energy requirements and training level. During the off-season or when you are training less, eliminate your dependence on sport drinks and focus on eating more whole foods. When you are in the heart of your season, enjoy the convenience of these products. Also keep in mind that the carbohydrate mix that works for you might not be the one preferred by your training partner or suggested by the food pyramid. Rather, what is important is that you meet your carbohydrate and nutrient needs by consuming a variety of grains, colorful fruits and vegetables, and, if desired, sport supplements in a mix that works for you. This will inevitably affect your health and your performance. Stay tuned, now, as we move on to fat.

4

Choosing Smart Fat Over No Fat

My training group had just ridden the century (160-kilometer bike ride) from hell. We were starved! One of my training partners, however, just sat there sipping her sport drink while the rest of us devoured a crawfish specialty (no sausage) prepared by the famous New Orleans chef Paul Prudhomme. It wasn't that she didn't like Cajun food; she just knew that the dish contained too much fat. She looked miserable. We had specifically traveled to this small-town Cajun festival to participate in the athletic events—it hosted a 5K run on Saturday morning followed by the century bicycle ride on Sunday—and enjoy the food and festivities. The weather in early June had been hotter and more humid than we had planned. Between that, a few wrong turns, and a flat tire, it had taken us a little longer than normal to finish the century. Now that the work was over, we had the afternoon to relax (before our drive home) and enjoy some local fare. I felt bad, however, that my training partner was unable to enjoy herself. Despite riding more than 100 miles (160 km) and competing in a 5K run the day before, she was afraid to eat a single gram of fat. On the way out of town, she made a beeline for the Wendy's drive-through and ordered two plain baked potatoes with broccoli.

Dietary fat has gotten a bad rap. The truth of the matter, however, is that you need it. You need it to help digest and absorb certain nutrients, to synthesize hormone-like regulators, and to help you enjoy the taste of your food. You also need fat as a fuel during exercise. Indeed, as useful as it is, consuming too much fat can displace valuable carbohydrate calories and, if it is saturated or even partially hydrogenated, it can elevate "bad" low-density lipoprotein (LDL) cholesterol levels and increase even an athlete's risk for heart and other vascular disease. This chapter directs you toward choosing smart fat over no fat. It reviews the importance of fat in an athlete's diet, provides information on how much of what type of fat vegetarian athletes need, and provides tips for getting the good fat sources into and the bad fat sources out of your diet.

Why Athletes Need Fat

Fat is a necessary component of the diet. It provides essential fatty acids and associated nutrients such as vitamins E, A, and D and aids in the digestion, absorption, and transport of these nutrients and all other fat-soluble phytochemicals found in plant foods. The essential fatty acids—alpha-linolenic acid and lenoleic acid—are the precursors for many regulatory compounds within the body and include the major regulators of the inflammatory process, which is discussed in chapter 11. The fat-soluble vitamins and phytonutrients—carotenoids and lycopene—are required for many essential metabolic processes and may even reduce the risk of many chronic diseases. In addition, dietary fat is a component of the protective barrier around all of the body's cells called the cell membrane and thus helps the skin and other tissues remain soft and pliable.

Fat also serves as a source of energy. As discussed earlier, fat and carbohydrate are the main energy fuels used during exercise. Emphasis is typically placed on dietary carbohydrate because carbohydrate stores in the body are limited and carbohydrate is the only fuel that can support intense bouts of exercise. This does not mean, however, that fat is unimportant. Fat serves as a necessary and constant fuel source during exercise and could theoretically supply most of the fuel needed during light to moderate efforts. Carbohydrate fuel simply makes up the difference between the level provided by fat and that needed for more-intense efforts. This is because fat cannot be broken down fast enough to support the rapid energy demands of more-intense efforts. Increasing the muscles' ability to burn fat as a fuel, which happens with endurance training, is thought to preserve or spare carbohydrate for use during quick or intense physical effort, which is required during most training and competitive efforts.

The source of fat used to fuel exercising muscle comes predominantly from fat stored both in adipose tissue—your body fat—and the exercising muscle itself. The small amount of fat that circulates in blood as triglycerides (serum triglycerides) is another possible fat source but contributes only a negligible amount even after a high-fat meal. The fat stored within exercising muscle as droplets (see figure 4.1) is the ideal source because it provides a direct source of fat to the mitochondria, the cell's ATP-generating powerhouse. In fact, many times in well-trained endurance athletes, the fat droplet appears to be completely encircled by the mitochondria, as can be seen in figure 4.1.

Fat stored in adipose tissue, on the other hand, has to do a lot of traveling. It must first be broken down to fatty acids, which is the chemical form used

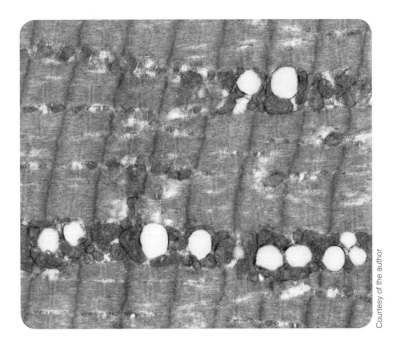

Courtesy of the author

FIGURE 4.1 **Electron microscopy of the muscle cell obtained from the thigh (vastus lateralis) of a male runner. The fat droplets (bright white circles) are in close contact with mitochondria (darker structures), which are the structure responsible for producing ATP from fat and carbohydrate fuel.**

for energy, be released from the adipose cell, travel in the blood bound to an escort protein called albumin, and then pass through the cell and mitochondria membranes escorted by other carriers (a transmembrane carrier and carnitine, respectively). And you thought your workout was tough! Although the amount of energy stored in adipose depots is large compared to the amount in other storage sites of the body, the energy content of the fat stored within the muscle cell is also significant and has been estimated to be slightly greater than that stored as glycogen (see table 4.1).

Until recently, the importance of muscle fat as a fuel source during exercise was largely ignored and is, in fact, still being investigated. This is in part because measuring muscle-fat stores and determining its oxidation or "burning" rate during exercise is technically difficult. Nonetheless, evidence collected over the last 20 years or so, using a variety of state-of-the-art techniques, has suggested that fat stored within the muscle cell may be more important than we had thought. For instance, it has been estimated in both men and women (as shown in figure 4.2) that muscle fat serves as an important source of fat fuel during moderate (65 percent $\dot{V}O_2max$) and intense exercise (85 percent $\dot{V}O_2max$)[25, 26] and is reduced by 20 to 50 percent after moderate to strenuous endurance exercise. Furthermore, endurance training increases the amount of fat stored within muscle and also the use of this fuel during exercise.

TABLE 4.1   Estimated Energy Stores of Fat and Carbohydrate in a 75-kg (165 lb) Male Athlete With 15% Body Fat

Energy fuel stores	Components	Energy (kcal)
Fat	Blood fat (free fatty acids and triglyceride)	40
	Adipose tissue	99,000+
	Muscle lipid droplets	2,600
	Estimated total	101,640
Carbohydrate	Blood glucose	80
	Liver glycogen	380
	Muscle glycogen	1,500-1,600
	Estimated total	1,960-2,060

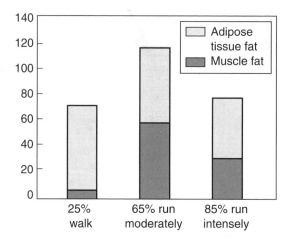

FIGURE 4.2   Contribution of fat from muscle fat stores, as droplets within the muscle cell, and adipose tissue breakdown, from delivery in blood as free fatty acids, to energy expenditure after 30 minutes of exercise at 25 percent, 65 percent and 85 percent of maximal oxygen uptake ($\dot{V}O_2$max).

Adapted from E.F. Coyle, 1995, "Fat metabolism during exercise," *Sports Science Exchange* 8(6).

Fat's Influence on Performance

Although not yet proven, some researchers question whether diets that are too low in fat, meaning less than 10 to 15 percent of energy, impair endurance performance by compromising fat stores in muscle. This concept is similar to the way diets lower in carbohydrate compromise muscle-glycogen stores. Studies from several groups[6, 7] and one from my research group,[15] found that the amount of fat stored in exercised muscles can be increased by eating a diet that is higher in fat. In our study, eight female runners completed a two-hour run on the tread-mill at 65 percent of $\dot{V}O_2$max. We then fed them a very low-fat (10 percent fat) and a moderate-fat (35 percent fat) vegetarian diet for three days, which they consumed in a randomly assigned order on two different occasions. We found that muscle-fat stores were reduced by an average 25 percent during the endur-ance run and that recovery depended on the fat content of the diet. Consuming the moderate-fat diet allowed muscle-fat stores to return to baseline the follow-ing morning (22 hours later) and to overshoot baseline values three days later, despite the fact that the runners continued to perform 45-minute training runs. Consuming the low-fat diet, in contrast, did not allow muscle fat to be restocked even three days after the run.

The pressing question is whether endurance performance can be enhanced by stocking the muscle full of fat, or alternatively, be compromised by overzealous fat restriction. Unfortunately, we do not yet know the answer. One study conducted by researchers at the State University of New York at Buffalo,[22] however, has produced compelling results. Researchers had male collegiate distance run-ners follow a diet for seven days that provided either more or less fat than their normal diet, which derived 22 percent of its calories from fat. The lower-fat diet provided 15 percent of energy and 9.6 grams of carbohydrate per kilogram of body mass, and the higher-fat diet provided 38 percent and 6.7 grams of carbo-hydrate per kilogram of body mass. Both diets provided 3,500 calories per day. At the end of the seven days, the runners were asked to run for 30 minutes at a relatively intense effort (85 percent of $\dot{V}O_2$max) before running to exhaustion at a more moderate effort (75 percent of $\dot{V}O_2$max). The researchers noted that the runners on the 38 percent fat diet, which still provided carbohydrate within the recommended range, were able to run 15 to 20 minutes longer than the runners on the lower-fat diet.

Although more research is needed, the suggestion is that you may be able to improve your performance during endurance efforts by increasing your muscle-fat stores through a slightly higher-fat diet. This implies, of course, that you do not lower glycogen stores at the same time. Hypothetically, the increased muscle fat would serve as a readily available fuel during exercise and be particularly advan-tageous during moderate to intense endurance exercise when fat delivery from adipose tissue is limited. The muscle would then be able to use more fat during less-intense effort and reserve carbohydrate for when it is really needed—for the sprint at the end of the race. Laboratory research supports this speculation. We know, for example, that if we bring an athlete into the laboratory and artifi-cially increase his or her blood-fat levels by directly infusing fatty acids along with a compound called heparin, which, as you might guess, is illegal in athletic competitions, we can force the muscle to use more fat and spare its glycogen stores.[9, 31]

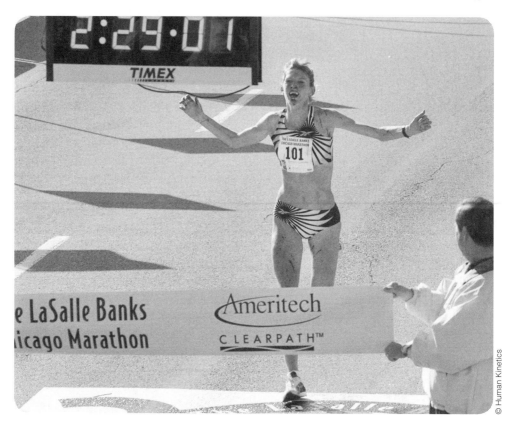

© Human Kinetics

A slightly higher-fat diet may help improve endurance performance by providing muscle fat as a ready fuel and reserving carbohydrate for the finishing sprint.

Determining Fat Needs

The amount of fat in your overall diet should make up the remainder of energy intake after your carbohydrate and protein needs are met. For many active people and athletes, this is 20 to 30 percent of daily energy intake, which is the recommendation of the American College of Sports Medicine, the American Dietetic Association, and Dietitians of Canada.[4] Specifying fat intake as a percentage of daily energy, however, can be complicated because it requires that the athlete know his or her daily energy requirements. Furthermore, the percentage can be misleading because you can consume a higher percentage of energy from fat (and still meet carbohydrate and protein needs) the higher your energy needs. Indeed, smaller athletes with lower energy demands may need to hover near the low end of the range and consume around 20 to 25 percent of daily energy intake as fat in order to meet their carbohydrate and protein requirements. But athletes with high energy needs could consume 35 percent or more of their daily energy intake from fat and still consume enough carbohydrate and protein. For example, a 75-kilogram (165 lb) endurance athlete whose energy needs are 4,500 calories

TABLE 4.2   Level of Acceptable Fat Intake for a 75-kg (165 lb) Male Endurance Athlete Whose Energy Needs Are 4,500 kcal/day

Total daily energy requirements		=	4,500 kcal/day (line a)
Estimated carbohydrate requirements (using 8 g/kg body mass)	600 g/day × 4 kcal/g	=	2,400 kcal/day from carbohydrate (line b)
Estimated protein requirements (using 1.2 g/kg body mass [see chapter 5])	90 g/day × 4 kcal/g	=	360 kcal/day from protein (line c)
Estimated fat intake in kcal/day (subtract lines b and c from line a)		=	1,740 kcal/day from fat (line d)
Estimated fat intake in g (divide kcal from fat by 9 kcal/g)	1,740 kcal/day ÷ 9 kcal/g	=	193 g fat (line e)
Estimated percentage of kcal from fat (divide kcal from fat [line d] by total kcal [line a] and multiply by 100)	1,740 ÷ 4,500 × 100	=	38.7% of daily energy as fat*

*By these calculations, fat intake is estimated as the remainder of energy after the athlete's carbohydrate and fat intake is met. If the athlete consumes 10 g carbohydrate/kg body mass rather than 8 g carbohydrate/kg body mass, the fat content of the diet would be 25% of daily energy.

per day (as shown in table 4.2), can eat a diet that provides 38 percent of daily energy intake from fat and still meet his or her carbohydrate and protein requirements. You can use this table to estimate your own dietary-fat range.

If you are wondering if dangers are associated with eating too much or too little fat, the answer is definitely yes. Diets that are too high in fat, or even protein for that matter, do not provide sufficient carbohydrate to keep glycogen stores stocked, and diets too high in saturated and trans fat, but not total fat, promote cardiovascular disease. But just because too much dietary fat is detrimental, athletes shouldn't severely limit fat, and in fact, some athletes with high energy demands can consume more than 30 percent fat (table 4.2) as long as the sources are low in saturated and trans fat. If a higher fat intake makes you nervous, you may find comfort in knowing that the most recent Dietary Reference Intakes (DRIs)[10] and guidelines from the National Cholesterol Education Program (NCEP)[2] and the American Diabetes Association (ADA)[1] no longer recommend eating a diet that provides less than 30 percent fat. The DRIs suggest that healthy adults consume between 20 and 35 percent fat, and the NCEP recommends 25 to 35 percent fat. The ADA boldly suggests that fat intake be individualized, with carbohydrate and monounsaturated fat together making 60 to 70 percent of the energy intake. All recommendations, however, suggest that saturated and trans fat intake be kept to a minimum.

In athletes, evidence suggests that diets that are too low in fat, typically defined as those providing less than 15 percent fat, are associated with dry flaky skin, compromised immune function,[30] and increased risk for amenorrhea or altered menstrual cycle function.[5, 8, 18] Low-fat diets are also known to raise serum triglycerides, even in athletes.[4, 15] Elevated serum triglyceride concentrations above 150 milligrams per deciliter are thought to be a risk factor for heart disease. Although slightly elevated triglycerides are not a problem for most athletes—who have low triglyceride concentrations to begin with—several healthy runners in my studies have exceeded the 150 milligrams per deciliter mark when placed on a research diet consisting of 10 percent fat. Furthermore, as discussed earlier, low-fat diets may even impair endurance performance by reducing fat storage in muscle.

Connection Between Dietary Fat and Body Fat

A final point to discuss—just in case it is lingering in the back of your mind—is whether consuming a little extra fat in your diet will result in body fat or body weight gain. Indeed, there are a handful of studies[20]—including a few of my own[16, 17]—that have found a positive relationship between dietary-fat intake (as a percentage of calories) and body fat percentage among nonathletes. Although these studies seem to suggest that eating more fat may go to your hips or your belly, I first need to point out that the reported relationship between dietary fat and body fat is very weak (accounting for approximately 10 percent or less of the variance in body fat), and in one of our studies, it completely disappeared when we accounted for the physical activity level of our participants.[16] In addition, the intake of polyunsaturated fat may have the opposite effect and be negatively correlated with body fat.[16, 29]

Nonetheless, many athletes (like my former training partner) are convinced that they need to eat as little fat as possible to stay lean. Although there is a grain of truth to this thinking, it appears that the danger is not that dietary fat slows metabolism or goes right to your hips,[19, 32] but that traditional higher-fat diets encourage overeating. Researchers discovered this when they manipulated the fat content of various omnivorous recipes and then allowed sedentary volunteers to eat as much as they wanted.[24] The research volunteers overate when the higher-fat versions of the same recipes were offered, which the researchers speculated was caused by both the higher energy density (9 kcal/g for fat vs. 4 kcal/g for carbohydrate and protein) and enhanced sensory qualities of dietary fats.[24] The participants tended to choose the same volume of food, which resulted in increased energy intake of the high-fat foods because of its higher energy density. Results from these studies in sedentary subjects, however, should not be taken to mean that vegetarian athletes will overeat and increase their body fat stores simply by being a little more liberal with their fat intake at the expense of carbohydrate. Studies in endurance athletes[4, 23] have found that body fat is not influenced by following self-selected higher-fat diets that provided up to 50 percent of energy intake for as long as 12 weeks.[4] The other side of the story is that athletes may eat more on a less-tasty low-fat diet simply because it does not provide as much satisfaction as a tastier fat-containing meal. Think, for example, of a person who consumes an entire package of fat-free cookies and still wants the taste of just one or two "real" fat-containing cookies.

Balancing Good Fat and Bad Fat for Health

In addition to thinking of fat exclusively as an energy source, dietary fat needs to be considered in terms of its effect on health. We have learned so much in this area lately, that if I had written this book five years ago, this chapter would have been about half the length. Although we have known for a long time that consuming too much saturated fat was "bad," we really did not appreciate that consuming certain types of fat, at the expense of others, might actually benefit health. Hence, this next section is devoted to increasing your understanding of the different types of fats and their food sources in an effort to help you adjust your diet as needed. Your overall goal—of course—is to get to know the "good guy" fats, avoid contact with the "bad guy" fats, and learn your tolerance for the "just OK" fats. Making smart fat choices should have an impact on your long-term health, but it may also reduce whole-body inflammation and potentially affect your life as an athlete. This will be discussed more in chapter 11. Results from nearly 150 epidemiological and clinical investigations,[13] including the Nurses' Health Study,[12] support the idea that eating smart fat over no fat may be more effective at preventing coronary heart disease and possibly other chronic diseases.

"Bad Guys"—Saturated Fats and Trans Fats

Unless you have been training in a box, you probably know quite a bit about saturated fats and trans fats (see box 4.1 for a review). Indeed, saturated fats are found mostly in animal products and tropical oils and should be limited in your diet because they increase your risk of cardiovascular disease, stroke, and other types of vascular disease. The most common recommendation of many major health organizations, such as the American Heart Association (AHA),[14] the American Diabetes Association (ADA),[1] and the National Cholesterol Education Program (NCEP),[2] is that saturated fat intake be limited to no more than 10 percent[14, 1] of energy. Another recommendation states that it should be less than 7 percent.[2] If your LDL is elevated (more than 100 milligrams per deciliter), you are limited by most guidelines to 7 percent[14, 1] of daily energy. Trans fats, on the other hand, are obtained mostly from processed foods in which partially hydrogenated oils are used in their preparation or processing. The DRI and the recommendations from most of the aforementioned health organizations are to keep the amount of trans fat in the diet as low as possible. The AHA, however, recommends more concretely that saturated and trans fats—the cholesterol-raising fats—not exceed 10 percent of energy. Although trans fats are probably not as effective as saturated fats at elevating LDL, they provide a double whammy by also decreasing high-density

Box
4.1

Classes of Dietary Fats

Dietary fats. The fat people are generally concerned about in their diet is found in a chemical structure called *triglycerides.* Triglycerides consist of a backbone molecule called glycerol that holds three fatty acids, thus the name triglycerides. Fatty acids are simply chains of carbon molecules with one acid end that attaches to the glycerol backbone and one stable methyl end. Most of the fatty acids in the diet are long chain (14 to 22 carbons), but some foods contain small amounts of short-chain (4 to 6 carbons) and medium-chain (8 to 12 carbons) fatty acids.

Saturated fats. Saturated fats include those fatty acids that have all their carbon chains saturated with hydrogen atoms. This saturation makes them solid at room temperature. In general, animal fats provide approximately 40 to 60 percent of their fats as saturated fats and plants provide only 10 to 20 percent of their fats as saturated fats (see figures 4.3 and 4.4).

Monounsaturated fats. Monounsaturated fats have one missing pair of hydrogen molecules. They are therefore unsaturated at one location and thus have one double bond. Monounsaturated fats are found in both animal and plant foods, but their richest sources are olive oil, canola oil, most nuts and peanuts, and avocado (see figures 4.3 and 4.4). A common monounsaturated fat found in the diet is oleic acid.

Polyunsaturated fats. Polyunsaturated fats have two or more missing hydrogen pairs, and thus have two or more double bonds. These fats are further classified by the position of the first double bond from the stable methyl end as omega-6s and omega-3s.

Omega-6 fatty acids. These polyunsaturated fatty acids have the first double bond positioned at carbon number 6. The most common omega-6 in the diet is the essential fatty acid linoleic acid, which is abundant in common plant foods: corn, sunflower, safflower, soybean, and cottonseed oils (see figure 4.4). Gamma-linolenic acid (found in evening primrose) is also an omega-6 fatty acid. Arachidonic acid is a longer-chain omega-6 found in animal products and is the form used to make the inflammatory eicosanoids. The body can convert linoleic acid to arachidonic acid.

Omega-3 fats. These polyunsaturated fatty acids have the first double bond positioned at carbon number 3. The plant version, alpha-linolenic acid (ALA) is found in specific plant foods, such as flaxseed, flaxseed oil, hemp oil, canola oil, soybean oil, and English (not black) walnuts (see figure 4.4). The longer fatty-acid versions, eicosapentaenoic acid (EPA) and docosahexaenoic acid (DHA) are found mostly in fatty fish, which include salmon, sturgeon, striped bass, and anchovies and in fish oil capsules. A vegan version (Martek vegetarian DHA) derived from microalgae, however, has recently entered the market and may soon be added to selected food products.[21] Obtaining omega-3s as DHA or EPA is thought to have some advantage as these versions are more biologically active. Alpha-linolenic acid has to be elongated in the body, which may be a slow or limited process, to more active DHA or EPA.

Hydrogenated fats and trans fats. Hydrogenation is a process practiced by the food industry in which hydrogen atoms are forced onto vegetable oil molecules under high pressure and temperature. This converts unsaturated fatty acids into saturated ones, thereby converting a liquid oil into a soft solid with improved stability. Partial hydrogenation, in which only some of the oil's unsaturated fatty acids become saturated, produces some unusual fatty acids that are called trans-fatty acids. Trans fat is found in vegetable shortenings, hard margarines, as well as crackers, cookies, snack foods, and many other foods made with or fried in partially hydrogenated oils. Margarines low in trans fat are now available.

Medium-chain triglycerides (MCTs). Medium-chain triglycerides are saturated fatty acids with a chain of 8 to 12 carbons. Some can be found naturally in milk fat, coconut oil, and palm kernel oil. They are also made commercially as a by-product of margarine production. Medium-chain triglycerides are water soluble and are more easily and rapidly digested, absorbed, and oxidized for fuel than are long-chain triglycerides. MCTs are commonly recommended for people who have problems digesting long-chain fats. Research has not found that MCTs benefit athletes.

lipoprotein (HDL) cholesterol, or "good" cholesterol.[3] HDL cholesterol helps keep cholesterol from building up in the arteries. In addition, the American Institute for Cancer Research also considers saturated fat intake a possible risk factor for certain types of cancer, including lung, colon, rectal, breast, endometrial, and prostate cancers. Furthermore, a not so obvious danger of trans fat is that scientists still do not know whether our bodies have the enzymes to fully oxidize them for energy. Yes, it is a little scary thinking where they might be lingering!

Being an athlete with a higher energy expenditure gives you a little more leeway to eat more saturated fat (if you follow the rules of less than 7 or 10 percent), but the unnatural trans fats—in my opinion—should be kept as low as possible no matter how much energy you expend. And as of January 1, 2006, the Food and Drug Administration (FDA) requires that trans fat be listed on food labels right under saturated fat. While this is great news for the most part, there are still loopholes in the regulation that allow products with less than 0.5 grams of trans fat per serving to claim "zero grams of trans" or "trans free." Although less than 0.5 grams doesn't sound like a lot, it can add up quickly, especially if you consume a lot of processed foods or eat a bigger serving than what is suggested (what athlete doesn't?). Thus, in addition to looking at the nutrition facts panel for trans and saturated fats, also check the ingredients list for partially hydrogenated oils, which contain trans fats.

Even though it is prudent to keep your combined intake of both below 10 percent of energy, it is probably not necessary to count saturated plus trans fat grams unless your LDL level is elevated. Rather, assess your diet for foods and specific brands of food products that may be too high in saturated fat or contain trans fat, and then work toward limiting sources of saturated fat and replacing trans-containing food products with trans-fat-free products. For example, replace trans-fat-containing margarines with a low-trans-fat version and bake homemade cookies with canola oil instead of buying those made with partially hydrogenated oils. If your LDL cholesterol is elevated, the information in table 4.3 should help you set your upper limit for the "bad guys."

"Good Guys"—Monounsaturated Fat and Omega-3s

Diets that are rich sources of monounsaturated and omega-3 fats (see box 4.1) are advocated for the prevention of heart and other vascular diseases. Monounsaturated fats, when substituted for saturated fats in the diet, lower LDL cholesterol and favorably influence other cardiovascular risk factors by lowering blood pressure, protecting against LDL oxidation, reducing blood clotting, and protecting the lining of the blood vessels. Omega-3 fatty acids, including both plant and fish forms (described in box 4.1), lower triglycerides, reduce inflam-

TABLE 4.3 Estimating Daily Maximum Goals for Saturated Fat and Linoleic Acid (Omega-6 Fat) and Minimum Goals for Omega-3 Fats

Enter total daily energy requirements (estimated in box 2.2 or table 2.1)		=	_____kcal/day *(line a)*
Estimate maximal intake from saturated fat and trans fat (based on recommendation to achieve less than 10% of total daily energy from saturated fats plus trans fat)	_____ kcal/day × 0.10 *(enter value line a)* Note: use 0.07 instead of 0.10 if your LDL cholesterol is high	=	_____kcal/day from saturated fat plus trans fat *(line b)*
Estimate maximal daily grams of saturated fat	_____ kcal/day ÷ 9 kcal/g *(enter value line b)*	=	_____ g/day from saturated fat *(line c)*
Estimate maximal intake from linoleic acid (omega-6 fat) (based on recommendation for an upper limit of 3% of daily energy from linoleic acid)	_____ kcal/day × 0.03 *(enter value line a)*	=	_____ kcal/day from linoleic acid *(line d)*
Estimated maximal daily grams of lenoleic acid	_____kcal/day ÷ 9 kcal/g *(enter value line d)*	=	_____ g/day from linoleic acid *(line e)*
Estimate minimal intake from omega-3 fats (based on recommendation to obtain at least 1.3% of total daily energy from omega-3s)	_____ kcal/day × 0.013 *(enter value line a)*	=	_____ kcal/day from omega-3s *(line f)*
Estimated maximal daily grams from omega-3 fats	_____ kcal/day ÷ 9 kcal/g *(enter value line f)*	=	_____ g/day from omega-3s

From *Vegetarian Sports Nutrition* by D. Enette Larson-Meyer, 2007, Champaign, IL: Human Kinetics.

mation, and improve immune function. All in all, they appear to reduce the risk for most chronic diseases.

The recommendation to increase the "good guys" is not as straightforward as the recommendation to decrease the "bad guys." Both the ADA[1] and the NCEP recommend that monounsaturates make up a large portion of energy intake. The NCEP[2] suggests up to 20 percent. The recommendation for omega-3s, however, comes with additional considerations. Because the omega-3s and their polyunsaturated counterparts, the omega-6s, both compete to be included as precursors for making a family of hormonelike substances called eicosanoids, it is recommended that you increase omega-3s in the diet and decrease their polyunsaturated partners. The eicosanoids are important and potent signal regulators, or mediators, of many biochemical functions such as blood clotting, blood pressure, vascular dilation, immune function, and inflammation. The mediators produced from the omega-3s tend to be more health promoting than the mediators produced from the omega-6s. The current recommendations for polyunsaturates are to limit linoleic acid (the parent compound of the omega-6 class) to 2 percent (or no more than 3 percent) of daily energy, and increase alpha-linolenic acid (the parent compound of the omega-3 class) to at least 1 percent of daily energy with at least an additional 0.3 percent from the longer (more biologically active) marine or microalgae omega-3s.[28] However, because vegetarians are able to produce the longer marine omega-3s from alpha-linolenic acid,[27] they may receive the same health benefits by increasing alpha-linolenic acid to at least 1.3 percent of their daily energy and by periodically incorporating longer marine omega-3s made from microalgae,[11] but this needs to be backed up by further research. To do this practically, begin adding foods that are good sources of monounsaturated and omega-3 fats in place of foods high in saturated fat, trans fat, and omega-6 fats (see figures 4.3 and 4.4). A simple way to accomplish this is to alter the oils you cook and bake with. For example, bake with canola oil (high in monounsaturated and omega-3s and low in saturated and omega-6 fats) and cook using olive oil or avocado oil (both high in monounsaturated fats). Also, try incorporating walnuts, ground flaxseed, and other nuts and healthy oils into your meals and snacks (see table 4.4) and at the same time limit intake of corn, safflower, sunflower, bean, and cottonseed oils along with butter, vegetable shortening, and most margarines. Table 4.3 can help you calculate your upper and lower limit for omega-6s and omega-3s based on your energy demands.

Striving for Smart Fat

As an active person, you can't ignore dietary fat. Fat has received a bad rap for many years, but you need it to maintain health and to enjoy your food. Therefore, achieving a healthy attitude toward smart fat requires you to do two things. The first is to enjoy eating fat. Fat sources have wonderful flavors (see table 4.4) and alert your taste buds to the flavors in your grains, vegetables, and fruits. The

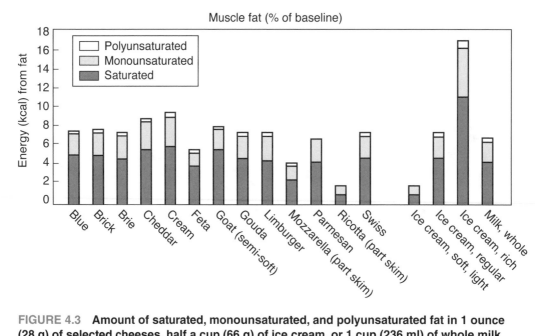

FIGURE 4.3 **Amount of saturated, monounsaturated, and polyunsaturated fat in 1 ounce (28 g) of selected cheeses, half a cup (66 g) of ice cream, or 1 cup (236 ml) of whole milk.** *Note:* Most cheese provides 8 grams of fat per serving, with about 5 of these grams coming from saturated fat.

Data from the USDA National Nutrient Database for Standard Reference. Available: http://www.ars.usda.gov/nutrientdata.

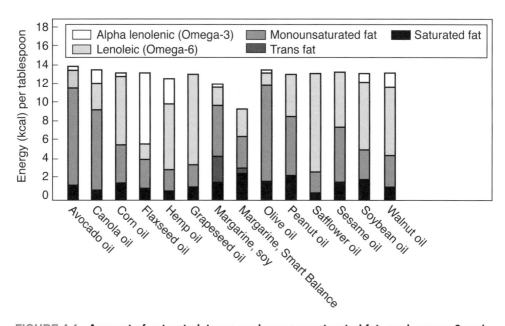

FIGURE 4.4 **Amount of saturated, trans, and monounsaturated fats and omega-6 and omega-3 polyunsaturated fats in 1 tablespoon (15 ml) of butter or vegetable oil.**

Data from the USDA National Nutrient Database for Standard Reference. Available: http://www.ars.usda.gov/nutrientdata.

Product information for hemp (seed) oil not contained in the USDA database.

TABLE 4.4 Characteristics and Recommended Uses for Selected Vegetarian Oils

Oil	Characteristics and recommended uses
Avocado	Made for high heat (when refined); perfect for frying, broiling, or wok cooking; smoke point is 510-520 °F (265-271 °C).
Canola	The ultimate all-purpose oil for cooking and baking, also works well for frying or wok cooking; has a high smoke point in general (400-425 °F [204-218 °C]), but "high" heat versions are available.
Flaxseed	Use without direct heat in finished dishes, including salads, grains, and soups or blended into dressings and smoothies. Combines well with tofu, garlic, and onions. Keep refrigerated. Smoke point is 225 °F (107 °C).
Grape seed	An all-purpose oil with a neutral taste to let other flavors take center stage. Best for short-term, medium-heat cooking, baking, or sauteing. Smoke point is 420-425 °F (204-218 °C).
Hazelnut, toasted	Has the distinctive flavor and aroma of toasted hazelnuts for use in salads and sauces and drizzled in soups. Especially good paired with bitter greens. For best results, use on finished dishes. Smoke point is 430 °F (221°C).
Hemp seed	Provides distinctive nutty flavor and can be added to most recipes. To preserve essential fatty acid content, do not use for frying. Best kept refrigerated. Smoke point is 330 °F (165 °C).
Olive	Suitable for most vegetarian fare, including salads, sautes, and sauces and to dip bread in. Light-flavored olive oil is also good for baking. Smoke point is 320 °F (160 °C) (unrefined), 400-420 °F (204-215 °C) (refined), and 468 °F (242 °C) (light). Do not use unrefined oils for frying at high heats.
Peanut	The unrefined version adds depth and intensity to any saute or stir-fry. Refined versions are perfect for high-heat applications such as frying or wok cooking. Smoke point is 320 °F (160 °C) (unrefined) and 440 °F (226 °C) (refined).
Pumpkin seed	An opaque oil with the robust flavor of roasted pumpkin. Delicious drizzled over root vegetables (with a little cheese if desired). For best results, use on finished dishes. Smoke point is not available.
Sesame	Great in Asian dishes and salad dressings. Refined versions are acceptable for wok cooking, cooking, or sauteing. Use unrefined and toasted versions for intense flavor, allowing the flavor of the oil into the finished dish. Smoke point is 350 °F (176 °C) (unrefined), and 410-450 °F (210-232 °C) (refined).
Tahini	Use as an ingredient in uncooked or already-cooked dishes, for example in hummus, tabouli, soups, grains, or salads or blended into dressings.
Walnut	Best for short-term, medium-heat cooking, baking, or sauteing. Try it drizzled over vegetables and toasted nuts and in salads or fruit muffins. Allow the flavor of the oil to be part of the finished dish. Smoke point is 320-400 °F (160-204 °C).

Note: The smoke point of the various oils is an approximation and may vary slightly from source to source. Oils should not be heated above the smoke point, which is the temperature at which the oil begins to break down and smoke. Heating above this temperature breaks down essential fatty acids and causes off-flavors. Corn, bean, safflower, and sunflower oils are not reviewed because of their commonality and high levels of omega-6 fatty acids.

second thing you must do is to consider the health aspects of fat. Limit the bad guys and focus on incorporating more of the good guys in your diet. By the same token, if you really love a food product such as brie cheese, coconut curry, cheese cake, or corn on the cob *with* butter, don't deprive yourself. Just remember to enjoy these foods on occasion. And by all means, get rid of the guilt associated with eating fat.

That said, you can choose smart fat by being more liberal in your consumption of whole foods containing monounsaturated fats and alpha-linolenic acid and limiting foods high in linoleic acid (see figure 4.4). You can accomplish this by snacking on nuts, sprinkling ground flaxseed or flaxseed oil in your cereal, smoothie, or salad (it tastes yummy), cooking regularly with olive or canola oil, and experimenting with different and even new oils. Once you stray from the common refined oils found in grocery stores (corn, sunflower, bean, safflower, and even soybean), you will discover that individual oils have unique properties and flavors. Some oils, such as canola, are better for baking or cooking at high temperatures, while others, such as olive oil, are perfect for sauteing or dipping and add immense flavor. Some, such as toasted hazelnut or flax, are best simply sprinkled on cooked food or cold salads. Enjoy, as we move on to learn more about protein.

Building Muscle Without Meat

H*e asked to sit with me at lunch the day I divulged that I was a sports nutrition-ist (sometimes it is easiest to keep this quiet). He was about 20 years old and a counselor at the family camp we were attending. He informed me that he was majoring in biochemistry but was interested in nutrition, both personally and as a career option. During the college year he trained with weights and dabbled rec-reationally in many sports. At camp, located in the heart of the Sangre de Cristo mountains of southern Colorado, he was just plain active chasing after kids and hiking up 13,000-foot (3,962 m) peaks.*

"I was vegetarian during the first two weeks of camp," he told me. "I really wanted to be vegetarian," he said "but I was not getting enough protein." "Really?" I asked. I thought about the camp, which had a reputation for providing nutritious meals. The cooking staff made their own bread daily and served a vegetarian entree at every meal. The camp provided better meals than my family currently ate at home. "It's OK for girls," he continued, "but guys need more protein." I paused for a second remembering my weightlifting days in college before I became addicted to endurance sports. I remember guys telling me—upon learning I was vegetarian—that I looked "too meaty to be vegetarian" (yes, they thought they were being cute). I would tell them, as I explained in detail to my counselor friend that day, that meat is not needed for building muscle strength or muscle mass.

Eating meat to achieve strength and victory has a history in athletics of more than 2,000 years. The diets of athletes in the ancient Olympic era—including the legend-ary wrestler Milo of Croton who earned five successive Olympic wins from 532 to 516 ʙ–reportedly contained large quantities of meat for "physical strength."[14] And those of laborers and athletes at the turn of the 20th century—including the renowned Harvard and Yale rowing teams—were high in protein because at the time protein was considered to be the primary energy source for exercise. In addition, many cultures also believed that consuming the muscle of an animal would result in the transfer of that animal's strength and prowess to the athlete.[9] Certainly, some of these myths still linger as many coaches and athletes continue to believe that large quantities of protein—particularly animal protein—are needed to produce strong and "meaty" athletes. Although protein does play a critical role in an athlete's health and performance, it can be adequately supplied by vegetarian and vegan diets. This chapter reviews the role of protein in the diet and discusses how you can easily build muscle strength and mass without meat.

Protein Primer

Dietary protein is necessary for sustaining life. It provides the amino acid building blocks needed to form the structural basis of most of the body's tissue including skeletal muscle, tendons, hormones, enzymes, red blood cells, and immune cells. Amino acids also serve as a source of energy, and certain amino acids can be converted to blood sugar in a process called *gluconeogenesis,* which is important during both prolonged exercise and starvation. Chemically, each of the 20 different amino acids is structurally distinct, but all contain at least one nitrogen-containing amino group attached to a similar skeleton of carbon, hydrogen, and oxygen.

Our body's requirement for protein is really a requirement for amino acids and nitrogen. Our bodies cannot produce 8 of these amino acids—called the essential amino acids—but are able to make the remaining 12 or so as long as enough nitrogen is consumed in the diet (see table 5.1). Together, the 20 essential and nonessential amino acids are arranged in various combinations to build the many proteins in the body. The arrangement of these amino acid building blocks is unique for each protein in the body as well as the diet. Closely related species,

TABLE 5.1 Essential and Nonessential Amino Acids

Essential amino acids (also called indispensable amino acids) cannot be made by the body and must be obtained through the diet.	Isoleucine* Leucine* Lysine Methionine	Phenylalanine Threonine Tryptophan Valine*
Conditional amino acids are made by the body but are essential in times of growth because they can't be made at a rate fast enough to support growth.	Arginine	Histidine
Nonessential amino acids (also called dispensable amino acids) can be made by the body, and thus it is not essential to obtain them through the diet.	Alanine Asparagine Aspartic acid Cysteine Glutamic acid	Glutamine Glycine Proline Serine Tyrosine

*Branched-chain amino acids.

such as humans and animals, tend to make proteins with a similar spectrum of amino acids, and those of very different species, such as plants compared to mammals, tend to have quite different spectrums. Protein building is initiated after a signal—typically a hormone or mechanical-stress signal—to the cell's genetic material, or DNA, is communicated to initiate gene transcription and ultimately protein synthesis.

Although the body can make the nonessential amino acids, the essential amino acids must be obtained through the diet. If the profile of the essential amino acids consumed in the diet does not match that required by the body, the amino acid or acids found in the shortest supply, relative to the amount needed for protein synthesis, are referred to as the *limiting amino acid or acids*. Diets based on a protein from a single plant food do not foster optimal growth because the diet does not supply enough of the needed building blocks for human protein synthesis. For example, maize is low in tryptophan, rice is low in lysine and threonine, wheat is low in lysine, and most legumes, except soy, are low in methionine or tryptophan or both. Diets based on soy protein and combinations of plant proteins, as well as meat protein, however, can easily supply enough of the right amino acid building blocks for human growth and muscle development.

Determining Protein Needs

As an athlete, your protein needs are most likely—but not necessarily—higher than those of your inactive friends. Whether they are higher, and how much higher, depends on your sport and current training program. For example, if you are a fitness enthusiast or a recreationally active athlete who exercises or plays sports several times a week, your needs should easily be met by the Recommended Dietary Allowance (RDA) of 0.8 grams of protein per kilogram of body mass per day. The same is true if you are in maintenance training during the off-season or are recovering from an injury. If, however, you are training intensely for 8 to 40 hours a week, your protein needs may be about twice the RDA, particularly during the start of the season or a new training regimen. The consensus of sports nutritionists—which is based on published research on the protein needs of male athletes—suggests that endurance athletes need 1.2 to 1.4 grams of protein per kilogram of body mass per day, whereas resistance and strength-trained athletes may require as much as 1.6 to 1.7 grams of protein per kilogram of body mass per day.[4] Female athletes may require slightly less protein per kilogram of body mass than male athletes,[15] but more research is needed before specific recommendations can be made. The rationale for the additional protein required during training is based on the need to repair exercise-induced microdamage to muscle fibers (all athletes know about this), the minimal use of protein for fuel during exercise, and, to a lesser extent, the need for additional protein to support muscle development.

In addition, inadequate intake of both energy and carbohydrate increases protein needs. Research has shown that during prolonged endurance activity,

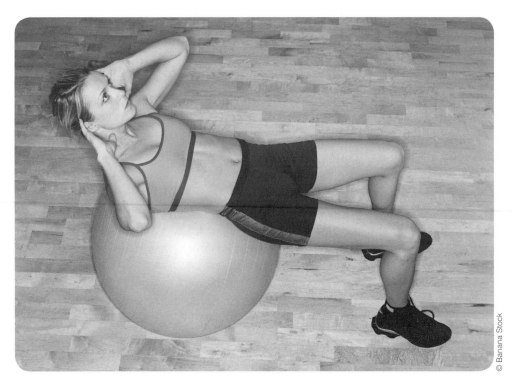

© Banana Stock

The amino acids needed for muscle development can be derived from soy protein and a variety of protein-rich plant foods.

athletes with low glycogen stores metabolize twice as much protein as those with adequate stores, primarily because of the increased conversion of amino acids to glucose to maintain blood sugar.[8] This, however, can be halted by adequately supplementing with carbohydrate before or during exercise or both. Furthermore, athlete or not, your protein needs are likely to be higher if you intentionally restrict calories to promote weight or body fat loss.

Although no research suggests that protein recommendations are different for vegetarian athletes, it has been suggested that vegetarians may need to consume approximately 10 percent more protein than omnivores to account for the lower digestibility of plant protein compared with animal proteins.[11] Accordingly, the protein requirements of vegetarian athletes (based on the aforementioned recommendations for athletes) would be approximately 1.3 to 1.8 grams per kilogram of body mass.[17] However, the additional requirement to account for lower digestibility is not true for all plant proteins. The protein in most soy products for example is readily digestible compared to protein from legumes, which is not as easily digested. Furthermore, in its release of the Dietary Reference Intake (DRIs) for protein, the Food and Nutrition Board of the National Academy of Sciences Institute of Medicine concluded that a separate recommendation for protein consumption was not required for vegetarians who consume dairy products or eggs and complementary mixtures of high-quality plant proteins.[5]

Finally, it is important to mention that not all scientists believe that the protein needs of athletes are higher than those recommended for the general population. Although many studies show that protein utilization, and therefore requirements, increases with the initiation of exercise training, most of these studies have been short term and may not have allowed enough time for adaptation to the training regimen.[3] Hence, it is possible that the protein needs are only temporarily elevated and return to baseline at some point after training initiation and adaptation.[3] For instance, a long-term study conducted in the early '70s found that people starting a cycling program experienced a negative nitrogen balance with initiation of training, but this negative nitrogen balance returned to neutral after 20 days of training with no change in diet.[7] In the recent release of the DRIs, the scientists on the panel did not feel there was enough compelling evidence to suggest that additional protein is needed for healthy adults undertaking resistance or endurance exercise.[5] You can estimate your daily protein needs using the calculations in table 5.2.

TABLE 5.2   Estimating Daily Protein Needs

Enter your body mass (weight) in kilograms (weight in pounds divided by 2.2).	_____ kg *(line a)*
Enter estimated range of protein needed to support your current level of training and performance (see table 3.1). • 0.8 g protein/kg body mass • 1.2-1.4 g protein/kg body mass • 1.6-1.7 g protein/kg body mass • 1.3-1.8 g protein/kg body mass	_____ to _____ g/kg *(line b_1) (line b_2)*
Multiply line a by line b_1 to get your estimated lower range.	_____ g protein/day
Multiply line a by line b_2 to get your estimated upper range.	_____ g protein/day

From *Vegetarian Sports Nutrition* by D. Enette Larson-Meyer, 2007, Champaign, IL: Human Kinetics.

Meeting Protein Needs

Despite the controversy over the protein needs of vegetarians and athletes, you can easily meet your protein needs—even if they are in the upper level recommended—on a vegetarian diet. This, of course, is provided that your diet contains both adequate energy and a variety of plant-based protein foods. The once-held belief that vegetarians need to eat specific combinations of plant proteins in the same meal has been dispelled, at least among nonathletic adults,[19] and replaced with the recommendation to simply consume a variety of plant-based protein-rich foods over the course of a day.[1, 19] Emphasizing amino acid balance at each meal is not necessary because the limiting amino acids in one meal can be buffered (at least over the short term) by small pools of free amino acids in the gut, skeletal muscle, and blood. Furthermore, although some plant foods tend to be low in certain amino acids, usual combinations of proteins consumed in the diets of many cultures tend to be complete by naturally providing all essential amino acids (see table 5.3).

That said, however, it is possible that vegetarian athletes in intense training should consume a protein-containing snack or meal soon after exhaustive exercise, when amino acid pools may be compromised. Examples of high-quality proteins are soy protein, which is comparable in quality to that of animal proteins,[6, 18] and dairy and egg protein. Another option is combinations of two or more vegetable proteins such as peanut butter on bread, nuts with toasted grains (in muesli), or a mini bean burrito. Most likely these are snacks you naturally select, maybe just not after exercise.

If you are concerned about your protein intake, my first thought is—don't be. Surveys of athletes have consistently found that most, simply by virtue of their high energy intake, meet or even exceed their protein requirements without even trying. This is true for vegetarian and vegan athletes as well. Vegetarian diets generally derive 12.5 percent of energy from protein, whereas vegan diets derive 11 percent from protein.[10] Therefore, according to these percentages, if you were an 80-kilogram (176 lb) male athlete consuming 3,600 calories, you would receive 1.41 grams of protein per kilogram of body weight from the average vegetarian diet and 1.2 grams per kilogram from the average vegan diet. If you were a 50-kilogram (110 lb) female gymnast consuming 2,200 calories, you would receive 1.38 grams per kilogram from a vegetarian diet and 1.21 grams per kilogram from a vegan diet.

Nevertheless, if you are concerned about your own protein intake, you can check yourself by counting your protein intake for a day or two using the information provided in tables 5.4 and 5.5. The information on the food labels should also be helpful. Remember also to count the protein in your bread, cereal, and grain foods, which can add up to a considerable amount. If you find your intake of protein is lacking compared to your estimated requirements, simply strive to

TABLE 5.3 Natural Food Combinations That Provide All Essential Amino Acids

Excellent combinations	Examples
Grains and legumes	Rice and beans, toast triangles with bean soup, tortillas with beans, peanut butter sandwich
Grains or vegetable with dairy or soy accent	Pasta with cheese, baked potato with dairy or soy sour cream, cream of vegetable soup, rice pudding
Legumes and nuts	Hummus made with chickpeas and tahini, lentil and nut "meat" balls
Soy protein	Tofu stir-fry, barbeque soybeans, tofu smoothie, vegetarian burgers, marinated tempeh

TABLE 5.4 Approximate Protein Content of Selected Food and Beverages

Food	Portion	Protein (g)
Bread, grains, rice, pasta	1 oz serving	2-3
Cheese, medium and hard	1 oz	7
Cheese, cottage	1/4 cup	7
"Cheese," soy or veggie	1 oz	6
Egg, whole	1 large	7
Legumes (most beans and peas)	1/2 cup cooked	7
Milk, cows'	1 cup	8
Milk, soy	1 cup	7
Nuts, most	2 Tbsp	7
Peanut butter	2 Tbsp	7
Quinoa, cooked	1 cup	11
Quorn (mycoprotein) Meat-Free Meatballs	4 meatballs (68 g)	14
Quorn (mycoprotein) Naked Cutlets	1 cutlet (69 g)	11
Quorn (mycoprotein) Turkey-Style Roast	1/5 roast (3 oz)	15
Seitan	4 oz	21
Soybean-curd cheese	1/4 cup	7
Soy protein isolate	1 oz	21
Tempeh	1 cup	31
Textured vegetable protein (TVP), cooked	1/2 cup	8
Tofu, soft	1 cup	10
Tofu, firm	1 cup	20
Vegemite sandwich spread	1 tsp	1.5
Vegetables, most	1/2 cup cooked	2-3
Vegetarian "burgers"	1 patty	6-16
Vegetarian "burger" crumbles	1/2 cup	7-11
Vegetarian "chicken" patties or nuggets	1 patty (~6 nuggets)	7-15
Vegetarian "dogs"	1 dog	9-12
Yogurt, dairy	1 cup	8
Yogurt, soy	1 cup	8

Data compiled from the Diabetic Exchange List for Meal Planning, 2003, The USDA National Nutrient Database for Standard Reference (http://www.ars.usda.gov/nutrientdata), and selected Food Labels, including those from Quorn™ (http://www.quorn.com) and CalorieKing Australia (http://www.thecalorieking.com.au).

TABLE 5.5 Sample Log for Counting Protein

1 1/2 cups cornflakes (3/4 cup = 1 oz serving)	4-6
1 cup 1% milk	8
12 oz (1 1/2 cups) orange juice	0
White bread, 2 slices	4-6
2 Tbsp peanut butter	7
1 can (~2 cups) fruit cocktail in light syrup	0
1 large handful (~1 cup) grapes	0
Jelly beans (~2 oz)	0
1/3 cup granola	2-3
1/4 cup almonds	14
2 cups vegetarian chili (contains ~1 cup beans and 1 cup onion, green peppers, and tomato sauce combined)	14
~2 oz cheddar cheese	14
15 saltine crackers	4-6
Total g	71-78
Total g/kg	1.11-1.22

Reported daily carbohydrate intake for a 141-lb (64 kg) female volleyball player involved in off-season training. Her protein goal based on the RDA of 0.8 g protein/kg body weight is 51 g/day. Although she is likely to exceed her needs, she needs to increase protein intake during periods of more-intense training. This should happen naturally by increasing caloric intake. For example, she could add half a cup of beans and another grain serving (10 additional g protein) to the intake shown above. *Note:* Protein counting is most accurate if portion sizes are accurately measured and food labels are used to supplement the information presented in table 5.4. Refer to appendix E for guidance on converting English units to metric.

add one to three servings of protein-rich vegetarian foods to your regular meals or snacks. For example, add soy milk to a fruit snack, lentils to spaghetti sauce, tofu to stir-fry, or chickpeas (garbanzo beans) to salad. In my experience, however, the only athletes who tend to lack protein are those who focus too much on carbohydrate (the bagel, pasta, banana athletes) or who consume too little food in general. Vegetarian foods that are particularly rich sources of protein are legumes, tofu, seitan, quinoa, soy protein isolate, and commercially available meat analogues, such as vegetarian hot dogs, burgers, and "chicken" made from soy or mycoprotein. Vegetarian athletes who are not particularly fond of many protein-rich plant foods or are allergic to them may also need to monitor their protein intake.

Role of Excess Protein

Improvements in both strength and muscle mass occur as a result of your training and are also dictated by your genetic makeup. Dietary protein simply provides the amino acid building blocks needed to make protein and facilitate neuroendocrine connections. Thus, you will not receive the training gains you deserve—muscle strength and muscle mass gains—if your diet is lacking in either energy or protein. On the other hand, you will not magically gain strength or functional muscle if you consume amino acid building blocks in excess. If this were true, your average male couch potato would look more like Arnold Schwarzenegger. A classic study conducted at McMaster University in Canada in the early 1990s nicely illustrates this point.[16] In this study, researchers randomly assigned both male strength athletes and sedentary subjects to receive one of three protein-modified diets for 13 days. One diet supplied approximately the U.S. RDA for protein (0.86 g protein/ kg body mass/day), one provided close to the current recommendation for athletes (1.4 g protein/kg body mass/day), and one provided an excessive amount of protein (2.4 g protein/kg body mass/day). The researchers found that the diet containing approximately the U.S. RDA for protein did not provide adequate protein for the strength athletes and impaired whole-body protein building compared to the other two diets. The diet providing 2.4 grams of protein, however, did not increase whole-body protein synthesis any more than the diet providing 1.4 grams of protein did. In contrast, the diet that followed the RDA recommendation supplied adequate protein for the sedentary men. Not surprisingly, increasing protein intake in the nontraining men did not increase protein synthesis.

What happens to excess protein intake? Quite simply, if you consume more than you need, the nitrogen group is removed and it is either used for energy or stored as fat. This makes for an expensive source of energy, both from a personal metabolic and ecological viewpoint. Although it is not known whether habitually high protein intake causes long-term detrimental effects, some nutritionists question whether such diets place added stress on the kidney (which is the organ responsible for eliminating the excess nitrogen) as well as the liver. One recent study found that an Atkins-style high-protein diet increased the risk for both kidney stones and calcium loss from bone.[13]

Considering Protein Supplements

Vegetarian and vegan athletes can meet their protein needs through diet alone. For convenience, however, many vegetarian athletes choose to supplement their diets on occasion with protein-containing nutrition beverages, such as Boost Breeze, and soy protein-isolate drinks, or protein bars, such as Genisoy. Although this is fine on occasion, these food products should not replace eating real food and real meals, despite some companies' marketing ploys to convince you otherwise. The latest supplemental trend suggests that certain isolated whole proteins, including isolated soy protein, isolated casein, or isolated whey,[2, 4, 12] promote greater gains in lean mass than do the whole protein found in foods such as tofu and milk, which contain casein and whey. Although some evidence suggests that isolated protein may be more rapidly digested and promote greater protein retention (at least over the short term), evidence that this affects the gain of muscle or strength in well-trained athletes in the long run does not exist. The

6

Optimizing Bone Health

I still vividly remember the day I gave up drinking cows' milk. I had been working late at the lab and came home a bit tired and hungry and poured a late-night glass of milk. As I stopped pouring, however, I thought I saw a string hanging between the carton and the glass. It lingered something like raw egg does from a cracked shell into a bowl. I thought I was seeing things, so I smelled the milk. It smelled fine. I took a drink, it tasted fine . . . at first, and then the feel in my mouth was not quite right, and as I stopped drinking that same string appeared between my lips and the glass. I dumped the milk out, closed the refrigerator, and went to bed hoping I just needed sleep.

The next day I learned that much of the milk from dairies in my area had developed what is commonly called ropiness, caused by the growth of certain harmless bacteria that had gone a little crazy during the unseasonably wet spring. After that, I found I could no longer tolerate milk, which at the time was my main source of calcium. I was completely unprepared. First, I nearly went broke drinking calcium-fortified soy milk and then found myself jumping on the bandwagon with those who believe that vegans and vegetarians who consume little dairy don't need as much calcium as meat-eating Westerners. Finally, after levelheaded research, I recognized that all vegetarians should strive to meet the recommended Dietary Reference Intake for calcium and that this intake can be achieved on a vegetarian diet without overdependence on dairy or fortified products. I also began to recognize that calcium is not the only nutrient responsible for keeping bones strong and healthy and that a properly selected vegetarian diet may even be advantageous for promoting healthy bone.

It is hard to argue the importance of bone health. As athletes, we know that we can't perform without a healthy skeleton and that our exercise training in turn helps us maintain healthy muscles and bone. Whether we are immediately concerned about the nutrients that promote healthy bone, however, is often another story. It seems that some athletes feel immune to bone problems, and others seem to think—perhaps as I once did—that getting adequate calcium is all that is needed. As vegetarians, many may also be antidairy—believing that calcium and bone-related research is tainted by the powerful dairy industry—which in the long run could come back to haunt them. Research, for example, has suggested that although the bone density of lacto–ovo vegetarians is equal to or greater than that of omnivores, the bone density of many vegans is lower than vegetarians or omnivores. This chapter is directed at helping vegan and vegetarian athletes understand the basics of bone metabolism and bone health and how bone health can be optimized on a vegetarian eating plan.

Bone Health Basics

Most of us think of bone simply as the rigid part of our skeleton that forms the levers upon which our muscles contract. Bone, however, is a living, growing tissue that is actively broken down and rebuilt, a process scientists call *bone turnover.* Bone turnover, also called *remodeling,* is the process of replacing existing bone structure—the matrix—with new bone structure. Remodeling occurs in both the developing skeleton of children and teens and in the nongrowing skeleton of adults. In fact, it is estimated that adult bone turns over at a rate of about 10 percent per year. This remodeling is thought to be necessary for maintaining healthy bone and normal calcium levels in the body. For example, one of the major functions of bone, apart from supporting our bodies, is to aid in maintaining blood calcium within the normal range. If bone could not be used as an immediate calcium reserve, the muscles in our body, including our heart muscle, would contract improperly, and our enzymes would operate uncontrollably. Obviously, the outcome would not be good. In addition, remodeling is probably also necessary for preventing the accumulation of microfractures, including stress fractures.

How bone remodeling occurs is fascinating. The process is directed by two types of key bone cells known as osteoblasts and osteoclasts. Osteoclasts erode the bone surface—forming small cavities—through a set of reactions known as resorption. Osteoblasts act at the site of the cavities to synthesize the new bone matrix. This is referred to as *formation.* The new bone matrix is then mineralized with calcium, phosphorus, and other minerals, resulting in new bone tissue. Bone health is maintained if resorption and formation are tightly coupled, whereas bone loss ensues if bone resorption occurs at a rate greater than bone formation.

Structurally, bone tissue is made up largely of collagen, a protein that gives the bone its tensile strength and framework, and the calcium phosphate mineralized complex that hardens the framework. The combination of collagen and calcium phosphate crystals, called *hydroxyapatite,* makes bone strong yet flexible enough to bear weight and withstand stress.

Bone tissue, however, is not just bone tissue. Rather, adult bone is made up of two major types of tissue: cortical bone and trabecular bone. Trabecular bone makes up approximately 20 percent of your skeleton and has a faster turnover rate than cortical bone. It is estimated that as much as 20 percent of trabecular bone can be undergoing active remodeling at one time. Cortical bone makes up the remaining 80 percent, but only 5 percent of its surface is in active remodeling at one time. Cortical bone is found primarily in the long bones, for example, those in the arms and legs. Trabecular bone is found mostly in the axial skeleton, the flat bones, and the ends of the long bones. Common fracture sites are thought to have a high trabecular content. Trabecular bone has a faster turnover rate because it has more metabolically active cells and greater blood supply. Hence, trabecular bone is more sensitive to hormones that govern day-to-day calcium deposits and withdrawals, which means it more readily gives up minerals whenever blood calcium starts to drop. Loss of trabecular bone can occur whenever calcium withdrawal exceeds calcium deposits, but loss typically begins around age 30, even for people who eat a healthy diet. Although cortical bone also gives up calcium, this occurs at a slower and steadier pace. Cortical bone losses typically begin at about age 40 and continue slowly but surely thereafter.

Factors That Influence Bone Health

Many factors regulate bone health, mainly by influencing bone turnover. These factors include physical activity, hormonal status, and nutrition. Participation in weight-bearing, impact-loading, and weight-training activities, which include running, racewalking, rope jumping, gymnastics, and weightlifting, promotes denser and stronger bones. Just how exercise does this is not completely understood, but the prevailing theory considers bone to react as a piezoelectric crystal that converts the mechanical stress—from the muscle or ground forces—into electrical energy.[25] The electrical charges created then stimulate bone formation by stimulating osteoblast activity. The stimulatory effect appears to be related to the magnitude of the applied force and its frequency of application, but it can be inhibited by hormone signals or lack of them. We know, for example, that certain male and female athletes are at risk for low bone density, and that those most at risk include females with altered menstrual function or low concentrations of circulating estrogen.

Hormones and More Hormones

The main hormones involved in bone remodeling and thus bone health include parathyroid hormone (PTH), vitamin D, calcitonin, and estrogen. However, the priority of most of these hormones is not to maintain healthy bone but to keep blood calcium in check (as discussed earlier), which ultimately affects bone-mineral content and density. PTH plays the major role in this effect, stimulating the release of calcium from bone into blood at the first sign of a lowered blood-calcium concentration. PTH also activates vitamin D, signals the kidneys to retain more calcium and excrete less in urine, and indirectly signals the intestines, through vitamin D, to increase calcium absorption. Calcitonin, on the other hand, decreases rising blood-calcium concentrations by inhibiting osteoclast activity, thereby suppressing bone resorption, and increasing both calcium and phosphorus loss in the urine.

The sex hormones estrogen and possibly testosterone, or male androgens in general, appear to regulate bone turnover in both men and women. Estrogen deficiency increases the rate of bone remodeling and the amount of bone lost with each remodeling cycle.[34] Androgen deficiency, as is noted in men undergoing removal of diseased testes, also results in more fractures,[42] but the specific mechanism and its relation to low bone density in men is not well understood. Testosterone replacement therapy, however, may improve bone health in men with reduced sex hormone status.

Nutrition—More Than Just Calcium

Several nutrients play a critical role in bone health. Thanks to marketing by the American Dairy Association, most Americans are aware that calcium is important for bone health. If you are a vegan athlete, you are also probably very aware that most Americans feel that if you don't "Got Milk," you don't "Got Calcium." Thus, in some sense we have been brainwashed to equate bone health with cows' milk (or other dairy products). Like most things, however, many dietary factors affect bone health. These include calcium, vitamin D, magnesium, vitamins A, C, and K—which favorably affect bone health—and phosphorus, caffeine, alcohol, animal protein, and even oxylates, which negatively affect bone when overconsumed. Other factors, such as fluoride, can optimize bone health but only if consumed in the right quantities. The next section reviews each of these nutrients and provides tips for making food choices from a plant-based diet to optimize bone health.

Calcium

Calcium is the most abundant mineral in the body and is necessary for bone formation, muscle contraction, nerve-impulse transmission, and enzyme activation. Calcium intake is thought to play a key role in bone health because it is the largest constituent of the bone crystals—made of hydroxyapatite—and has been found in many studies to be directly associated with a person's bone density. For example, previous calcium intake from milk during childhood and adolescence is found to be associated with greater bone density in young women.[19, 38] Adequate calcium intake from both food and supplements in early adulthood has also been shown to retard loss of bone-mineral content.[32]

To this end, however, most vegetarians may have already heard that calcium balance is influenced by factors other than dietary calcium intake. These include calcium absorption in the intestines and calcium excretion in the urine and feces. On the intake side, 20 to 40 percent of the calcium eaten is absorbed by the intestines, but the absorption rate can vary considerably depending on the food source (as will be discussed later). On the excretion side, large amounts of dietary sodium and protein, particularly meat protein, increase calcium loss through urine. Although it is often argued that the effect of sodium and protein on increasing calcium loss is small, experimental evidence suggests that the combined effect of a diet with excessive animal protein and sodium has a more pronounced effect.[21] In sedentary people, sodium and protein intakes typical of the Western diet (7,100 mg sodium, 2 g protein/kg body weight) were found to almost double daily calcium excretion (152 vs. 257 mg calcium lost per day) when compared to a diet lower in both nutrients (3,200 mg sodium, 1 g protein/kg body weight)[21] and more reflective of a vegetarian diet. Consequently to account for the additional 105 grams of calcium lost on the high-sodium, high-protein diet, it would be necessary to consume an additional 263 to 525 milligrams of calcium daily, assuming an absorption rate of 20 to 40 percent.

Based on these and other findings, it is often argued that vegans and vegetarians consuming small amounts of animal foods may have daily calcium requirements that are lower than those proposed by the Dietary Reference Intakes (DRIs) for calcium. The argument holds that because the vegan diet is lower in animal protein and most likely sodium, less calcium is needed daily to replace the resulting lower calcium loss through urine. Although I must admit that the argument is intriguing, supporting research is not available. Thus, your best bet as an athlete is to strive for the recommended DRI, which is 1,000 milligrams of calcium per day for adults ages 19 to 50. Those older than 50 should strive for 1,200 milligrams per day, and those under 18 should strive for 1,300 milligrams per day. Evidence suggests that amenorrheic athletes (those who have not experienced a menstrual cycle for at least three months) may require up to 1,500 milligrams per day to retain calcium balance.[11] Low calcium intake has been associated with an increased risk of stress fractures[29] and decreased bone density, particularly in amenorrheic athletes.[45] Regular exercise, however, has not been shown to increase calcium requirements above that of the general population.

If you are a male or regularly menstruating female athlete, you can meet your calcium requirements by including several servings of dairy products or approximately five to eight servings of calcium-containing plant foods daily. Plant foods that are rich in easily absorbable calcium are listed in table 6.1 and include low-oxalate green leafy vegetables (collard, mustard, and turnip greens), tofu (set with calcium), tahini, certain legumes, fortified orange juice, almonds, and blackstrap molasses. Research has suggested that calcium absorption from most of these foods is as good as or better than milk,[14, 43, 44] which has a fractional absorption rate of 32 percent (see figure 6.1). Recent evidence, however, found that the calcium-absorption rate from calcium-fortified orange juice, and thus likely other juices, varies considerably by fortification system, with the fractional absorption being nearly 50 percent greater for calcium citrate malate than for tricalcium phosphate/calcium lactate.[15] On the other hand, the calcium in fortified soy milk, most legumes, nuts, and seeds is slightly less well absorbed. The fractional

TABLE 6.1 Calcium, Calcium-to-Phosphorus Ratio, and Magnesium Content of Selected Vegetarian Foods

Food	Portion	Calcium (mg)	Calcium-to-phosphorus ratio	Magnesium (mg)
GRAIN EQUIVALENTS				
Bread, enriched	1 oz slice	43	1.5:1	7
Bread, whole wheat	1 oz slice	20	0.3:1-0.5:1	24
Cereal, calcium-fortified	1 serving (1 oz)	125-1,000	>1:1	Varies
VEGETABLES AND LEGUMES, INCLUDING SOY				
Beet greens	1 cup cooked	164	2.8:1	98
Black beans	1 cup cooked	46	0.2:1	120
Broccoli	1 cup cooked	62	0.6:1	32
Cabbage, Chinese (bok choy)	1 cup cooked	158	3.2:1	19
Cabbage, head	1 cup cooked	46	4.2:1	12
Chickpeas (garbanzo beans)	1 cup cooked	80	0.3:1	79
Collard greens	1 cup cooked	266	4.7:1	38
Kale	1 cup cooked	94	2.6:1	23
Lentils	1 cup cooked	38	0.1:1	71
Mustard greens	1 cup cooked	104	1.8:1	21
Okra	1 cup cooked, sliced	62	2.4:1	58
Pinto beans	1 cup cooked	79	0.3:1	86
Red kidney beans	1 cup cooked	50	0.2:1	80
Southern peas (black-eyed, crowder)	1 cup cooked	41	0.2:1	91
Soybeans	1 cup cooked	175	0.4:1	148
Sweet potato	1 medium, baked	43	0.7:1	31
Tofu, firm (calcium set)	1/2 cup	861*	3.6:1	73
Tofu, regular (calcium set)	1/2 cup	434*	3.6:1	37
Turnip greens	1 cup cooked	197	4.7:1	32
FRUITS				
Grapefruit juice, calcium fortified	1 cup	350	9.5:1	30
Orange juice, calcium fortified	1 cup	350	7:1-8:1	27
NUTS AND SEEDS				
Almonds	1 oz	70	0.5:1	78
Cashews, peanuts, pecans, pine nuts, sunflower seeds	1 oz	5-20	>0.1:1	22-71
Pumpkin seeds	1 oz	12	0.04:1	151
Tahini	1 Tbsp	64	0.6:1	14
Walnuts	1 oz	28	0.3:1	45

Food	Portion	Calcium (mg)	Calcium-to-phosphorus ratio	Magnesium (mg)
MILK, SOY MILK, AND CHEESE				
Soy milk, calcium fortified	1 cup	368*	1.6:1	39
Cows' milk, skim	1 cup	306	1.2:1	27
Cows' milk, 2%	1 cup	285	1.2:1	27
Cheddar cheese	1 oz	204	1.4:1	8
Mozzarella	1 oz	207	1.4:1	7
Swiss	1 oz	224	1.4:1	11
OTHER				
Molasses	1 Tbsp	41	6.8:1	48
Blackstrap molasses, plantation	1 Tbsp	200	N/a	N/a

*Varies by brand.

Data from the USDA National Nutrient Database for Standard Reference. Available: http://www.ars.usda.gov/nutrientdata.

Calcium absorption	Food
>50%	Bok choy, broccoli, Chinese/Napa cabbage, collards, kale, okra, turnip greens, TVP, blackstrap molasses
~30%	Milk, calcium-set tofu, calcium-fortified orange juice (with calcium citrate malate)
20%	Fortified soy milk, most nuts and seeds, most legumes, fortified orange juice (with tricalcium phosphate/calcium lactate)
≤5%	Spinach, Swiss chard, beet greens, rhubarb

FIGURE 6.1 **Calcium absorption from vegetable and dairy sources.**

Values represent fractional absorption or percent of calcium intake absorbed in the intestines.

Data from C.Weaver and K. Plawecki, 1994, "Dietary calcium: Adequacy of a vegetarian diet," *Am J Clin Nutr.* 59: 1238S-1241S; C.M. Weaver, W.R. Proulx and R. Heaney, 1999, "Choices for achieving adequate dietary calcium with a vegetarian diet," *Am J Clin Nutr.* 70: 543S-548S; R.P. Heaney, M.S. Dowell,K. Rafferty and J. Bierman, 2000, "Bioavailabilty of the calcium in fortified soy milk with some observations on method," *Am J Clin Nutr.* 71: 1166-1169; E.R. Monsen and J.L. Balintfy, 1982, "Calculating dietary iron bioavailability: Refinement and computerization," *J Am Diet Assoc.* 80: 307-311.

absorption of these foods is in the range of 17 to 24 percent. Foods with a high oxalate or high phytate content, including rhubarb, spinach, Swiss chard, and beet greens, are poorly absorbed sources of calcium.

If after reading this section, you or your coach are still nervous about shaking the dairy habit—a recent clinical study may set you at ease. Researchers in Germany measured calcium balance and bone turnover in eight young adults placed on an energy-balanced vegan and vegetarian diet for 10 days each.[20] They found that although calcium intake was lower on the vegan (843 ± 140 mg) compared with the lacto vegetarian diet (1,322 ± 303 mg), all participants were able to maintain a positive calcium balance and appropriate rate of bone turnover on both diets. The calcium provided in the vegan diet was from well-absorbed foods and calcium-rich mineral water.

Although it is possible to maintain calcium balance on a plant-based diet,[1, 20, 44] some active vegetarians may find it more convenient to use fortified foods or calcium supplements to help meet their requirements. Calcium carbonate and calcium citrate are well-absorbed sources used in supplements, but calcium carbonate is generally less expensive. Long-term supplementation with calcium carbonate does not compromise iron status in iron-replete adults[27] (as was once thought), but it is best to take calcium supplements several hours after a meal, for example, at bedtime, rather than with meals.[10] Because vitamin D is also required for bone health, your calcium source should also contain vitamin D.

Vitamin D

Healthy bones also depend on vitamin D, a versatile nutrient that functions both as a vitamin and a hormone. As you may know, an early form of vitamin D, called vitamin D_3, is made in the skin upon stimulation by the sun's UV light. Vitamin D_3 is then turned into calcidiol, the main storage form, by the liver and later activated as needed to its active form calcitriol by the kidney. Calcitriol's main function is to maintain blood calcium, but in doing so, it also promotes intestinal calcium absorption and provides adequate quantities of calcium and phosphorus for bone formation. Research clearly suggests that adequate vitamin D along with calcium are imperative for healthy bones.[17, 34]

Some athletes may be at risk for poor vitamin D status, which some researchers consider to be an unrecognized epidemic.[17] Vitamin D deficiency can manifest in unexplained muscle pain or weakness and compromised calcium balance. Those at risk include athletes with low intakes of fortified foods or supplements, limited sun exposure (especially in northern climates), dark-pigmented skin, and chronic use of sunscreen.[16] Vitamin D is found in a limited number of foods, which mainly include fortified cows' milk; certain brands of soy milk and rice milk; calcium-fortified orange juice, breakfast cereals, and margarines;[1] and in fatty fish (see table 6.2). Although spending just a few minutes outside in your exercise shorts several times a week is enough to meet your vitamin D needs in the late spring, summer, and early fall if you are Caucasian, taking in vitamin D in food or as a supplement is wise in the winter. This is also a wise idea if you are dark skinned,

TABLE 6.2 Selected Vegetarian Sources of Vitamin D

Food	Portion	International units (IU)
Cereal, all varieties fortified with 10% DV	3/4 cup	40-50
Cereal grain bar, fortified with 10% DV	1 bar	40
Egg	1 whole	25
Margarine, fortified	1 Tbsp	60
Milk, vitamin D fortified (nonfat, reduced fat, and whole)	1 cup	98
Milk, rice, vitamin D fortified	1 cup	100*
Milk, soy, vitamin D fortified	1 cup	100*
Orange juice, vitamin D fortified	1 cup	100

The Daily Value (DV) for vitamin D is 400 IU. The Vitamin D Council, however, feels that the DV should be increased. Refer to appendix E for guidance on converting English units to metric.

*May be a source of D_2 rather than D_3.

because research shows that dark-skinned people do not produce adequate vitamin D from sunlight exposure.[8]

Just how much vitamin D you should take is not known, but the Vitamin D Council suggests that 2,000 international units (IU) is a good general recommendation.[4] This amount is currently the tolerable upper intake level; however, it is too low to permit optimization of vitamin D status in the general population.[13] Because this value is much higher than what you can obtain from natural or supplemented food sources, a vitamin D supplement containing vitamin D_3 (cholecalciferol) is recommended, but may be needed only in the winter. Vegans, however, should know that the vitamin D_3 used to fortify some products is of animal origin[1, 26] and that the vitamin D_2 form (ergocalciferol)—often called vegetarian vitamin D—may not be as effective as vitamin D_3 at increasing vitamin D status.[40] In fact, the Vitamin D Council has recently warned that ergocalciferol may partially block the action of vitamin D.[4] To be most effective, supplements should contain real vitamin D (vitamin D_3 or cholecalciferol) rather than vitamin D_2 (ergocalciferol), and they shouldn't contain Vitamin A, which can interfere with vitamin D's function. If you are vegan, however, please stay tuned to the vitamin D_2 issue, because research is currently evolving.

Magnesium

Magnesium is the third most abundant mineral in bone—after calcium and phosphorus—and is also involved in the bone mineralization process. As with calcium, magnesium in bone can act as a reservoir to ensure that adequate magnesium is available to the body when needed. Both dietary intake of magnesium and the magnesium concentration in blood have been found to be positively correlated with bone mineral content, an indicator of bone strength or overall bone health.

In one large study conducted in more than 2,000 men and women in their 70s who were enrolled in the Health, Aging, and Body Composition Study, higher magnesium intake from foods and supplements was found to predict a higher bone-mineral density.[35] In this study, however, the researchers found that the relationship between dietary magnesium and bone health was apparent in Caucasian but not black volunteers, which the researchers speculated was caused by differences in either calcium regulation or nutrient reporting.

Although true deficiencies of magnesium are rare, research seems to indicate that consuming adequate magnesium may be important for optimal bone health.

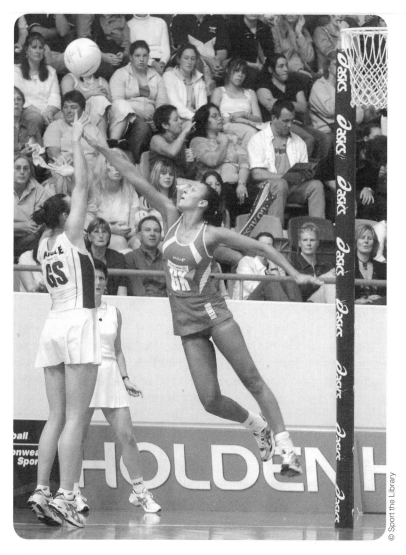

© Sport the Library

Although athletes, particularly female athletes, often come up short of the recommended intake of magnesium, vegetarians are more likely to get enough of this nutrient through seeds, nuts, legumes, and dark green vegetables.

Indeed, surveys of various groups of athletes have found that intake of magnesium is often insufficient,[39] particularly among female athletes,[22] and possibly also among athletes who restrict energy intake. As a whole, however, vegetarian athletes may be at an advantage when it comes to dietary magnesium because seeds, nuts, legumes, unmilled cereal grains, and dark-green vegetables as well as dark chocolate, are high in magnesium. Refined foods or dairy products, on the other hand, tend to be low in magnesium. The magnesium content of selected foods is listed in table 6.1, along with the calcium content of these foods. A listing of the 20 best sources of magnesium is also found in chapter 11. The DRI for magnesium is listed in appendix D.

Fluoride

Adequate fluoride plays a critical role in strengthening bone as well as teeth. Fluoride is incorporated into the hydroxyapatite crystals of bones and teeth after mineralization, specifically replacing some of the chemical "hydroxyl" group. This makes bones stronger and teeth more resistant to decay.[31] The most significant sources of fluoride in the United States are green and black teas, seafood, and fluoridated water, and in some countries, fluoride is added to salt and milk.[18] Significant sources of fluoride are not found in other food sources; however, fluoridated toothpaste can provide a source for teeth and bone if small amounts are swallowed. Although low-dose fluoride supplementation in postmenopausal osteoporotic patients has been shown to increase bone-mineral density in the spine,[30] long-term treatment with fluoride is not recommended[31] because excess fluoride can have the opposite effect on bone, inducing the formation of large, abnormally placed mineral crystals that decrease bone strength and quality.[37] Excess fluoride also discolors teeth and large doses are toxic.

Although no hard-and-fast rules exist for ensuring that you get adequate, but not too much, fluoride, one of the first steps is to ensure that the water you drink or cook with contains appropriate levels of fluoride. In the United States, an estimated 67 percent of the public water supply is fluoridated, but this varies by state. Within the United States you can check the status of your area by calling your local water utility company. You may also find helpful information about the fluoride content of your state's water supply from the Centers for Disease Control and Prevention (CDC) Web site.[5] Fluoride concentrations are expressed as parts per million (ppm), which is equal to one milligram fluoride per liter. Fluoride is generally added to tap water at the rate of approximately one ppm; however, the CDC recommends 0.7 ppm for warmer climates and 1.2 ppm for cooler climates to account for the tendency of people to drink more water in warmer climates.[5] Thus, depending on the content of your water, you may want to adjust your water sources and even toothpaste selection to ensure that your fluoride intake is close to the recommended adequate intake (AI) of three milligrams per day for adult women and four milligrams per day for adult men. For example, if your tap water contains 1.2 milligrams per liter and you consume two liters of tap water and tap water mixed with Gatorade during your morning workout session (1.2 mg/l × 2 l = 2.4 mg), plus an additional 1.5 liters in coffee and drinking water throughout the day (1.2 mg/l × 1.5 l = 1.8 mg), you would easily be taking in more than the AI for fluoride and may want to avoid using fluoridated toothpaste. If you drink exclusively bottled water, remember that most do not contain fluoride. Many brands—such as Dannon Fluoride to Go—offer fluoridated versions of their water.

Phosphorus

Phosphorus is the second most abundant mineral in bone and also plays a role in energy regulation and acid–base buffering. Unlike calcium, however, dietary phosphorus is readily absorbed, at an efficiency of 60 to 70 percent, and too much phosphorus—rather than not enough—is a concern for bone health. Excessive phosphorus intake relative to calcium intake increases the hormones PTH and calcitriol (active vitamin D), which ultimately results in removal of both calcium and phosphorus from bone. Although somewhat controversial, high phosphorus intakes over a long period may result in bone loss. According to a study of bone fractures in active teenage females conducted by Harvard researchers, a strong association was found between phosphate-rich cola beverage consumption and bone fractures.[46] Other epidemiological studies have found that excessive phosphorus negatively affects bone health in elderly vegetarian and omnivorous men and women.[41]

Although phosphorus is found in most foods, common sources in a Western diet are grains, meats, legumes, nuts, seeds, dairy products, soda pop, and phosphorus additives to foods—mostly in the form of phosphates. Table 6.1 lists the calcium-to-phosphorus ratio of selected calcium-containing foods. This ratio is high in leafy greens, dairy, and calcium-fortified soy products and low in grains, nuts, and seeds. The ideal calcium-to-phosphorus ratio in the diet is not known, but according to the 1997 recommendations for calcium of 1,000 milligrams and phosphorus of 700 milligrams, it should be approximately 1.43:1. Because most Americans take in too much phosphorus, both from foods and soda, and many do not meet the recommendations for calcium, the calcium-to-phosphorus ratio of the average American diet tends to be less than ideal. Because this issue is still relatively controversial, the simple message may be to pack those leafy greens into your diet (a high calcium-to-phosphate ratio is just one more reason), avoid consuming too much soda and other foods with phosphate additives, and strive to get your calcium from a variety of vegetarian sources.

Vitamins K, C, and A

Vitamins K, C, and A also can affect bone health. Vitamin K has gained more attention lately because it is required for synthesis of a bone-specific protein called *osteocalcin*. Ostoecalcin is produced by the osteoblasts and is involved in bone formation. Like vitamin D, vitamin K can be obtained from food and nonfood sources, which in this case includes vitamin K made by intestinal bacteria. In fact, about half of your daily vitamin K needs can be obtained as a result of bacteria that synthesizes this vitamin in your gut. Food sources of vitamin K include green leafy vegetables, avocado, cruciferous vegetables (broccoli, brussels sprouts, cabbage, and cauliflower), and eggs. Although we still have a lot to learn about vitamin K and bone health, vitamin K intake appears to play a part in reducing the risk of hip fractures. In a study conducted on more than 70,000 women—as part of the Nurses' Health Study cohort—those who had low intakes of vitamin K (mainly from green vegetables) were at greater risk for hip fractures.[9] Many calcium supplements marketed to women now contain vitamin K as well as vitamin D. As an athlete, you should once again strive to eat your green leafy vegetables. Also, be aware that regular use of antibiotics decreases the number of vitamin K–producing bacteria in the gut.

Vitamins C and A play important—and often overlooked—backstage roles in bone health. Vitamin C is involved in the formation of collagen, which forms the matrix for all connective tissue in the body, including bones, teeth, skin, and tendon. Vitamin A's role is related to its function in cell growth, cell differentiation, and bone resorption, which is an essential step in bone growth and remodeling. Although it appears that only a severe deficiency of either vitamin is likely to affect bone health in adults, vegetarian athletes should consider bone health another reason to meet the needs of both of these vitamins. Food sources of vitamin C are listed in table 7.4 on page 91 and sources of vitamin A in table 8.5 on page 107.

Other Nutrients

Several other nutrients, including caffeine, alcohol, and soy isoflavones, may also influence bone-mineral density and bone health. Caffeine consumption is thought to increase calcium excretion by the kidneys and is associated with reduced bone-mineral density in some epidemiological studies. The effect of lifetime caffeine intake, however, seems to be weak; 10 cups (2,360 ml) of coffee every day for 30 years was associated with only a 1.1 percent reduction in bone mass.[3] In studies of postmenopausal women not on estrogen therapy, as little as two cups (472 ml) of coffee were found to accelerate bone loss in women who did not regularly drink milk[2] (or perhaps get adequate calcium). In addition, too much alcohol contributes to bone loss by inhibiting osteoblasts in their job of forming new bone.[6] Heavy drinkers may lose bone mass in just a few years. Similar to the case of caffeine, it is not clear how much alcohol is too much, but there is evidence that people who have three to four drinks a day are at increased risk for bone loss. Small amounts of alcohol may have the opposite effect by actually promoting bone formation.

Soy isoflavones, on the other hand, may have a beneficial effect on long-term bone health.[36] In a study conducted at the University of Illinois at Urbana-Champaign, supplementation of soy isoflavones (at a level of 90 mg/day) for six months increased both bone-mineral content and bone-mineral density in healthy postmenopausal women.[33] The magnitude of the effect of soy and the specific mechanism of action are not known. Similarly, it is also not known whether limiting caffeine (to a certain unknown level) or packing in the isoflavones influences bone health in athletic vegetarians. The isoflavone content of selected soy foods is presented in table 6.3.

TABLE 6.3   **Total Soy Isoflavone Content in Selected Soy Products**

Food	Portion	Value (mg)
Soybeans, cooked	1 cup cooked (172 g)	221
Soy flour, full fat	2 Tbsp (10 grams)	18
Soy milk	1 cup (236 ml)	23
Soy protein concentrate (water extracted)	1 oz (28.35 grams)	29
Soy protein concentrate (alcohol extracted)	1 oz (28.35 grams)	4
Soy protein isolate	1 oz (28.35 grams)	28
Soy bars (Revival brand)	1 bar	160
Soy chips (Revival brand)	1 oz package	15
Soy dog	1 dog (70 g)	10.5
Soy shake (Revival brand)	8 oz mixed	160
Tempeh	1/2 cup (83 grams)	35
Tofu, soft	1/2 cup (124 grams)	36
Tofu, firm	1/2 cup (126 grams)	29

Total isoflavones (daidzein and genistein) extrapolated from the USDA-Iowa State University Database on the Isoflavone Content of Foods, Release 1.3, 2002. Available: http://www.nal.usda.gov/fnic/foodcomp/Data/isoflav/isfl_tbl.pdf.

Bone Health and the Vegetarian Diet

Whether vegetarian athletes are at risk for poor bone health depends on many factors including genetics, training, and diet. Overall, research in small groups of vegetarians has found that the bone-mineral densities of lacto–ovo vegetarians is similar to and in some cases higher than in omnivores.[43] In a larger-scale investigation conducted in Seventh-Day Adventists, a vegetarian diet appeared to be somewhat able to defend against bone-mineral loss in aging women[24] but not men.[23] The investigators found that although bone-mineral density was not different between younger lacto–ovo vegetarians and omnivores, increasing differences in bone mass appeared at age 50, and by age 89, nonvegetarians had lost 35 percent of their bone mass, whereas the vegetarians had lost just 18 percent.[24] Limited research in vegans, however, has found that bone mineral densities of vegans is often suboptimal.[7, 43] The main difference between the diets of lacto–ovo vegetarians, omnivores, and vegans in these studies was that the vegans took in less protein and had a lower protein-to-calcium ratio in their diet, which may be a predictor of bone density. Higher bone-mineral densities are desirable because the incidence of fragility fractures is inversely proportional

Box
6.1

Tips for Optimizing Bone Health

› Obtain adequate calcium from a variety of plant and, if appropriate, dairy sources.

› Maintain adequate levels of vitamin D in the blood by spending just a few minutes outside in your exercise shorts several times a week, if you are Caucasian. In the winter, or year-round if you are dark skinned, make an effort to consume foods fortified with vitamin D or take a vitamin D supplement. The Vitamin D Council recommends 2,000 IU (more than the RDA) of vitamin D_3 for those whose exposure to sunlight is inadequate.[4]

› Incorporate leafy greens into the diet regularly, if not daily. Most leafy greens are well-absorbed sources of calcium and also contain vitamin K and vitamin A. Leafy greens also are low in phosphorus.

› Reduce the phosphorus content of your diet by limiting the intake of regular and diet soda and foods with added phosphates. However, do not limit plant foods high in phosphates in an effort to improve the calcium-to-phosphate ratio because many of these foods, such as nuts, seeds, grains, and legumes, are excellent sources of other nutrients, including magnesium.

› Ensure that the water you cook with contains adequate fluoride. And remember that both too little and too much fluoride can compromise bone health.

› Consume adequate energy. Low intakes of energy and protein can compromise bone and also compromise the intake of important nutrients, including calcium and magnesium.

› Limit caffeine intake to one to two cups (236-472 ml) of caffeine-containing beverages per day. Even this amount may increase calcium loss if calcium intake is not adequate.

› Consider regularly consuming soy foods containing isoflavones. The jury is still out, however, concerning how much is needed daily to benefit bone health, particularly in people who are active.

› If you drink alcohol, do so in moderation. Excessive drinking not only keeps you from performing your best, but may also impair bone health.

to bone-mineral content. However, no studies—either short or long term—have been done with vegetarian athletes.

To maintain optimal bone health, your main concerns should be ensuring that you consume adequate calcium, receive a reliable source of vitamin D, and avoid taking in too much phosphate from soda and other processed foods. Tips for optimizing bone health are summarized in box 6.1. In addition, you should evaluate your training and—if you are female—ensure that you are menstruating normally (see box 2.3 on page 20). Weight-bearing activities like running, jumping, and resistance training promote bone density, which is great if you are a runner, ballplayer, dancer, gymnast, or power lifter, but not so great if you are a swimmer, cyclist or table tennis player. Athletes in these and other non-weight-bearing sports—no matter their performance or fitness level—need to incorporate regular weight-bearing activities into their in-season and off-season training, even if it is simply walking briskly a few miles several times a week. Speaking from experience, I forced myself to jog 6 to 10 miles (10-16 km) a week back in my days as a rather competitive recreational distance cyclist. Although my motivation was partially to use weight-bearing activity to induce a piezoelectric effect, in the end, I found it was great cross-training. The rest of the story is that I eventually became a runner, but that's another topic of discussion.

Indeed, a vegetarian diet packed with appropriate food choices can adequately support bone health—with or without dairy products—just as it can maintain a normal iron status, which is discussed in the next chapter.

Boosting Iron Intake and Absorption

A friend of a good friend is what you might call a fitness enthusiast. She became vegetarian in college for health reasons and did fine nutritionally while living and dining in her sorority house. Upon graduation, however, she faced a demanding new job as an accountant and then, having to cook for herself, began noticing that she just did not feel right. She became increasingly fatigued and lethargic and finally went to her doctor, who diagnosed her with iron deficiency anemia. His recommendation was for her to start eating meat. To this day, I hear she is a semi-vegetarian because she is convinced—based on this misinformation—that she needs to eat chicken breast and turkey to maintain her iron status. In reality, what she needs is a little education on how to maintain iron status on a vegetarian diet. Believe me, if we lived in the same state, this would have already happened.

You have probably been informed at least once during your athletic career that you need to watch your iron consumption either because you are vegetarian or because you are an athlete. Indeed, nearly every source you read implies that vegetarians and athletes need to take a supplement or include a little flesh in their diet to achieve normal iron status. Although you should take threats of poor iron status seriously, you can easily maintain adequate iron stores by consuming a vegetarian diet alone—hold the fish, chicken breast, and supplements. This chapter reviews the basics of iron metabolism and why iron is important to athletes, and provides suggestions for boosting iron intake and absorption on a vegetarian diet.

What Is So Important About Iron?

Every living cell—whether plant or animal—contains iron. Most of the iron in your body is found as part of two proteins called hemoglobin, which is found in red blood cells, and myoglobin, which is found in muscle cells. Hemoglobin in blood carries the oxygen you breathe into your lungs to all tissues throughout the body, and myoglobin in muscle holds and stores oxygen for use during exercise. Myoglobin is particularly important for aerobic muscle fibers that are also called slow-twitch red (or type I) fibers. In fact, it is the myoglobin that makes endurance muscle reddish in color and may help explain why chickens, with white muscle in their breasts, are able to fly just a few feet, but ducks, with dark muscle in their breasts, can fly for hours.

The iron in hemoglobin and myoglobin is key because it has special chemical properties that allow it to carry oxygen and then release it to the tissues as needed. Your cells—particularly your working muscle cells—need a regular supply of oxygen to produce energy. Iron-containing hemoglobin is also needed to assist in the elimination of carbon and hydrogen atoms released during the use of carbohydrate and fat fuels for energy, forming carbon dioxide and hydrogen. Thus, having adequate iron stores is particularly important during exercise when the hemoglobin-rich red blood cells shuttle between your lungs and exercising muscle, bringing in fresh oxygen and eliminating carbon dioxide.

In addition to its vital role in oxygen and carbon dioxide shuttling, iron helps many enzymes in the energy-generating pathways. Iron is also needed to make new cells, hormones, neurotransmitters, and amino acids.

Iron is so important to your body that is has been referred to as the body's gold: a precious mineral to be hoarded. Following absorption in the intestines, a protein called *transferrin* escorts it to various tissues. Iron is stored primarily in the liver and bone marrow as part of two other proteins called *ferritin* and *hemosiderin.* Some storage also occurs in the spleen and in muscle. A small amount of the storage protein ferritin also circulates in the blood. Serum ferritin can be used to assess iron storage because blood levels typically reflect iron stores in the body, although there is some evidence that this might not be true in endurance-trained athletes because serum ferritin is also influenced by factors other than iron stores.[28] Only a very small amount of unescorted iron circulates in the blood.

The liver packs iron, sent from bone marrow or from its own stores, into new red blood cells, also made in bone marrow, and releases them into the blood.[22] Your red blood cells typically live for three to four months. When they die, the spleen and liver salvage the iron and send it back to the bone marrow for storage and reuse. In this way, iron is truly hoarded. Small amounts of iron, however, are lost daily through the shedding of cells in your skin, scalp, and gastrointestinal (GI) tract and through your perspiration. The greatest loss of iron, however, occurs through bleeding. Normal average daily iron loss is approximately 1 milligram for men and nonmenstruating women, and approximately 1.4 to 1.5 milligrams for menstruating women. Monthly menstrual losses account for the higher average iron loss in women.

Athletes in training may also lose iron through GI bleeding, the destruction of red blood cells, urinary loss, and heavy sweating. GI bleeding is a recognized problem that occurs in endurance runners, cyclists, and triathletes[14, 19, 21] and is thought to be related, at least in part, to regular use of aspirin and anti-inflammatory medications. These medications may have a toxic effect on the gut lining, leaving it raw and bleeding.[7] Red cell destruction, called *hemolysis,* is thought to be caused by the stress of repetitive foot contact with the ground during prolonged running or marching[8, 25] or by the rapid propulsion of blood cells through the blood vessels that can occur with intense muscular training. This excess force can then rupture some of the red blood cells, which, although not dangerous, can increase iron requirements. Loss of hemoglobin in urine, called *hematuria,* usually follows hemolysis because the kidneys' capacity to hoard the hemoglobin released from ruptured blood cells, is temporarily overwhelmed. Iron loss in urine can also occur if muscle cells are ruptured during intense training, resulting in the release of stored myoglobin, or if the inner lining of the bladder becomes irritated, resulting in loss of red blood cells in the urine. Blood loss in urine may occur in any athletic situation that places stress on the bladder and may include prolonged running and running during pregnancy. Finally, iron loss in sweat is also thought to be significant for some athletes during prolonged effort, although not all experts agree. Research in this area suggests that iron loss through sweating increases with exercise duration, particularly in males, and may be as high as 0.3 to 0.4 milligrams of iron lost per liter (4 cups) of sweat.[26] Although very few studies have cumulatively assessed total iron losses in athletes, data collected from endurance-trained athletes indicate that iron losses from feces, urine, and sweat were approximately 1.75 milligrams for men and 2.3 milligrams for women.[27]

Iron Needs of Athletes

Daily iron requirements for humans varies by sex and age and are shown in appendix D. The recommended intake is roughly 10 times the estimated average daily loss to account for the relatively low absorption of iron by the intestines. On average, only 10 percent of the iron consumed on a diet containing both meat and plant foods is absorbed. The recommended intake for iron, however, does not account for either the additional loss that may occur during heavy training or for the lower iron absorption from plant sources. Several sources have suggested that the iron requirement for athletes in training would need to be approximately 75 percent higher in male athletes and about 65 percent higher in female athletes to account for their increased daily loss,[27] and those of vegetarians would need to be 80 percent greater than nonvegetarians to account for the lower absorption rate of iron from a vegetarian diet.[9] Although it is impossible to extrapolate these recommendations to a recommended value for vegetarian athletes, you should consider that your iron needs may be higher than the daily recommendation—particularly during intense training—but that your needs are likely to vary depending on your food choices, which will be discussed later. You should also recognize that some degree of adaptation occurs in athletes and vegetarians, which over the long run enhances your ability to absorb and retain iron. An example of this adaptation is the increase in iron absorption in people with low iron reserves. One study in male runners also found that iron absorption was significantly higher in male distance runners compared to a control population.[19]

As a final note, iron needs may also be temporarily increased in vegetarian athletes who relocate to or begin training at high altitudes. At altitude, the body must adapt to the reduced air pressure by increasing production of hemoglobin-rich red cells, which draws upon body iron reserves. Inadequate iron intake during this period may lengthen the altitude-adaptation period, ultimately reducing training quality.

Results of Iron Deficiency

Quite simply, if you don't get enough iron in your daily diet to replace your losses, your ability to transport adequate oxygen for energy generation will be impaired. Ultimately, this is felt as a lack of "get up and go" both on and off the playing field.

As you would expect, athletic performance is impaired if the body becomes so deficient in iron that hemoglobin production stops and its concentration in the blood drops below the normal range—a condition called *anemia*. It is imperative, however, to also recognize that impairments in athletic performance[6] and aerobic training adaptation[5, 12] can occur even in the early stages of iron deficiency when iron stores in the liver and body tissues are lowered, but blood hemoglobin is still within the normal range (see box 7.1). Researchers at Cornell University recently followed 42 iron-depleted, but not anemic, women for six weeks.[5] The women, who were initially untrained, first cycled 15 kilometers (9.3 miles) to determine how quickly they could complete the bout before training. Tissue iron status was assessed through a technique that measures the concentration of serum transferrin receptors, which becomes elevated as tissue stores become depleted. Half then took an iron supplement containing 100 milligrams of ferrous sulfate per day, and the other half took a placebo. After four weeks of bicycle training, the women cycled the 15-kilometer distance again. Somewhat surprisingly, the researchers found that the women who had had low tissue iron stores but normal blood hemoglobin levels at the beginning of the training—and were not allowed to replenish these stores with an iron supplement—failed to show an improvement in the cycling time trial. The group who had had normal tissue iron stores but depleted liver iron stores experienced the expected training improvement whether they received the iron supplement or the placebo.

Research conducted at Pennsylvania State University further indicates that cognitive function may be impaired with moderate iron depletion.[18] In this study, young, nonathletic women who had low iron stores and normal hemoglobin levels were tested for several cognitive functions both before and after supplementation

Box
7.1

Stages of Iron Deficiency

Iron deficiency occurs when the body's iron stores are depleted and a restricted supply of iron to various tissues becomes apparent. If not corrected, iron deficiency can lead to iron deficiency anemia, which is a condition defined by a low hemoglobin concentration in the blood. Iron deficiency commonly occurs in three stages.

Stage 1: Diminished total-body iron content. This stage is identified by a reduction in serum ferritin. Serum ferritin concentration typically correlates well with total-body iron stores. However, within this stage, there may be varying degrees of depletion. Typically, a reduction in athletic performance is not apparent when iron stores in the liver are low but may likely occur when iron stores are depleted in the skeletal muscle or other tissues.[5] If you suspect your iron is low, ask your health care provider to measure the concentration of your serum transferrin receptors as well as serum ferritin. Keep in mind, however, that serum ferritin is often elevated in endurance athletes[28] and is not by itself a good indicator of body iron stores in athletes.

Stage 2: Reduced red blood cell formation. This stage occurs when the iron supply is insufficient to support the formation of red blood cells. High levels of a blood marker called zinc protoporphyrin (ZPP) can indicate this stage. When iron is not readily available, zinc is used in its place, producing ZPP. To help diagnose this stage, your physician might measure your transferrin saturation. Transferrin is a protein that carries iron in the blood. This test indicates iron deficiency if less than 15 percent of this protein contains iron.

Stage 3: Iron deficiency anemia. In this final stage, hemoglobin concentration is affected and drops below the normal range, which is typically 12 to 15 grams per deciliter for women and 14 to 16.5 grams per deciliter for men. The normal range, however, will be slightly higher for athletes living at higher altitudes.

with iron or a placebo for 16 weeks. Iron supplementation in this group resulted in significant improvements in attention, short-term and long-term memory, and performance on cognitive tasks. Taking the placebo did not.

The performance impairment associated with iron depletion without anemia is not well understood but may be caused by the lowered levels of iron-containing enzymes in various tissues. Many of these enzymes are involved in the energy-generating pathways of muscle and brain cells. What is important to you as a vegetarian athlete is to recognize that even mild iron deficiency may impair both physical and mental performance. Mild iron deficiency, or tissue depletion, is not detected by measuring the hemoglobin concentration, which may still be within the normal range, and is not likely to induce the classic symptoms of iron deficiency anemia, which include fatigue, weakness, lethargy, abnormal temperature regulation, and impaired immune function. These classic symptoms typically are not apparent until the hemoglobin concentration drops and the athlete becomes anemic.

Risk Factors for Iron Deficiency

Quite frankly, almost everyone is at risk for iron deficiency. Iron deficiency is the most common nutrition deficiency worldwide and is thought to affect nearly 15 percent of the world's population,[3] being particularly apparent in women of childbearing age. It is not known, however, whether vegetarian athletes are at greater risk for iron deficiency than either the general population or their meat-eating teammates. Some experts[3, 28] feel that those at risk of deficient body-iron stores are young athletes, female athletes, distance runners, and vegetarian athletes. The prevalence of iron deficiency is also thought to be higher in vegetarians who restrict food intake, but numerous studies in vegans and vegetarians have found that iron deficiency anemia is no more common among vegetarians than among the general population.[1, 2, 10, 15] Certainly, any athlete or vegetarian can be prone to iron deficiency anemia if he or she restricts food intake or makes poor food choices.

What is not well understood is whether reduced iron stores without anemia are indeed more prevalent in vegetarian athletes, and if they are, whether they are severe enough to cause tissue depletion and impaired exercise performance. Several studies conducted mostly in nonathletes have found rather consistently that vegetarians have lower total-body iron stores, or lower serum ferritin levels, than nonvegetarians despite reporting similar or higher intakes of dietary iron.[1] These lower iron stores, nevertheless, are usually within the normal range. Similar results were noted in a study conducted on female runners. In this study, the athletes who followed a modified vegetarian diet had a similar iron intake but lower iron status than their meat-eating teammates.[24] There were, however, no apparent differences in the maximal aerobic capacity or performance between the vegetarian and nonvegetarian runners.

Certainly, more research is needed to determine whether athletes following a supplement-free vegetarian diet for several years, or longer, are able to maintain normal iron stores when selecting a healthy diet. Although we know that the body's total iron stores can vary over a wide range without impairment in body function and performance and that iron supplementation does not improve performance unless tissue stores are depleted,[5] we do not know how iron status changes over time with training and a vegetarian diet. Although I do believe each person's genetics and food preferences can affect his or her iron status, I also believe that vegetarian athletes, in most cases, can achieve adequate iron status without depending on iron supplements or an occasional chicken breast. It has been my experience that it is not impossible, and in fact is quite easy, to do so. I have not taken an iron-containing supplement for 15 years, except on rare occasion for just a few weeks. I discovered—after becoming anemic *during* my dietetic internship—how to boost my iron intake and absorption. I believe, based on the literature and my own personal and professional experience, that vegetarian athletes who eat well and do not restrict their energy intake are likely to maintain iron stores that are just within the range considered normal or slightly greater than borderline, but that this is not a bad thing. Maintaining iron stores on the lower end of the normal range may be one factor that contributes to a reduced risk of cancer and other chronic diseases. In having borderline stores, however, vegetarian athletes may need to supplement occasionally—for example after giving blood, experiencing an excessively heavy menstrual cycle, or relocating (as I recently did) from sea level to 7,220 feet (2,200 m). Just as an aside, over the last 15 years I have maintained normal iron status while averaging 150-plus miles (241 km) a week on a bicycle, training for two marathons, and running during pregnancy with a singleton and twins. Yes I refused the prenatal vitamin, but I was confident I was eating well and had my iron status checked regularly—just in case.

Ensuring Sufficient Iron Intake and Absorption

Research suggests that the most common causes of iron deficiency among athletes are insufficient iron intake, reduced absorption, and, in females, menstrual blood loss. Thus, to avoid the pitfalls of poor iron status, you need to include a variety of iron-rich foods in your daily diet and ensure that the iron you consume is well absorbed. Education on plant sources of iron and on the dietary factors that enhance and inhibit iron absorption is all you need to get started. After that, you just need to make sure you make good choices and, as always, that you meet your energy intake needs.

First, good sources of iron are typically found in whole and enriched grains, cereals and pasta, root and leafy-green vegetables, dried fruits, legumes, and nuts and seeds. These are listed in table 7.1. Chances are that if you are eating a well-balanced vegetarian diet and are not restricting your calories, you are already getting enough iron. If you think your diet may be lacking, make an effort to add more iron-rich foods. You can also try cooking in an old-fashioned iron skillet or tossing an iron "egg" or "stone" into soups and sauces. The iron obtained from the skillet or stone can add to the iron content of cooked foods, particularly when the foods cooked are slightly acidic, such as tomato sauce. This is an old trick used by populations throughout the world living on a plant-based diet. Iron eggs, however, are hard to find in the United States but may be more readily available in other countries.

Next, ensure that the iron that you have consumed is absorbed. As you most likely know, the iron found in plant foods, eggs, and dairy is in a form called nonheme, or elemental, iron which is not absorbed as well (2 to 20 percent that is consumed is absorbed) as the heme iron form found in meat (15 to 35 percent that is consumed is absorbed). *Heme* refers to iron in the form of myoglobin and also hemoglobin (just like in the body), which is why dark meat has a higher iron content than whiter meat. In fact, heme iron is better absorbed because it is

TABLE 7.1   Approximate Iron Content of Selected Plant Foods

Food	Portion	Iron (mg)
GRAIN EQUIVALENTS		
Bread, enriched	1 slice or 1 oz	0.7-1.2
Bread, whole wheat	1 slice	0.8
Cereal, ready to eat and fortified	1 serving (1 oz)	2.0-22.4
Brown rice	1 cup cooked	1.0
Oatmeal	1 cup cooked	1.6
Pasta, enriched	1 oz uncooked	0.7-1.2
VEGETABLES AND LEGUMES		
Beet greens*	1 cup cooked	2.7
Black beans	1 cup cooked	3.6
Broccoli*	1 cup cooked	1.1
Brussels sprouts*	1 cup cooked	0.7
Cabbage, Chinese (bok choy)	1 cup cooked	1.8
Collard greens*	1 cup cooked	2.2
Chickpeas (garbanzo beans)	1 cup cooked	4.7
Kale	1 cup	1.2
Lentils	1 cup cooked	6.6
Mustard greens*	1 cup cooked	1.0
Peas, green*	1 cup cooked	2.4
Pinto beans	1 cup cooked	3.6
Potato*	1 medium, baked	2.2
Red kidney beans	1 cup cooked	5.2
Southern peas (black-eyed, crowder)	1 cup cooked	4.3
Soybeans	1 cup cooked	8.8
Sweet potato*	1 medium, baked	1.1
Tofu, firm (calcium set)	1/2 cup	3.4
Tofu, regular (calcium set)	1/2 cup	6.7
Tomato (year-round average)*	1 cup raw	0.5
Turnip greens*	1 cup cooked	1.2
Winter squash*	1 cup cooked	0.9-1.4
FRUITS		
Apricots	5 halves, dried	0.9
Raisins	1/4 cup	0.7
Raspberries, frozen*	1 cup	1.6
Strawberries*	5 large	0.4
Watermelon*	1 wedge	0.7

Food	Portion	Iron (mg)
NUTS AND SEEDS		
Almonds	1 oz	1.2
Cashews	1 oz	1.7
Peanuts	1 oz	0.6
Pecans	1 oz	0.7
Pine nuts	1 oz	1.6
Pumpkin seeds	1 oz	4.2
Sunflower seeds	1 oz	1.1
Tahini	1 Tbsp	1.3
Walnuts	1 oz	0.8
OTHER		
Molasses	1 Tbsp	0.9
Blackstrap molasses	1 Tbsp	3.6

*Also a good source of vitamin C.

Data from the USDA National Nutrient Database for Standard Reference. Available: http://www.ars.usda.gov/nutrientdata.

treated as a protein and is not affected by meal composition or gastrointestinal secretions. Nonheme iron, on the other hand, must be released from its binding to various plant structures by digestive enzymes and enters the small intestine in a specific chemical form. Nonheme iron is subject to attack by many different chemical reactions, which include oxidation and binding with other dietary components, which reduces absorption.

Iron absorption from plant sources can be both enhanced and inhibited by various dietary factors (see tables 7.2 and 7.3). By far the most potent plant-based factor is vitamin C, which aids in the absorption of iron from most plant sources. Research has shown that ingesting 25 to 75 milligrams of vitamin C—roughly the amount in half a cup (118 ml) of most fruit juices—increases the absorption of iron from foods consumed in the same meal threefold to fourfold.[17] Consuming other organic acids, such as citric, malic, lactic, and tartaric acids, also increases iron absorption, but their effects are not as powerful as vitamin C's.

On the other hand, iron absorption from plant sources can be inhibited by excessive intake of plant phytates, plant polyphenolics, bran, cocoa, coffee, tea (including some herbal teas), soy, egg and milk protein, and foods with high dietary concentrations of calcium, zinc, and other minerals. Fortunately, much of the natural processing that happens to foods, including soaking beans and fermenting soy products, helps reduce the inhibitory effects of many of these factors (see tables 7.2 and 7.3). Also fortunate is the fact that many vegetables and fruits that are high in iron are also high in vitamin C (see table 7.4). In addition, commonly eaten combinations, such as beans with tomato-based sauce, stir-fried tofu and broccoli, and orange juice with toast or cereal, also result in generous levels of

TABLE 7.2 Dietary Factors That Enhance Iron Absorption

Factor	Source
Vitamin C	Citrus fruits and juices, melons, berries, pineapple, tomatoes, bell peppers, broccoli, potatoes (see table 7.4)
Citric, malic, and tartaric acids	Fruits, vegetables, and vinegars
Lactic acid	Sauerkraut
Retinol and carotenoids (not yet proven)	Dark-green, red, and orange fruits and vegetables
Specific food-processing methods	Leavening and baking bread; soaking and sprouting beans, grains, and seeds; fermentation process for making some soy foods (miso, tempeh, natto); coagulation with a gluconic acid derivative in making silken-style tofu
Sulfur-containing amino acids	Many plant protein foods
Tissue-protein factor (TPF)	Flesh foods (TPF is a factor other than heme found in meat, poultry, and fish that promotes the absorption of nonheme iron from other foods consumed in the same meal.)

TABLE 7.3 Foods and Their Factors That Affect Iron Absorption

Food	Hindering factor (if known)	Enhancing factor (if known)
Bran, whole-grains, legumes, nuts, and seeds	Phytates	Leavening and baking bread (hydrolyzes phytates); soaking and sprouting beans, grains, and seeds
Soy products	Soy (phytate or protein)	Fermentation process for making some soy foods (miso, tempeh, natto); coagulation with a gluconic acid derivative in making silken-style tofu
Tea, coffee	Polyphenols (tannins)	—
Some vegetables, some herbal teas, red wine	Polyphenolics	—
Calcium-rich antacids, calcium phosphates, supplements	Calcium, zinc, other minerals (divalent ions)	—
Eggs, milk	Egg or milk protein; factor not known	—
Spices		Enhancing factors not established

TABLE 7.4 Approximate Vitamin C Content of Foods That Contain Iron

Food	Portion	Vitamin C (mg)
Asparagus	1 cup cooked	44
Beet greens	1 cup cooked	36
Broccoli	1 cup cooked	101
Brussels sprouts	1 cup cooked	71
Cabbage, all varieties	1 cup cooked	20-45
Cantaloupe	1 cup	59
Cauliflower	1 cup cooked	56
Collard greens	1 cup cooked	35
Cranberry juice cocktail	1 cup	90
Grapefruit	One half	39
Grapefruit juice	1 cup	94
Honeydew	1 cup	31
Kale	1 cup	53
Kiwi	1 medium	71
Kohlrabi	1 cup cooked	90
Lemon juice	From 1 lemon	31
Mango	1 cup	46
Mustard greens	1 cup cooked	35
Okra	1 cup cooked	26
Orange juice	1 cup	97-124
Oranges	1 medium	70
Papaya	1 cup	87
Peas, fresh or frozen	1 cup cooked	77
Peppers, green	1 cup cooked	120
Peppers, red	1 cup cooked	233
Pineapple	1 cup	56
Plantains, raw	1 medium	33
Potato	1 medium	19
Raspberries	1 cup	32
Strawberries	1 cup	98-106
Tangerine	1 medium	22
Tomato or vegetable juice	1 cup	44-67
Tomato sauce	1 cup	66
Tomato, raw or canned	1 cup	22-23
Turnip greens	1 cup cooked	40
Watermelon	1 wedge	23
Winter squash	1 cup cooked	19

Refer to appendix E for guidance on converting English units to metric.

Data from the USDA National Nutrient Database for Standard Reference. Available: http://www.ars.usda.gov/nutrientdata.

iron absorption. Not so fortunate is the fact that many of the foods and beverages we enjoy tend to inhibit iron absorption. Tea is a great example. The tannins in tea bind tightly with iron in the intestines so less iron is available for absorption. The way around this is to consume these and other iron inhibitors between meals. See box 7.2 for a summary of how to boost iron intake and absorption.

Considering Iron Supplements

Athletes concerned about their iron status should first try to boost their intake and absorption of iron from foods. However, there are times when vegetarian athletes may require iron supplements to maintain or replenish iron stores. An athlete allergic to or who dislikes legumes, nuts, and seeds, for example, will likely struggle to take in enough iron. A female endurance athlete with excessive menstrual blood loss on top of heavy endurance training may also find it difficult to maintain iron status during the preracing and racing seasons.

Box
7.2

Tips for Boosting Iron Intake and Absorption

➤ Inventory the iron-rich foods in your diet. If your diet lacks them, include more iron-rich foods daily (see table 7.1). If desired, cook in an iron skillet or use an iron "egg" or "stone." Remember, as a vegetarian athlete, your iron needs may be elevated.

➤ Include a source of vitamin C or other organic acids in most meals. Consider foods that are good sources of vitamin C and iron as well as food combinations that provide both. You can almost never go wrong by adding a small glass of citrus juice or topping foods with chopped tomatoes, tomato salsa or sauce, or a splash of flavored vinegar. One recent study found that iron absorbed from tofu was increased significantly when it was consumed with 10 ounces (295 ml) of orange juice.[13]

➤ Assess your regular consumption of inhibitors. Try to limit their consumption or consume them between meals. For example, instead of drinking milk or iced tea with a bean burrito or lentil soup, replace the beverage with citrus juice to enhance the iron absorbed from that meal. Or drink water and top the meal with chopped tomato or a splash of vinegar. Enjoy your milk or tea with a between-meal snack that is lower in iron. Also, consume tofu with vegetables or fruit. At breakfast, don't drink tea or coffee while eating iron-rich cereal, whole grain toast, or a bran muffin. Instead, drink a glass of orange juice or bowl of fresh melon to enhance the iron absorption. Depending on your training schedule and preference, morning tea or coffee should then be consumed an hour or so before or after your iron-rich breakfast.

If you want to supplement, you should first check with your personal or team physician to ensure that you are indeed iron depleted or iron deficient. Your physician can determine whether your iron status is truly compromised by checking your serum ferritin level or serum iron-binding capacity (see box 7.1). Some physicians may also be able to check your zinc protoporphyrin or serum transferrin receptor concentrations, which may be better indicators of iron status in athletes, pending their cost and availability. Reduced hemoglobin, hematocrit, and red blood cell levels do not indicate good iron status in endurance athletes[22] because of the exercise-induced plasma volume expansion (see box 7.3). Taking iron supplements on your own, except in the form of a multivitamin, is not advised because they may not be necessary and could unknowingly lead to hemochromatosis, an iron overload disease, in genetically susceptible people.

If iron supplementation is needed, low-dose iron supplements are probably the best bet because they will be less likely to cause side effects and will provide a dose of iron that is more easily absorbed than a multivitamin plus iron supplement.[3] The side effects of taking iron tablets are not pleasant and include stomach upset, burning gut, constipation, and diarrhea. After you have replenished the depleted stores—which may take several months—or develop "I can't stand it anymore" side effects, you can switch to a multivitamin and begin focusing on diet. Eventually, you can drop the multivitamin plus iron supplement. Alternatively, you may be able to take a low-dose iron supplement intermittently when needed—for example during menstrual bleeding or after giving blood—rather than regularly. The main advantage of intermittent supplementation is that it reduces side effects associated with high doses of iron.[4] Intermittent supplementation is somewhat controversial, however, and specific protocols are not available.

Problems With Too Much Iron

Recent research has found that high levels of iron in the blood are associated with an elevated risk of many chronic diseases, including heart disease, Parkinson's disease, cancer, and cancer mortality.[11] Iron may help form products called free radicals (discussed in the next chapter), which can attack many of the stable molecules in the body. Attack by free radicals is thought to promote the formation of oxidized low-density lipoprotein (LDL) particles (elevating the risk for cardiovascular and other vascular diseases, tumors, and even nerve cell death). In addition, the prevalence of hereditary hemochromatosis, an iron storage disease, is high in the United States and many countries but is not well recognized.[11] Hereditary hemochromatosis is a common genetic disorder in Caucasians.[16] The storage of excess iron in these people can be the underlying cause of liver disease, increased skin pigmentation, diabetes, heart disease, arrhythmias, arthritis, and hypogonadism. Clearly, excess iron in the diet or in the body is nothing to mess with. And unless you supplement, it is something a vegetarian may be immune to.

Box
7.3

Is It Really Anemia?

You are feeling fine and stop by your physician's office for another matter only to learn—surprisingly—that your hemoglobin is low. You are told you are anemic.

If you are an endurance athlete or athlete who has just initiated the season, chances are you are experiencing something called *dilutional anemia, sports anemia,* or *athletic anemia.* This type of anemia is not really anemia and is caused by the normal expansion in the volume of plasma fluid that occurs with training. Dilutional anemia is noted in endurance athletes during the precompetition or competition season (particularly when the weather is hot). It is also commonly noted at the beginning of the season for some athletes but then disappears when red blood cell formation catches up with fluid-volume expansion. In this case, many markers of iron status, including hemoglobin, hematocrit, and red blood cell concentrations are falsely lowered and are not good indicators of iron status.[22] On the other hand, serum ferritin may be elevated in endurance athletes and also inaccurately reflect iron storage.[28]

Dilutional anemia is not something to worry about because it will not impair performance or health. You should, however, determine that you are indeed experiencing dilutional rather than true anemia. You can do this by having your serum ferritin concentration checked or, better yet, by repeating the test after you have taken two or three days off from training. The training effect of volume expansion is short lived and will return to normal if you rest for several days. Don't worry, your plasma volume expands again as soon as you resume exercising and is beneficial. It helps you maintain your fluid volume for longer while sweating during exercise. Often, athletes experiencing volume expansion notice its effects in funny ways. For example, the ring you picked out during the off-season suddenly becomes tight, or the strap on your sport watch has to be loosened one or two slots.

I hope that after reading this chapter you understand how you can boost iron absorption and achieve normal iron status—without supplements—on a vegetarian diet. The next chapter addresses how you can make better choices to avoid dependence on vitamin and mineral supplements in general.

Breaking Free of Multivitamin Dependence

A collegiate tennis player came to see me about the nutritional quality of his diet. He had been a vegetarian in Germany as a teenager, but his parents encouraged him to eat meat after a blood test revealed some abnormal values. He told me he had quit eating meat again. "But this time I want to do it properly," he added. His diet appeared to contain adequate energy and carbohydrate (mainly from grains), some vegetables, and an occasional piece of fruit. At the time he was still eating fish, had been trying meat analogues (mainly vegetarian burgers), but had not yet discovered legumes. He was also religiously taking a multivitamin. My assessment of his diet was that it was not too bad overall, but he could improve it by increasing the variety of his food choices. We discussed the importance of eating an assortment of plant foods, including colorful fruits and vegetables, as well as legumes and nuts. I sent him off with "Vegetarian in a Nutshell" (a handout published by Vegetarian Resource Group) and the immediate goal of increasing his fruit and vegetable intake and trying dishes that contain legumes. My long-term plan was to help him discover new foods and ways to incorporate them into his diet so that he would feel more confident in his food choices and less dependent on his multivitamin supplement.

As an athlete who is a vegetarian, you are targeted twice with the message that you need to take a vitamin and mineral supplement of some sort in order to maintain nutritional status. Vegetarians, as the claims go, need vitamin and mineral supplements because of their meatless diet. And athletes need supplements because of their poor diets and excessive nutrient losses, purportedly caused by the increased breakdown and excretion of nutrients during training. These claims, however, neglect the simple fact that vegetarians are more likely than omnivores to choose diets rich in a wider variety of plant foods packed with vitamins and minerals, particularly if they make good food choices. They also ignore the fact that athletes are more likely to meet their vitamin and mineral needs than less-active people simply through their volume of food intake. In general, athletes do not need higher levels of vitamins and minerals than inactive people, with the possible exception of iron, riboflavin, vitamin C, and sodium. Although some vegetarian athletes should monitor certain "red flag" nutrients with a watchful eye, this need is based more on food choice and energy intake than on being a vegetarian athlete.

This chapter shows you how to meet your vitamin and mineral needs through your diet rather than depending on unnecessary vitamin and mineral supplements. Although you may not be comfortable completely giving up your daily multivitamin and mineral supplement, the information presented in this chapter should help you understand how vitamins and minerals affect your general health and performance and how your needs for the major vitamins and minerals can be met by making better food choices. Iron and the nutrients involved in bone health are not emphasized because they were the focus of previous chapters.

Vitamin and Mineral Primer

Getting adequate amounts of vitamins and minerals is important for health and performance. Both vitamins and minerals are key regulators of numerous bodily functions, many of which are critical for exercise and performance. Vitamins and minerals are classified as micronutrients, in contrast to the macronutrients carbohydrate, protein, fat, and water, because the body needs them in much smaller quantities. Macronutrient requirements are expressed in grams, whereas micronutrient requirements are expressed in micrograms to milligrams. And micronutrients also perform different functions than macronutrients. Macronutrients provide sources of energy, maintain cellular hydration, and provide the body structure for performing work. Micronutrients aid in the body's use of macronutrients during many processes, including energy generation and maintenance of skeletal health. Many vitamins and minerals also play a role in immune function and help protect cells from oxidative damage.

The body's need for macronutrients and micronutrients depends on whether the nutrient is used up or conserved for use and reuse, and whether the nutrient is stored in the body and in what quantity. For example, carbohydrate is used for energy, whereas iron is hoarded and reused. Thus, the daily carbohydrate need for athletes is close to 500 grams per day and the daily requirement for iron is 18 milligrams per day for menstruating females and 11 milligrams for adult males. Because only a small percentage of the minerals consumed are absorbed into the body, nutrient requirements are also influenced by how efficiently the intestines can absorb them.

If you are wondering if there is a difference between vitamins and minerals, the answer is yes. Vitamins are organic substances found in food. Organic means that they contain the elements carbon, oxygen, and hydrogen. Vitamins aid the essential biochemical reactions by catalyzing, or speeding, them. Without vitamin catalysts, many chemical reactions would occur too slowly to allow us to live. Vitamins are needed regularly in the diet because the body cannot make them. There are 13 known vitamins: four fat-soluble vitamins (A, D, E and K) and nine water-soluble vitamins (vitamin C, and the eight B-complex vitamins). In general, the body is able to store enough fat-soluble vitamins to last for months but only enough water-soluble vitamins to last a few weeks or less.

Minerals, on the other hand, are not organic and serve more as structural or helper components of enzymes rather than as catalysts. Fifteen minerals—calcium, phosphorus, magnesium, fluoride, iron, sodium, potassium, chloride, zinc, iodine, copper, selenium, chromium, manganese, and molybdenum—are considered essential.

Getting Your Vitamins and Minerals on a Vegetarian Diet

Most vegetarian athletes can meet their need for vitamins and minerals by consuming a diet that provides adequate energy and consists of a variety of wholesome foods, including whole grains, legumes, leafy greens and other vegetables, fruit, and, if acceptable, dairy products. Because of hectic training and work or school schedules, however, some athletes make poor food choices, resulting in a deficient intake of many vitamins and minerals. Others may be at risk for deficiencies simply because they restrict food intake to maintain low body weight. This is often the case with athletes involved in gymnastics, dancing, diving, distance running, figure skating, and wrestling. Surveys of various groups of athletes have suggested that intake of iron, calcium, zinc, copper, and magnesium are often insufficient,[49] particularly among female athletes.[32] Research in vegetarian and vegan populations has found that vitamin B_{12}, vitamin D, riboflavin, and iodine status are occasionally compromised.[1]

Better Food Choices for Improved Vitamin and Mineral Nutrition

Despite what supplement companies and vitamin gurus want you to believe, it is always best to improve your nutritional status through better food choices. The reason is simply that Mother Nature wanted us to eat food. Food is packed not only with vitamins and minerals but also with many known and unknown factors that aid in nutrient absorption and utilization. These factors—often called phytochemicals—may even reduce the risk of chronic diseases. Great examples include the bioflavins found in citrus fruits and vegetables that help the body absorb vitamin C; and the many anticancer substances including isoflavones, lutein, isothiocyanates, saponins, and allium compounds that trap free radicals (see box 8.1) or deactivate cancer-causing substances.[46]

Isolating one compound from a fruit or vegetable and putting it in a pill is probably appealing to those who would rather skip the spinach and simply gobble a

Box 8.1 Free Radicals and Antioxidants

Free radicals are produced by normal bodily processes that include the oxidation reactions required for energy generation from carbohydrate; fat, and protein (as described in chapter 2) during rest and particularly during exercise. Environmental factors such as ultraviolet light, air pollution, and tobacco smoke also produce free radicals. Free radicals are problematic because they are unstable and can attack and damage cellular proteins, unsaturated fatty acids located in cellular membranes, and even DNA. Their ability to damage DNA and genetic-related material explains why they may play a role in cancer promotion. In addition, free radicals are thought to be responsible for exercise-induced protein oxidation and to possibly contribute to muscle fatigue[39] and soreness.

Antioxidants can stabilize free radicals and protect against oxidative stress. In this role, they may have a protective effect on cognitive performance, aging, cancer, arthritis, cataracts, and heart disease. Although high intake of fruits and vegetables has been shown time and time again to have a protective effect on many age-related diseases, including cancer[4, 46, 47] and heart disease,[21] the specific factors responsible are not known. Known vitamin and mineral antioxidants are beta-carotene, other carotenoids, vitamin C, vitamin E, copper, and selenium. An assortment of other components in plants, called phytochemicals, have been implicated but have not been proven. It is known, however, that the antioxidant vitamins actively scavenge and quench free radicals, often becoming oxidized and inactive themselves in the process. Vitamin C is particularly important for the parts of the body that consist of water, whereas vitamin E is important in the cell membrane. Copper and selenium, on the other hand, serve as important cofactors for enzymes involved in the body's internal free radical–defense system.

It is not yet known whether antioxidants influence muscle recovery and enhance performance. Although studies have found that antioxidant supplements may reduce lipid peroxidation, they do not appear to enhance exercise performance.[6, 18, 39, 51] Research, however, is needed to determine whether a plant-based diet naturally high in antioxidants and phytochemicals would enhance recovery and make less severe the oxidative damage that occurs with heavy training. A recent study found that consuming a drink containing black grape, raspberry, and red currant concentrates before a bout of strenuous exercise reduced oxidative stress and possibly also muscle damage.[35] So keep eating those whole grains and colorful fruits and vegetables.

pill, but it defies nature. In fact, we are learning more and more that supplementing with isolated vitamins[8, 22, 37] often does not yield the same protective benefits of simply eating fruits and vegetables.[23, 47] Taking beta-carotene supplements, for example, has been shown to increase rather than decrease the risk of lung cancer and cardiovascular disease,[8, 22, 37] promoting particularly adverse effects in smokers and those exposed to asbestos.[8, 37] Taking folic acid supplements was recently found, somewhat surprisingly, to increase the risk of artery reclogging in heart patients following coronary stenting, an operation that unclogs arteries.[22] Eating plenty of fruits and vegetables high in these and other nutrients, on the other hand, appears to protect against most chronic diseases. Supplements made from concentrated fruit and vegetable extracts also do not provide the full benefits of whole foods. These supplements lack soluble and insoluble fiber and other structural components that help keep bowel functions regular and also have a protective influence on gut health and blood sugar regulation.

Tackling Vitamins With Less Reliance on Supplements

The bottom line is that supplements—even if they are pure extracts of real foods—do not provide the same benefit as consuming the real thing. Indeed, the nutrient content of whole real foods can be lost or destroyed through cooking, processing, or improper storage—either on your part or the growers' and food distributors'—but these factors can be minimized. To retain the nutrient content of food, don't overcook it, cook it in a minimal amount of water and with as low a heat as possible, purchase more locally grown foods, and eat fresh foods shortly after purchase. Storing fresh produce and grains in a dark, cool place away from direct sunlight, and in airtight containers, if appropriate, also preserves their nutrient content. Finally, educating yourself about good sources of the major nutrients and consuming a variety of foods containing these nutrients should help you meet your nutrient needs and maybe even feel secure enough in vegetarian eating to eliminate your dependence on supplements. The following section briefly discusses the vitamins that either are important to active vegetarians or that may be low in poorly selected vegetarian diets.

B Vitamins

The B-complex vitamins are a set of eight vitamins: thiamin, riboflavin, niacin, biotin, pantothenic acid, vitamin B_6, folate, and vitamin B_{12}. Collectively, these vitamins function as catalysts or coenzymes involved in the release of energy from carbohydrate, fat, and protein and also in the development, growth, and repair of all body cells. Therefore, requirements for some, but not all, B vitamins are tied to energy intake.

Surveys of athletes in general have noted that riboflavin, folate, and vitamin B_6 are frequently low in the diet of some female athletes,[32] most likely because of inadequate consumption of fruits, green leafy vegetables, legumes, and dairy products. Clinical studies have also noted that active people who restrict their energy intake or make poor dietary choices are at risk of poor thiamine, riboflavin, and vitamin B_6 status.[31]

Athletes who follow vegetarian diets and do not restrict energy intake should easily be able to meet their requirements for most B vitamins, which are widely distributed in plant foods (see table 8.1). In fact, many of the best sources of B vitamins, such as folate, are provided by plant rather than animal foods.

TABLE 8.1 B Vitamins and Vitamin C for Vegetarian Athletes

Vitamin	Recommended intake for athletes	Major vegetarian sources	Noted problems with excessive consumption
Thiamin (B_1)	DRI = 1.2 mg men, 1.1 mg women; recommendation of 0.6 mg/1,000 kcal may be more appropriate for athletes	Whole-grain products, enriched breads and cereals, legumes	No known toxicity
Riboflavin (B_2)	DRI = 1.3 mg men, 1.1 mg women; recommendation of 0.6 mg/1,000 kcal may be more appropriate for athletes	Milk and dairy products, enriched grain products, green leafy vegetables, legumes (table 8.2)	No known toxicity
Niacin	DRI = 16 mg men, 14 mg women; recommendation of 6.6 mg/1,000 kcal may be more appropriate for athletes	Whole-grain products, enriched breads and cereals, legumes	Headache, nausea, flushing of face, burning and itching skin (nicotinic acid)
Biotin	Adequate Intake (AI) = 30 mg for adults	Legumes, milk, egg yolk, whole-grain products, most vegetables	No known toxicity
Pantothenic acid	AI = 5 mg for adults	Milk, eggs, legumes, whole-grain products, most vegetables	No known toxicity
Vitamin B_6	DRI = 1.3 mg for adults ages 19-50; athletes may need values higher than the DRI because of increased protein intakes	Protein foods, legumes, green leafy vegetables (table 8.4)	Loss of nerve sensation, impaired gait
Folic acid	DRI = 400 mcg	Green leafy vegetables, legumes, nuts, enriched grain products (table 8.3)	Prevents detection of B_{12} deficiency
Vitamin B_{12}	RDA = 2.4 mcg	Animal foods only: fish, milk, eggs; also nutrition-support formula and fortified vegan products	No known toxicity
Vitamin C	DRI = 90 mg for men, 75 mg for women; athletes may need 100 mg	Fruits and vegetables particularly bell peppers, citrus fruits, broccoli (table 7.4)	Diarrhea, kidney stones, scurvy (when ceasing mega-doses), reduced copper absorption

However, riboflavin and vitamin B_{12} are potential exceptions. Both vitamins are of special interest to athletes and intake of both tends to be low in vegetarian diets that contain little or no dairy or animal products.

Riboflavin   Riboflavin is important for the formation of enzymes known as flavoproteins, which are involved in energy production from carbohydrate and fat. Several studies have found that riboflavin needs are increased with the initiation of an exercise program[3, 45] and possibly also with an abrupt increase in training volume, such as at the beginning of the preseason. Although riboflavin is widely distributed in foods, major sources include milk, other dairy products, meat, and eggs. An 8-ounce (236 ml) glass of milk, for example, contains 20 percent of the RDA for riboflavin. Because some studies have found that vegans take in less riboflavin than nonvegetarians,[33] vegan and vegetarian athletes who consume little or no dairy foods should make an effort to consume riboflavin-containing plant foods. This is particularly important when increasing training volume or when restricting energy intake. Good plant sources of riboflavin include whole-grain and fortified breads and cereals, legumes, tofu, nuts, seeds, bananas, asparagus, dark-green leafy vegetables, avocado, and sea vegetables, such as seaweed, kombu, arame, and dulse (see table 8.2).

Vitamin B_{12}   Vitamin B_{12} has been of interest in the athletic community for years. In fact, injections of B_{12} are popular with some athletes, trainers, coaches, and even referees because of their belief that the vitamin will increase energy, enhance endurance, and give the user an "energy high." Research has never supported the existence of performance-enhancing benefits of B_{12} injections[48] or of high-dose B_{12} supplementation with a multivitamin in the absence of an actual deficiency.[44] Severe deficiencies of Vitamin B_{12} and folate can result in anemia and reduce oxygen-carrying capacity and endurance performance.[29]

The major function of B_{12} is as part of a coenzyme complex that is essential in the synthesis of DNA, the body's genetic code, and red blood cells and in the formation of the protective sheath, called *myelin,* that surrounds nerve fibers. Although some believe that athletes may require more B_{12} because of their higher turnover of red blood cells, no scientific evidence supports this assumption.[33]

Vitamin B_{12} is of interest to vegan populations because cobalamin, the active form, is found exclusively in animal products.[13] Thus, vegan athletes need to regularly consume foods fortified with B_{12}. These include Red Star T6635 nutritional yeast, soy milk, breakfast cereals, margarines, and some meat analogues. I have not included a comprehensive list of fortified foods because the B_{12} content varies by brand and product, and sometimes manufacturers change the ingredients in their products. For example, Morningstar Farms Chik Patties provide 20 percent of the Daily Value (DV) for B_{12}, and their Veggie Breakfast Sausage Links provide 50 percent of the DV (neither are vegan). Boca meatless burgers (which are vegan) contain no added vitamin B_{12}, at least at the time of this book's publication. Red Star T6635 nutritional yeast, however, is a reliable source. Two teaspoons (10 ml) supplies nearly the adult RDA of 2.4 micrograms and is delicious sprinkled on many foods. Carefully check the labels of your favorite brands or write or call the

TABLE 8.2 Riboflavin, Zinc, and Copper Content of Selected Vegetarian and Dairy Foods

Food	Portion	Riboflavin (mg)	Zinc (mg)	Copper (mcg)
GRAIN EQUIVALENTS				
Bread, enriched	1 oz slice	0.09	0.2	70
Bread, whole wheat	1 oz slice	0.06	0.55	80
Cereal, fortified	1 serving (1 oz)	0.42	1.2-3.8	varies
VEGETABLES AND LEGUMES, INCLUDING SOY				
Asparagus	1 cup cooked	0.25	1.1	370
Avocado	1/4 avocado	0.06	0.3	100
Beet greens	1 cup cooked	0.42	0.72	360
Black beans	1 cup cooked	0.10	1.9	360
Broccoli	1 cup cooked	0.10	0.35	95
Cabbage, Chinese (bok choy)	1 cup cooked	0.11	0.3	40
Collard greens	1 cup cooked	0.20	2.5	70
Chickpeas (garbanzo beans)	1 cup cooked	0.09	0.3	580
Kale	1 cup cooked	0.09	0.3	200
Lentils	1 cup cooked	0.15	2.5	500
Mustard greens	1 cup cooked	0.09	0.15	120
Peas, green	1 cup cooked	0.24	1.9	280
Pinto beans	1 cup cooked	0.11	1.7	370
Red kidney beans	1 cup cooked	0.10	1.9	430
Southern peas (black-eyed, crowder)	1 cup cooked	0.10	2.2	460
Soybeans	1 cup cooked	2.0	0.5	700
Tofu, firm (calcium set)	1/2 cup	0.13	2.0	480
Tofu, regular (calcium set)	1/2 cup	0.06	1.0	240
Turnip greens	1 cup cooked	0.10	0.2	360
FRUITS				
Banana	1 medium	0.09	0.2	90
NUTS AND SEEDS				
Almonds	1 oz	0.23	0.95	330
Cashews	1 oz	0.06	1.6	630
Peanuts	1 oz	0.03	0.9	190
Pecans	1 oz	0.04	1.3	330
Pine nuts	1 oz	0.06	1.8	380
Pumpkin seeds	1 oz	0.09	2.1	390
Sunflower seeds	1 oz	0.07	1.5	520
Tahini	1 Tbsp	0.07	0.7	240
Walnuts	1 oz	0.04	0.9	450

Food	Portion	Riboflavin (mg)	Zinc (mg)	Copper (mcg)
MILK, SOY MILK, AND CHEESE				
Soy milk, calcium fortified	1 cup	0.53	0.5	200
Cows milk, skim	1 cup	0.45	1.0	30
Cows milk, 2%	1 cup	0.45	1.1	30
Cheddar cheese	1 oz	0.11	0.9	9
Goat, hard	1 oz	0.34	0.45	180
Mozzarella, low moisture	1 oz	0.09	0.9	8
Parmesan, hard	1 oz	0.09	0.8	9

Values for most vegetables and legumes are for those that have been cooked, boiled, and drained and without salt. Values for most nuts are for dry-roasted varieties without added oil or salt. Note: The RDA is 1.6 mg for riboflavin, 15 mg for zinc, and 900 mcg for copper. Refer to appendix E for guidance on converting English units to metric.

Data from the USDA National Nutrient Database for Standard Reference. Available: http://www.ars.usda.gov/nutrientdata.

manufacturers for nutritional information. Contrary to information recently published in the public press, nori and chlorella seaweeds are not a reliable source of well-absorbed B_{12}.[40]

Because of the irreversible neurological damage that can occur with vitamin B_{12} deficiency, vegans should have their B_{12} status monitored regularly by their personal or team physician.[13] The typical symptoms of B_{12} deficiency (usually apparent in the red blood cells) can be masked by high intake of folate, which is abundant in plant foods.

Vegetarians who consume dairy products or eggs are likely to take in adequate amounts of vitamin B_{12}.[1, 13] For example, one cup of milk (236 ml) contains approximately one microgram of vitamin B_{12} and one ounce (28 g) of low-moisture, part-skim mozzarella cheese contains 0.65 micrograms. However, athletes who are concerned should have their B_{12} status tested. Senior athletes may also be at risk for vitamin B_{12} deficiency because of the reduced absorption rate of this vitamin in the gut that occurs with aging.

Other B Vitamins Maintaining adequate levels of other B vitamins is generally not a problem for vegetarian athletes, unless, of course, they restrict energy intake or avoid grains and pulses (beans, peas, and lentils), which are excellent sources of most of the B vitamins. Nevertheless, a brief discussion of folate and vitamin B_6 may be of interest, particularly to female athletes.

Although folic acid is most likely abundant in the diet of vegetarian athletes, it is worth discussing here because of its recent media attention. Like vitamin B_{12}, folic acid is an essential factor in DNA synthesis and new-cell formation. It has received considerable attention because it may help reduce the risk of heart disease and cancer and prevent birth defects. Because many American adults do not get enough folic acid, the government now mandates that 140 micrograms of folic acid be added to every 100 grams of enriched grain products such as pasta, breakfast cereals, and flour. Folic acid, however, was first found in leafy green vegetables, which is how it got its name. The word folate, the name of the plant form of folic acid, is derived from the Latin word for leaf: *folium.*

The richest sources of folate—the natural form of the vitamin—are legumes and dark-green leafy vegetables and certain fruits such as oranges. The most abundant sources of folic acid—the synthetic form—are fortified grain products, which provide 15 to 100 percent of the DV. See table 8.3 for a list of the top 20 vegetarian sources of folate. Although vegetarian athletes in general are likely to meet folate requirements easily, even without including fortified foods,[43] you should still keep in mind that folate is easily destroyed by heat and oxidation (for example after cutting) and interactions with medications, including antacids and aspirin. Also, synthetic folic acid appears to be better absorbed than natural folate.

The other B vitamin worth discussing is vitamin B_6. Because women, both active and inactive, often take in insufficient amounts, it is commonly targeted as a vitamin to supplement. Vitamin B_6 has been purported to benefit those with mental depression, premenstrual syndrome (PMS), arthritis, carpal tunnel syndrome, sleep disorders, and the like, but supplementing with vitamin B_6 has received mixed and mostly negative reviews. Unlike some of the other B vitamins, however,

TABLE 8.3 Top 20 Natural Vegetarian Sources of Folate

Food	Portion	Value (mcg)
Lentils	1 cup cooked	358
Southern peas	1 cup cooked	358
Pinto beans	1 cup cooked	294
Okra	1 cup cooked, sliced	269
Spinach	1 cup cooked	263
Black beans/navy beans	1 cup cooked	256
Asparagus	1 cup cooked	243
Red kidney beans	1 cup cooked	230
Green soybeans	1 cup cooked	200
Great northern beans	1 cup cooked	181
Collard greens	1 cup cooked	177
Turnip greens	1 cup cooked	170
Broccoli	1 cup cooked	168
Chickpeas	1 cup cooked	161
Brussels sprouts, frozen	1 cup cooked	157
Lima beans	1 cup cooked	156
Beets, red	1 cup cooked	136
Split peas	1 cup cooked	127
Papaya	1 cup chopped	116
Corn, canned	1 cup cooked	115

The DRI for folate is 400 mcg for adults. Refer to appendix E for guidance on converting English units to metric.

Data from "Reports by Single Nutrients," *USDA National Nutrient Database for Standard Reference, Release 18.* Available: http://www.ars.usda.gov/Services/docs.htm?docid=9673.

regular supplementation with doses higher than two to three times the RDA may cause neurological symptoms. Thus, your best bet is to forget B_6 supplements and strive for adequate B_6 intake in the diet. Vitamin B_6 is widely distributed in foods; the best sources are protein foods, including vegetarian protein sources (see table 8.4).

TABLE 8.4   Top 20 Vegetarian Sources of Vitamin B_6

Food	Portion	Value (mg)
Ready-to-eat cereals, fortified	1 oz (3/4-1 1/3 cup)	0.50-3.6
Chickpeas	1 cup cooked	1.14
Chocolate malted drink mix, fortified	3 heaping tsp	0.92
Rice, long grain, parboiled, enriched	1 cup cooked	0.84
Hash browned potatoes	1 cup prepared	0.74
Baked potato	1 medium	0.63
Prune juice	1 cup	0.56
Banana	1 cup sliced	0.56
Stewed prunes	1 cup	0.54
Plantain	1 medium	0.54
Mashed potatoes, home prepared	1 cup	0.52
Carrot juice	1 cup	0.50
Sweet potato, canned	1 cup cooked	0.48
Brussels sprouts	1 cup cooked	0.45
Scalloped potatoes, home prepared	1 cup	0.44
Spinach	1 cup cooked	0.44
Peppers, red	1 cup	0.43
Marinara sauce, commercially prepared	1 cup	0.43
Soybeans	1 cup cooked	0.40
Pinto beans	1 cup cooked	0.39

The DRI for vitamin B_6 is 1.3 mg for adults ages 19-50. Refer to appendix E for guidance on converting English units to metric.

Data from "Reports by Single Nutrients," *USDA National Nutrient Database for Standard Reference, Release 18.* Available: http://www.ars.usda.gov/Services/docs.htm?docid=9673.

Vitamin C

Vitamin C provides many important health and performance functions. Vitamin C is probably best known for its roles in collagen synthesis and the prevention of scurvy, a disease caused by vitamin C deficiency and characterized by spongy gums and weak muscles. Vitamin C is needed for the synthesis of carnitine, which transports long-chain fats into the mitochondria for energy generation, as well as several hormones produced during exercise, including epinephrine, norepinephrine, and cortisol. Vitamin C also aids in the uptake of nonheme iron and is a potent antioxidant that helps trap free radicals and keep vitamin E in its active form.

Vitamin C depletion can induce fatigue, muscle weakness, and anemia and can decrease the ability to train because of recurrent injuries to connective tissue.

Vegetarian athletes are likely to have an abundance of vitamin C in their daily diets. Vitamin C is found in most fruits and vegetables, including bell peppers and citrus fruits (see table 7.4 on page 91), and is an additive in many fruit and juice products. Surveys of nonactive vegetarians have found that they typically consume at least twice the current recommendation for vitamin C[33] and display plasma concentrations of vitamin C higher than those of omnivores.[21, 41] Some suggest, however, that the recommended daily intake may not be adequate for most athletes because of vitamin C lost from foods exposed to heat and light, as well as the increased use of vitamin C to fight damage to body cells from smog, environmental pollutants, and free radicals produced during exercise.[18] In fact, some experts feel that people who consistently exercise may require 100 milligrams of vitamin C per day to maintain normal vitamin C status. And those competing in ultraendurance events may require up to 500 milligrams per day. The recommended intake in the United States is 75 milligrams per day for adult females and 90 milligrams per day for adult males.

Many athletes take vitamin C supplements with the belief that it will prevent colds and other acute illnesses and aid in the recovery from exercise. Although some research suggests that vitamin C supplementation reduces the risk of developing an upper-respiratory infection following a tough endurance race,[9, 38] no evidence suggests that it will prevent the common cold when taken either preventively or after symptoms develop.[9] In one study conducted by researchers in South Africa, endurance-trained men consuming a diet containing 500 milligrams of vitamin C received either 600 milligrams of vitamin C or a placebo for the three weeks before a 42-kilometer (26 miles) running race.[38] During the 14 days after the race, the runners who supplemented with vitamin C had fewer upper-respiratory-tract infections than did those without the supplement (33 compared to 68 percent).

Vitamin C may also facilitate recovery from intense training by enhancing immune function, trapping free radicals produced during exercise, and enhancing collagen repair. Studies demonstrating that vitamin C supplementation prevents muscle damage or oxidative stress, however, are scarce. A study conducted at the University of North Carolina at Greensboro found that supplementing with either 500 or 1,000 milligrams of vitamin C per day for two weeks reduced blood markers for oxidative stress following a 30-minute run at moderate intensity in a group of relatively fit nonathletic men.[11] Although more studies are needed to determine whether excessive vitamin C provides additional benefits, the take-home message for vegetarian athletes may simply be to keep eating fruits and vegetables, particularly during periods of high-volume training.

Vitamin A and the Carotenoids

Vitamin A is important for normal vision, gene expression, growth, and immune function. Technically, vitamin A is found only in animal products, but it can be made easily from beta-carotene and several other carotenoids, which form the beautiful red, orange, and yellow pigments in fruits and vegetables. Some dark-green fruits and vegetables also contain carotenoid pigments, but they're masked by chlorophyll, which is green. Although surveys of various athletic groups have indicated that most athletes easily consume enough vitamin A in their diets, those at risk of insufficient vitamin A levels tend to be younger athletes participating in wrestling, ballet, and gymnastics.[29] Vegetarians as a group typically take in adequate amounts of vitamin A and also have high blood levels of beta-carotene[41] and usually the other carotenoids as well. Because of their heartier appetites, vegetarian athletes are also likely to meet, if not exceed, the RDA for vitamin A and have an abundance of healthy carotenoids circulating in their blood. You can meet the RDA for vitamin A just by consuming one carrot, and carrots are not even the richest source (see table 8.5).

No research is available to suggest that marginal intakes of vitamin A or the carotenoids influence exercise performance. Nevertheless, the carotenoids found naturally in plant foods likely reduce the risk of many types of cancer[46] and several age-related diseases, including macular degeneration, a degenerative eye disease that leads to blindness.[5, 52] A diet high in carotenoids may also lessen the severity of the oxidative damage associated with heavy training (see box 8.1). The best strategy for ensuring adequate intake is to eat dark-green and red-orange fruits and vegetables daily. Good sources of beta-carotene, lutein, and zeaxanthin include leafy greens, pumpkin, sweet potatoes, carrots, and winter squash. Good sources of lycopene are tomato products, watermelon, and pink grapefruit. Taking a daily antioxidant supplement may provide some of the carotenoids, but it is not likely to provide as much nutritional impact as getting them straight from the source. Taking doses greater than the RDA of vitamin A is not recommended because vitamin A can cause headache, nausea, fatigue, liver and spleen damage, peeling skin, and joint pain. Supplementation with the carotenoids does not have the same toxic effect.

TABLE 8.5   Top 10 Vegetarian Sources of Vitamin A

Food	Portion	RAE* (mcg)
Carrot juice	1 cup	2,256
Pumpkin, canned	1 cup	1,906
Sweet potato, baked in skin	1 cup	1,922
Carrots, frozen	1 cup cooked	1,342
Spinach, frozen, chopped	1 cup cooked	1,146
Carrots, raw	1 cup chopped	1,076
Collards, frozen, chopped	1 cup cooked	978
Kale, frozen, chopped	1 cup cooked	956
Turnip greens, frozen, chopped	1 cup cooked	882
Beet greens, frozen, chopped	1 cup cooked	552

Refer to appendix E for guidance on converting English units to metric. The DRI for vitamin A is 900 mcg RAE/day for men and 700 mcg RAE for women (3,000 and 2,333 IU respectively).

*RAE = Retinol activity equivalents because of preformed retinol and beta-carotene.

Data from "Reports by Single Nutrients," *USDA National Nutrient Database for Standard Reference, Release 18.* Available: http://www.ars.usda.gov/Services/docs.htm?docid=9673.

Vitamin E

Vitamin E is a nutrient we need to learn a lot more about. Vitamin E is actually a generic term for eight naturally occurring compounds of two classes designated as alpha-tocopherols and gamma-tocopherols. The most active is RRR-alpha-tocopherol. The main function of vitamin E is to protect the polyunsaturated fats found in the cells from oxidative damage by free radicals. This includes protecting the membranes surrounding the muscle cells and the mitochondria.

As far as scientists know, vitamin E needs do not increase with physical training. Athletes, however, may need more vitamin E because of their higher intake of polyunsaturated fats, which increases with increased energy needs. Athletes may also benefit from higher intakes in the initial stages of training to increase vitamin E stores in the muscle cells. The principal sources of dietary vitamin E (both the gamma and alpha forms) include vegetables, nut and seed oils, wheat germ, and whole grains (see table 8.6). Some nuts are high in one form but not the other, which highlights the importance of variety. Animal products are generally poor sources of vitamin E.

TABLE 8.6 **Top 20 Vegetarian Sources of Vitamin E (Alpha Tocopherol)**

Food	Portion	Value (mg)
Ready-to-eat cereals (Total and Product 19)	1 oz (3/4-1 1/3 cup)	13.5
Sunflower seeds	1 oz	7.4
Almonds	1 oz	7.3
Spinach, frozen	1 cup cooked	6.7
Turnip greens, frozen	1 cup cooked	4.4
Hazelnuts or filberts	1 oz	4.3
Dandelion greens	1 cup cooked	3.6
Soy milk	1 cup	3.3
Nuts, mixed	1 oz	3.1
Carrot juice	1 cup	2.7
Turnip greens	1 cup cooked	2.7
Pine nuts	1 oz	2.7
Beet greens	1 cup cooked	2.6
Pumpkin or sweet potato, canned	1 cup cooked	2.6
Broccoli, frozen	1 cup cooked	2.6
Canola oil	1 Tbsp	2.4
Pepper, red	1 cup	2.4
Mango	1 fruit	2.3
Papaya	1 fruit	2.2
Peanuts	1 oz	2.2

Data from "Reports by Single Nutrients," *USDA National Nutrient Database for Standard Reference, Release 18.* Available: http://www.ars.usda.gov/Services/docs.htm?docid=9673.

Studies assessing both the dietary intake of vitamin E and the levels of vitamin E in the blood in nonathletes strongly suggest that vegetarians are likely to have both a higher intake and higher blood level than omnivores.[41] However, vitamin E status should be assessed by looking at the ratio of tochopherol to cholesterol in blood because a significant portion of the alpha-tocopherol is transported as part of the low-density lipoprotein (LDL), or bad cholesterol, (and vegetarians typically have lower LDL cholesterol concentrations).[41] Studies indicate that vegetarians have a much higher ratio of alpha-tocopherol to cholesterol in the plasma, which protects against LDL oxidation.[21, 41] Research also indicates that absolute vitamin E concentrations in the blood of vegetarians often exceed the suggested value deemed optimal for cancer prevention.[41] Hence, you are likely to get ample vitamin E in its many naturally occurring forms if you eat a well-rounded diet containing whole grains, nuts, seeds, and vegetable oils.

Whether you could benefit from taking a vitamin E supplement that provides levels far greater than the RDA is a different story and currently cannot be adequately addressed. Because of its role as an antioxidant, there is evidence that taking large doses of vitamin E may reduce the risk of heart disease and certain cancers and even reduce exercise-associated muscle damage and soreness. Currently, however, the evidence supporting the need to supplement is not compelling. Most recent studies suggest that consuming high levels of vitamin E has a negligible effect on reducing the risk of heart disease,[19] enhancing recovery, and improving athletic performance.[28] There is a chance, however, that vitamin E may improve performance during mountain climbing or other activities at altitudes greater than 1,000 meters (3,281 feet).[10] Vitamin E may eventually be shown to reduce the risk of developing cancer or Alzheimer's disease.[50] Please stay tuned. If you decide to give supplements a try, look for those containing natural vitamin E, which may be absorbed at about twice the rate of the synthetic forms.[25]

Tackling Red Flag Minerals: Are You Getting Enough?

The following section discusses the minerals that may be low in the diets of active vegetarians and vegetarian athletes (other than those discussed in chapters 6, 7, and 11) and briefly touch on others that are likely to be adequate in the diet of vegetarian athletes.

Zinc

Zinc is a component of many enzymes in the body, including those involved in protein synthesis, DNA synthesis, reproductive function, and immune function. Several of these enzymes are also involved in the major pathways of energy metabolism, including lactate dehydrogenase, which is important for the rapid generation of energy from carbohydrate (often incorrectly called anaerobic metabolism).

Zinc is commonly suggested as a red flag nutrient for vegetarian athletes[2, 12] because zinc intake is often low in both athletes and vegetarians in general,[34, 49] and its absorption rate is lower in a vegetarian diet than in a mixed omnivorous diet. Zinc is less well absorbed from a vegetarian diet because of the higher phytate concentrations in plant foods (phytates bind zinc and limit its absorption) and the lower intake of animal foods, which tend to enhance zinc absorption.[16] In addition, lower zinc concentrations, which are thought to indicate zinc status, are consistently noted in vegetarian and nonvegetarian athletes during heavy training.[26, 34]

However, just because zinc is a red flag nutrient does not mean that you cannot meet your zinc needs without supplements on a vegetarian diet. Rather, it means that you should ensure you are taking in enough absorbable zinc. A recent study from the U.S. Department of Agriculture found that nonathletic women were able to maintain normal zinc status on a lacto–ovo vegetarian diet, even though this diet was lower in total zinc and higher in phytate and fiber than the control meat-containing diet.[15] The key to their success was incorporating legumes and whole grains. Athletes in training should find it easier than their sedentary vegetarian counterparts to regularly consume enough legumes, whole grains, and other zinc-rich foods to maintain zinc status without supplementation, unless, of course, they are restricting energy intake. In addition to legumes and whole-grain products, other plant sources of zinc include fortified cereals, nuts, hard cheeses, soy products, and meat analogues (see table 8.2). Check the label on your favorite meat analogues because zinc content varies considerably. One serving of Yves brand vegetarian burgers contains 7.8 milligrams of zinc, and its vegetarian sandwich analogues contain 4.5 milligrams. As with iron, some food preparation

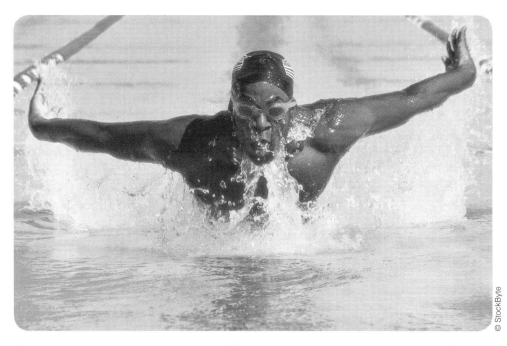

© StockByte

Zinc status is often low in vegetarian athletes, especially during training, but a diet that includes legumes, whole grains, nuts, hard cheeses, and soy should provide enough zinc to preclude supplementing.

techniques, such as soaking and sprouting beans, grains, and seeds as well as leavening bread, can reduce the binding of zinc by phytate and increase the absorbability of zinc.[1]

The significance of the low or slightly compromised zinc status noted in athletes during training[26, 34] is not yet understood. In fact, some studies have found that zinc supplementation does not influence zinc levels during training[30, 44] and appears to have no benefit on athletic performance.[44] This may suggest then that lowered serum zinc levels do not indicate zinc status in athletes, but reflect altered storage sites. For example, zinc storage may shift from the blood into skeletal muscle or other tissues during training. Nevertheless, to ensure that your zinc level is not compromised, strive to meet or slightly exceed the dietary recommendations for zinc of 11 milligrams per day for adult men and 8 milligrams per day for adult women. A recent well-controlled clinical trial conducted at the United States Department of Agriculture's Grand Forks Human Nutrition Research Center found that inadequate zinc intake (4 mg/day for 9 weeks) significantly impaired peak oxygen uptake.[27]

Iodine

The body's main use for iodine is as a component of thyroid hormone. Thyroid hormone is an important regulator of energy metabolism and protein synthesis and is the hormone best known for preventing a sluggish metabolism.

Several recent studies[20, 24, 42] have noted that iodine may be a red flag nutrient for some vegans and vegetarians. Although iodine status is not generally a concern for athletes living in industrial countries—because of the fortification of table salt—these studies found a high prevalence of iodine deficiency among vegans and vegetarians compared to nonvegetarians. This deficiency was related to the consumption of plant foods[20] grown in soil with low iodine levels,[42] limited consumption of cows' milk,[24] limited intake of fish or sea products,[20] and reduced intake of iodized salt.[20, 42] In one of these studies conducted near Bratislava, Slovakia, an area where the iodine content of soil is likely low, a striking 80 percent of vegans and 25 percent of vegetarians were found to be deficient in iodine compared to 9 percent of those on a mixed diet.[20] What is particularly problematic—and an emerging area of interest—is that perchlorate pollutants in the food and water supply can inhibit iodine uptake by the thyroid and the synthesis of thyroid hormone. Perchlorate comes from solid fuels used to power high-energy devices such as rockets, flares, fireworks, and air bags and appears to be a problem only in those with low iodine intakes.[7]

Because vegetarian athletes can get by with and in fact may need more sodium and salt than is recommended for sedentary people (as discussed in chapter 11), vegetarian athletes can ensure adequate iodine status by regularly using iodized salt in cooking and baking. Half a teaspoon (3 g) of iodized salt provides the RDA for iodine. Unfortunately, the iodine content of plant foods varies depending on the soil content. And processed foods and sea salt are not reliable sources of iodine because the salt used in processing and sea salt generally are not iodized. Reliance on iodized salt, on the other hand, is probably not necessary if you regularly include sea vegetables in your diet.

Copper

Copper is an essential mineral that—like many minerals—we need to better understand. Copper plays a role in iron metabolism and hemoglobin production and like iron is also important for energy metabolism. Unlike iron, however, copper is an antioxidant rather than a pro-oxidant and is a cofactor for superoxide dismutase, one of the body's enzymes that protect cells against oxidative damage. Copper is also thought to be important in collagen formation.

Copper may be a red flag nutrient for some vegetarian athletes. Studies suggest that both copper intake and blood markers of copper status may be low in vegetarians compared to omnivores,[17] which may be because copper from plant foods is not as well absorbed.[53] Other studies have found insufficient copper intake among athletes actively attempting to lose weight.[26] A vegetarian diet, however, has the potential to supply adequate amounts of copper [41] (see table 8.2), and, in fact, vegetables are a major source of dietary copper.[53] Copper, like zinc and iron, can also be made more readily available by soaking, fermenting, or sprouting copper-containing foods.[53] As with iron, mineral-to-mineral interactions, especially competitive binding between zinc and copper, can decrease copper availability, whereas organic acids (except vitamin C) can increase availability. Unlike iron absorption, high intakes of vitamin C impair copper absorption, which is one reason vitamin C supplementation above 1,000 milligrams is not recommended.

Although it is currently not known whether marginal levels of copper influence performance or health, actual copper deficiency can lead to anemia. Copper is found in most vegetables, legumes, peanut butter, nuts and seeds, and seafood. Selected vegetarian sources are listed in table 8.2. The recommended intake for copper is 900 micrograms per day for adults.

Other Key Minerals

Although several other minerals are required for health and possibly for performance (see table 8.7), these minerals are not typically a problem for the general population or for vegetarian athletes. The content of several of these minerals, including selenium, copper, and iodine, however, varies in the food supply depending on soil conditions. While most soil conditions are generally favorable, you may want to check conditions in your area, particularly if you purchase locally grown produce or grow your own. Although selenium is of interest to scientists because of its role as a cofactor in one of the body's internal defense systems, glutathione peroxidase, selenium supplementation is not recommended unless you live in an area with selenium-deficient soil (e.g. areas in China, New Zealand, and Africa). General supplementation of any of the other minerals is also discouraged.

Considering Vitamin and Mineral Supplements

To date, no evidence suggests that extra vitamins or minerals taken either as a multivitamin and mineral supplement or alone will enhance athletic performance, increase endurance or strength, or build muscle, unless of course you are deficient

TABLE 8.7 **Trace Mineral Intake for Vegetarian Athletes**

Mineral	Recommended intake for athletes	Major function	Major vegetarian sources	Problems with excessive consumption
Magnesium	420 mg men; 320 mg women	Involved in protein synthesis, oxygen delivery, energy metabolism, and muscle contraction; also a component of bone	Whole-grain products, legumes	Nausea, vomiting, diarrhea
Chromium	35 mg men; 25 mg women ages 19-50	Enhanced insulin action (part of glucose tolerance factor)	Whole grains, nuts, beer, egg yolks, mushrooms	Not known
Selenium	55 mcg for adults	Defends against oxidation; regulates thyroid hormone; may protect against certain types of cancer	Whole grains, nuts, and vegetables grown in selenium-rich soil	Hair and nail loss, skin rash, fatigue, irritability
Manganese	2.3 mg men; 1.8 mg women	Cofactor for several metabolic reactions, including bone formation; deficiencies are rare	Widespread in food supply	Weakness, nervous system problems, mental confusion
Molybdenum	45 mcg for adults	Works with riboflavin in enzymes involved in carbohydrate and fat metabolism	Whole-grain products, legumes	Rare

to begin with. Certainly, a vitamin or mineral deficiency can impair performance, but deficiencies generally occur in athletes who restrict energy intake or make poor food choices. Deficiencies are unlikely in athletes with robust appetites. The exceptions to the rule include vitamin B_{12} for vegan athletes, iodine and selenium for those obtaining food grown in deficient soils, and vitamin D for those not getting adequate sunshine or with dark skin. More research is needed to determine whether intake of vitamins C and E beyond what can be obtained in a normal diet is beneficial during training. There is insufficient scientific evidence to recommend vitamin or mineral supplements as a way to prevent cancer or heart disease.[36]

In certain cases, however, a multivitamin and mineral supplement may be necessary or prudent to improve overall micronutrient status. Typically, supplementation with a multivitamin is recommended for dieters or people consuming fewer than 1,200 calories a day, those with food allergies or intolerances, and those who are pregnant or planning to get pregnant. With respect to the latter, the Centers for Disease Control and Prevention recommend that every woman who could possibly get pregnant take 400 micrograms of folic acid daily in a multivitamin or in foods that have been enriched with folic acid, in addition to a healthy diet, to prevent neural tube defects.

In addition, people who find it necessary to supplement may be better off supplementing with a standard multivitamin and mineral supplement than with individual nutrients. The multivitamin and mineral supplement should provide no more than 100 percent of the RDA for the essential nutrients and should contain only components that are universally accepted by nutritionists. In most cases, the local store brand is as good as and costs less than a nationally recognized brand. In all cases, vegetarian athletes should strive to improve eating habits and not rely on the multivitamin; supplementation should not provide an excuse to choose tortilla chips over spinach for dinner. Also keep in mind that because many products are enriched and fortified in the United States and other countries, taking vitamin and mineral supplements may be unnecessary.

Food—The Best Source

I am a firm believer that vegetarian athletes should stay as independent from vitamin supplements as possible. Food is indeed the way you were meant to get your vitamins, minerals, and phytochemicals. To accomplish this, you must ensure that you meet your energy needs and select a variety of wholesome foods, including whole grains, legumes, leafy greens and other vegetables, fruit, and, if acceptable, dairy. The information presented in chapters 12 and 14 put these recommendations into practice. The information presented in this chapter (as well as chapters 6 and 7) should help you inventory your intake of the red flag vitamins and minerals and understand how easy it is to meet the vitamin requirements that increase with training, such as vitamin C and riboflavin. Although there are times when you regularly or occasionally need a supplement—such as vitamin B_{12} or vitamin D if you are dark skinned—you will be a much better advocate of the vegetarian diet if you live, train, and perform as free from multivitamin and mineral dependence as possible. In the next chapter we talk about the importance of nutrition and nutrient timing before, during, and after exercise.

Prioritizing Eating Before, During, and After Events

About a year after our twins were born, my husband and I decided to run a marathon to help us get back into shape. The trouble was, we had a lot less time than we had been used to. But as it goes with athletes, we somehow managed to keep decent training schedules that included regular long, tempo, and marathon-paced runs. I even maintained a higher weekly mileage than my first (prechildren) marathon. And my husband managed to sneak in weekly grueling interval runs. Overall, our training went well, and we arrived in the marathon city the day before the event—both feeling as if we might set personal records.

Our mistake, however, started with our ignoring the basics of preevent nutrition planning. Rather than hitting a grocery store to stock up on high-carbohydrate foods and reading through our race packet information to learn where the water and sport drink stops would be, we went sightseeing with the kids and the in-laws, who were along to help. When deciding what to do for our premarathon breakfast, I told my husband we could grab something from the coffee shop near the hotel, which was two blocks from the starting line, and supplement it with the two bananas I had brought and a few glasses of the race's "official sport beverage" that I assumed would be available at the starting line. I made too many assumptions.

Race morning, our hungry early-rising twins ate the bananas, we discovered that the bakery did not open until after the marathon start time, and that there was no "official sport beverage" at the starting line. A volunteer told us, however, that there would be plenty available at mile five (8 km) and at every water station thereafter (information that was most likely covered in our race packet). I also could not find the sport gels I thought I had packed. Nevertheless, we ran but had kissed our chances of a personal record goodbye. I began feeling zapped just after the 10-mile mark (16 km) and crawled in 22 minutes slower than my anticipated time. My husband, who typically finishes in less than three hours, finished in 3:22.

Consuming the right food and fluid before, during, and after exercise is important for optimal training and performance. Nutrition during these times provides fuel for the brain and exercising muscles, prevents dehydration, and provides the building blocks for recovery. This is so important that neglecting proper nutrition during these times can negate all your hard training and all your efforts to eat healthy at other times. Thus, this chapter will help you optimize your performance by teaching you how to take in the right amount of the right foods at the right time before, during, and after your training and competitions. It also reviews some of the exciting new sport science that has evolved in these areas and what these results mean to a vegetarian athlete.

Prioritizing Preevent Nutrition

The meal you eat before exercise is as important during your regular training and practice sessions as it is before your most important game or race of the season. This meal should provide just the right amount of carbohydrate and fluid and possibly also protein to prevent hunger, low blood sugar, and stomach or intestinal discomfort, and it should be low in fat. The nutrition provided by the preevent meal may also improve your performance. If consumed three to four hours before exercise, a high-carbohydrate meal can restock glycogen stores in the liver (which have been lowered by the overnight fast) and even top off glycogen stores in the muscles. If consumed half an hour to two hours before exercise, the ingested carbohydrate is used as a fuel to supplement your muscle- and liver-glycogen stores. The only potential disadvantages to consuming a meal too close to exercise is that it may cause stomach discomfort or, in sensitive athletes, lead to rebound low blood sugar, or hypoglycemia, which can result in fatigue in the early periods of exercise. However, you can prevent rebound hypoglycemia by avoiding the consumption of carbohydrate 20 to 60 minutes before you start to exercise (see box 9.1).

Improved Performance With a Preexercise Meal

Just how much improvement you can expect from eating a preevent meal depends on many factors, including how long and intensely you exercise, how well you have eaten in the preceding days, whether you plan to supplement during exercise, and your choice of carbohydrate. Research has shown that

Box
9.1

Special Concerns for Preevent Meals

Rebound hypoglycemia. Although rare, some athletes experience a condition called rebound hypoglycemia (low blood sugar) during exercise when carbohydrate foods are consumed within 20 to 60 minutes of exercise. This is caused by elevated levels of the hormone insulin (released in response to the carbohydrate-containing meal) whose job it is to facilitate the entry of glucose into the muscle and other tissues. Symptoms specifically associated with low blood sugar include lightheadedness, fatigue, tiredness, and shakiness. Sensitive athletes who experience rebound hypoglycemia should consume their preexercise meal 90 to 120 minutes before exercise. Selecting mostly carbohydrate foods with a low glycemic index before exercise may also help. In addition, two cups (472 ml) of a carbohydrate-containing fluid replacement beverage can also be consumed 5 to 10 minutes before exercise without ill effects.

Hunger. Fluid-replacement beverages, or sport drinks, consumed 10 minutes before practice or competition may delay feelings of hunger and provide benefits similar to those of carbohydrate consumption during exercise. These beverages are readily absorbed and appear in the bloodstream 5 to 10 minutes after ingestion. When consumed in this fashion, fluid replacement beverages do not contribute to rebound hypoglycemia.

Nausea. Preevent emotional tension or anxiety may delay digestion and contribute to nausea and even vomiting before a practice or competition. Research has suggested that liquid meals are better tolerated and more easily digested under these conditions. Beverages with lower concentrations of sugar, such as fluid-replacement beverages rather than fruit juice, and that are free of fructose may also be better tolerated. Athletes who experience preexercise nausea should attempt to consume one or two cups of a liquid supplement or smoothie as tolerated instead of a regular meal about 45 to 90 minutes before exercise. These athletes should also avoid foods and beverages containing high amounts of fructose. Sipping slowly rather than gulping these beverages may prevent you from swallowing excessive air, which can contribute to nausea. Finally, a few soda crackers or a piece of dry toast are also options. Consume water as tolerated.

Heartburn. Athletes, particularly those involved in stop-and-go sport activities, often experience heartburn, or gastrointestinal reflux. Heartburn is caused when the ring of muscles located at the bottom of the esophagus, called the lower esphophageal sphincter, becomes too relaxed. These muscles keep the food you have swallowed into your stomach from being regurgitated back up. Research had consistently shown that coffee, chocolate, peppermint, and a high-fat meal relax the sphincter muscles and contribute to heartburn. Other foods such as milk; raw sulfur-containing vegetables such as onions, garlic, and green peppers; and even bananas are believed to cause reflux in some people. To avoid heartburn, avoid high-fat meals and culprit food products before exercise.

(continued)

(continued)

> **Diarrhea, intestinal cramping, and bloating.** Noninfectious diarrhea and cramping and bloating during exercise can be caused by eating high-fiber, high-residual, or gas-producing foods (which include whole grains, fruits with skin, small seeds, legumes, lactose-containing dairy products, and poorly absorbed sugars) too soon before exercise. It can occur when regular defecation habits are hindered by travel, stress, or competition. Athletes who experience these problems during exercise should monitor their intake of whole grains and cereals, legumes, high-fiber fruits, olestra, and sugar alcohols in the preevent meal. Sensitive athletes should avoid these foods in the days leading up to major competitions or events. Ensuring that defecation habits are regular is also imperative. However, because games, races, or even training sessions are not always held at the same time, drinking a half to three-quarters of a cup (118-177 ml) of coffee, tea, or plain hot water with the preevent meal may prevent intestinal problems by promoting defecation before starting to exercise.

carbohydrate-rich meals consumed three to four hours before exercise can improve race time (during a lab-simulated race) by 15 percent,[23] prolong time to fatigue by approximately 26 percent,[21, 35] and improve work output toward the end of exercise by approximately 10 percent. For those involved in stop-and-go sports a recent study also found that a carbohydrate-rich meal consumed three hours before exercise improved endurance during an interval-running protocol that involved moderately paced running interspersed with 30-second sprints every five minutes until exhaustion.[18]

Carbohydrate-containing meals consumed 30 to 90 minutes before exercise also have been shown to improve endurance performance by 7 to 27 percent. However, research has not shown the consistent performance-enhancing effects when carbohydrates are ingested during this window as compared to three to four hours before exercise. Nevertheless, consuming a carbohydrate-containing preexercise meal is most practical during this time frame if you participate in early-morning practices or training sessions, and it should not hinder performance unless you experience stomach upset or a rare low blood sugar. A limited amount of research has also found that consuming preexercise foods with a low glycemic index (GI) such as lentils, bran cereal, steel-cut oats, peaches, or apples may sustain blood sugar levels during extended exercise better than foods with a high GI, including white bread, mashed potatoes, and cornflakes, and also may improve endurance performance.[15, 24, 27] Other research, nonetheless, has found no difference in performance between low- and high-GI meals eaten between 30 and 60 minutes before exercise. In theory, consuming low-GI foods the hour or so before exercise should provide a slower-release source of glucose for use during exercise, as compared to high-GI foods, and may make personal sense for vegetarian athletes despite the lack of solid scientific evidence. A list of the glycemic index of common foods can be found in appendix C.

When and What to Eat Before Exercise

Exactly how much carbohydrate and fluid you should consume and at what time depends on your sport and individual tolerances. The general guidelines for both fluid and carbohydrate intake are summarized in table 9.1 and suggest that athletes drink approximately 1.5 to 2.5 cups (354-590 ml) of fluid two to three hours before exercise and consume either a large carbohydrate meal (providing 3 to 4 grams of carbohydrate per kilogram of body mass) three to four hours before exercise or a smaller meal or snack (providing 1 to 2 grams of carbohydrate per kilogram of body mass) one to two hours before exercise. As an example, a 90-kilogram (198 lb) male track athlete who eats breakfast 90 minutes before exercising should

TABLE 9.1 Carbohydrate and Fluid Recommendations Before, During, and After Exercise

	Carbohydrate	Fluid
Before exercise: 24 hrs	Consume a carbohydrate-rich diet that provides 6-10 g carbohydrate/kg body weight.	Drink generous amounts of fluid to ensure that you are well hydrated. Monitor the color of your urine, which should be pale to light yellow.
Before exercise: 1-4 hrs	Consume a meal or snack that provides 1-2 g carbohydrate/kg body mass if taken 1-2 hrs before exercise OR 3-4 g carbohydrate/kg body mass if taken 3-4 hrs before exercise.	Drink 354-590 ml (~1 1/2-2 1/2 cups) of fluid 2-3 hrs before exercise. This should allow enough time for excess fluid to be excreted as urine before starting exercise.
Before exercise: 5-10 min	If desired, 15-30 g carbohydrate may be consumed with water or as part of a fluid-replacement beverage.	If possible, drink 150-350 ml (~3/4-1 1/2 cups) immediately before or at the start of exercise.
During exercise	Consume approximately 0.7 g carbohydrate/kg body mass/hr (or 30-60 g/hr) for exercise lasting longer than 90 min. Initiate this shortly after the start of exercise. New evidence suggests that intake of up to 100 g/hr may be beneficial during intense, prolonged effort if the sugar sources are varied. A small amount of protein along with carbohydrate may also offer some performance advantages.	Drink enough fluid to maintain body weight. If you cannot accomplish this, drink as much as you can tolerate. In general, optimal hydration can be facilitated by drinking 150-350 ml every 15-20 min. You should never gain weight during exercise as this indicates you are drinking too much fluid.
After exercise	Consume a mixed meal providing carbohydrate, protein, and fat soon after a strenuous competition or training session.	Drink up to 1 1/2 liters for every kg of body mass lost during exercise (or 3 cups for every pound lost). Including sodium in or with the fluid prevents urinating much of this water intake.

Summarized from the American College of Sports Medicine Position Stand on Exercise and Fluid Replacement and the American College of Sports Medicine, the American Dietetic Association, and the Dietitians of Canada Joint Position Statement on Nutrition and Athletic Performance.

consume between 90 and 180 grams of carbohydrate in his preevent meal. A 60-kilogram (132 lb) female cyclist should consume between 60 and 120 grams of carbohydrate one to two hours before an early-morning training ride, and between 180 and 240 grams four hours or so before a late-afternoon training ride. A sample preevent meal that provides 90 grams of carbohydrate and focuses on low-GI foods is provided in table 9.2. In addition, evidence shows that consuming a well-tolerated carbohydrate source, such as a fluid-replacement beverage or piece of fruit with a few sips of water, 5 to 10 minutes before exercise will further benefit performance during prolonged or intense exercise. Research has shown that carbohydrate consumed with adequate water immediately before exercise provides benefits similar to carbohydrate consumption during exercise.

Another guideline for the preevent meal is to consume only familiar, well-tolerated, high-carbohydrate foods that are low in sodium, simple sugars, and fiber and don't contain excess spice.[26] Experimenting with a new food or product is fine as long as you experiment during training or practice and preferably not an important one. If you are accustomed to eating gas-producing foods such as legumes and they offer no ill effects—go for it! Again, these and other low-GI foods may offer a performance advantage over higher-GI foods by providing a slowly

TABLE 9.2 **Preexercise Meals Providing 90 Grams of Carbohydrate**

Early-morning	Estimated carbohydrate (g)
1 cup oatmeal, Irish or steel cut	30
1 Tbsp raw or brown sugar	15
1 cup fresh peaches	30
1 cup soy milk	12-15
1 cup water	
Total	87-90
Later in the day	
Macaroni salad made with 1 cup macaroni, 1/3 cup chickpeas, mixed vegetables, and a light vinegar and oil dressing	40-55
1 slice bread	15
1 thin slice (3/4 oz cheese or soy cheese)	—
1 large apple	30
1 cup water	
Total	85-100

Based on the approximate carbohydrate content of foods provided in table 3.2. The carbohydrate content of foods per serving listed on food labels is also useful in planning a preevent meal. Refer to appendix E for guidance on converting English units to metric.

released form of glucose during exercise. On the other hand, gas-producing and high-fiber whole-grain foods may not be as readily emptied from the gut and may contribute to nausea or diarrhea. This is particularly a concern if you get a "nervous stomach" or typically have problems defecating before competitions. Guidelines for special circumstances, such as rebound hypoglycemia, heartburn, nausea, gas, and diarrhea, are presented in box 9.1.

Fasting and Early-Morning Workouts

It would be unfair to leave you with the idea that your performance will be absolutely impaired if you skip breakfast before an early-morning workout. Indeed, it is crazy to think you should get up at 4 a.m. to eat before your 5 a.m. training run (at least the women's soccer team told me it was). Oh, better make that 3 A.M. so you can have time to adequately hydrate.

In truth, eating before an early-morning workout is not always necessary. Research and intuition hold that the preevent meal is more likely to make a difference the longer and more intense your training session or race and if you paid little attention to your nutrition for a couple of days before the event.

I have established what I call the three-to-four flat rule for my early-morning runs. If I have eaten well the day before and am adequately hydrated, I can run an easy three to four miles (5-6 km) on just a few sips of water and feel fine. If I run a little harder, a large glass of a fluid-replacement beverage or diluted fruit juice holds me over. But if I run four miles or more, I need to get out of bed a little earlier so I have time for a light carbohydrate breakfast 45 to 60 minutes before I run. The same goes for hilly workouts. Figuring out a similar rule or set of personal guidelines might be beneficial. It lets you know your limitations and may even give you a few extra moments of valuable sleep.

Carbohydrate Loading and Nutrition the Week Before Competition

No chapter discussing preevent nutrition would be complete if it failed to discuss carbohydrate loading. *Carbohydrate loading,* or *glycogen supercompensation,* as it is also called, is practiced by many endurance athletes and sometimes other athletes for the purpose of elevating their muscle-glycogen stores above normal before a major competition or event. Indeed, this practice has been found to improve performance in male athletes performing endurance exercise lasting more than 90 minutes. Performance improvement in female athletes has also been noted but not as consistently as in male athletes.

Glycogen supercompensation is different from simply eating a high-carbohydrate diet before competition in that it requires the athlete to follow a diet-and-exercise protocol for five to seven days before the chosen competition. The early classic carbohydrate-loading protocol of the 1960s and 1970s included a depletion phase that typically required the athlete to exercise until near exhaustion the week before competition and then eat a diet very low in carbohydrate (less than 10 percent of energy) for three days. This was followed by three days of a high-carbohydrate (approximately 80 to 90 percent of energy) diet. Modified protocols that include a training taper, which may or may not begin with a depletion bout of exercise, have been developed more recently because the three-day low-carbohydrate phase produced negative side effects, including weakness, irritability, carbohydrate cravings, and susceptibility to infection. The modified protocols simply involve following a typical carbohydrate diet (55 to 60 percent of energy) until three days before competition and then switching to a high-carbohydrate diet while at the same time tapering. Although omitting the depletion phase and simply following a high-carbohydrate diet, compared to a lower-carbohydrate diet, for several days before competition has been noted to improve performance during running,[34] soccer,[3] and other sports, this type of regimen is not truly carbohydrate loading because it simply ensures that glycogen stores are adequate rather than supercompensated at the start of exercise.

As an endurance athlete, then, how do you carbohydrate load? Unfortunately, there is no definitive answer. Despite numerous studies, there is no set and agreed-on protocol for muscle-glycogen loading. Two recent studies have also produced nearly conflicting conclusions about the correct diet and training regimen for glycogen loading. One study found that an exhaustive taper is necessary in order to maximize the glycogen supercompensation effects. Male athletes in this study either performed a glycogen-depleting exercise (120 minutes of moderate cycling followed by 1 minute sprints to exhaustion) or a nondepleting exercise (20 minutes of moderate cycling) before following a high-carbohydrate diet that provided 9 grams of carbohydrate per kilogram of body weight for seven days.[10] The muscle-glycogen content of the athletes in the glycogen-depleting exercise group was elevated by 138 percent of baseline on day three and by 147 percent on days five through seven; whereas, the muscle glycogen in the group that exercised for 20 minutes was elevated by 124 percent of baseline on day three and declined between days three and seven to a value similar to baseline. The athletes were allowed to exercise for just 20 minutes daily during the weeklong loading phase. The second study found that a short-term bout of high-intensity exercise followed by a high carbohydrate intake enabled athletes to attain supercompensated muscle-glycogen levels within 24 hours.[7] In this study, male athletes performed a short sprinting regimen on a stationary bike, consisting of 150 seconds of above-maximal effort followed by 30 seconds of all-out cycling, and then one day of a high-carbohydrate diet that emphasized high-GI foods and provided 10.3 grams of carbohydrate per kilogram of body weight. Muscle-glycogen stores were found to increase on the order of 80 percent in all muscle fibers during this 24-hour regimen. This was comparable to or higher than those reported during two- to six-day regimens.

As you can see from these two studies—one stating that a long taper is necessary for glycogen supercompensation and the other stating that supercompensation can be achieved in 24 hours after intense exercise and high carbohydrate intake—it is difficult to make specific suggestions. And this is particularly true for females because both of the studies were conducted on men. Because both protocols seem to have an influence on supercompensating glycogen stores, athletes may want to select the most convenient protocol. However, it is still believed that athletes should not perform true glycogen-loading regimens more than a few times a year. This is because the enzymes in the body seem to adapt and lose their ability to respond to the loading protocols by packing in extra glycogen. Thus, you should use glycogen loading only before your most important competitions. Furthermore, because glycogen loading can result in a small amount of weight gain (0.5 to 1 kg [1-2 lb]), it may not help athletes in events where even a small amount of excess body weight can impair performance, for example, during shorter running events. The weight gain concern does not apply during endurance events because benefits gained from the extra fuel offset any negative effects from the small weight gain, which is usually lost as exercise progresses.

Prioritizing Nutrition and Fluids During Exercise

The goals of your nutrition strategy during practice, training, or competition are to consume enough carbohydrate (if necessary) to optimize performance and to consume an appropriate amount of fluid to maintain hydration. Research has shown almost unequivocally that consuming 30 to 75 grams of carbohydrate per hour during exercise will benefit performance during both prolonged and intermittent, high-intensity activities. Carbohydrate supplementation extends endurance and improves race time during simulated endurance races or trials and also improves sprinting ability and power output at the end of races or sporting events. Although less is known about team sports, a few relatively recent studies have found that carbohydrate intake during exercise improved tennis stroke quality during the final stages of prolonged play[31] and physical and mental function during intermittent shuttle running that mimicked that of many competitive team sports.[33] Carbohydrate ingestion most likely exerts these performance benefits by maintaining blood glucose concentration, thereby ensuring a continuous source of carbohydrate for the working muscle. These benefits are most noted during the latter stages of a race or after half-time when liver and muscle glycogen are compromised, and—with prolonged events—are in addition to those gained by consumption of a preexercise carbohydrate meal.[6]

Fluid intake, with or without carbohydrate, also ensures optimal performance. Research in this area has shown—without a doubt—that fluid ingestion during exercise improves endurance performance and that the performance-enhancing effects of carbohydrate and fluid are independent but additive. For example, one study conducted in the late 1990s at the Chichester Institute of Higher Education in the United Kingdom found that male and female runners were able to run 33 percent longer before exhaustion when they consumed 180 milliliters (0.75 cup) of water every 15 minutes compared to when they consumed no fluids.[8] Their actual time to exhaustion during the treadmill test was 133 minutes when they consumed water and 78 minutes when they did not. Another study conducted at the University of Texas in Austin found that male athletes experienced a 6 percent improvement in sprinting performance when they consumed 1,330 milliliters (5.6 cups) of water, enough to replace about 80 percent of their fluid lost through sweat, compared to when they ingested just 200 milliliters (0.85 cup) of water.[4] In this study the athletes cycled for 50 minutes at a relatively intense effort before completing a sprint to the finish that took approximately 10 minutes. Not surprisingly, the athletes experienced a 12 percent improvement in performance when they consumed 1,330 milliliters of carbohydrate-containing sport drink rather than water.

Although dehydration from inadequate fluid consumption can impair performance, both dehydration and overhydration can result in severe, life-threatening health consequences that are worth mentioning here. Briefly, varying degrees of dehydration are common during exercise because athletes typically drink enough to satisfy their thirst but do not drink enough to offset the fluid losses that occur during sweating. This is primarily because thirst is not an adequate guide to fluid replacement, but it is also caused by factors such as water availability; game rules and regulations; intense focus on playing, training, or racing; and even drinking skill during exercise. Dehydration can lead to increased core temperature, headache, dizziness, gastrointestinal discomfort, poor concentration, and reduced performance. All of these symptoms are a result of decreased blood flow, which reduces the escape of heat through the skin and the absorption of ingested fluid and foods. If not corrected, dehydration can lead to heat injury, exhaustion, heatstroke, and death.

In contrast, hyponatremia, or "water intoxication," has emerged as a cause of life-threatening illness and race-related death in endurance competitions such as the marathon and ultramarathon. Hyponatremia occurs when excess water, relative to sodium, accumulates in the blood and is defined by an abnormally low concentration of plasma sodium (less than 135 mmol/l). In athletes, it is called water intoxication because it seems to result from drinking an excessive amount of low-sodium fluids during prolonged endurance exercise. A recent report found that hyponatremia occurred in approximately 13 percent of runners completing the 2002 Boston Marathon, and of those 13 percent, slightly less than 1 percent experienced severe hyponatremia (sodium concentration less than 120 mmol/l).[1] In this event, the strongest indication of hyponatremia was weight gain during the race of one kilogram to almost five kilograms (2.2-11 lbs) caused by fluid intake that far exceeded the sweat rate. This and other studies also seem to indicate that those at greatest risk for hyponatremia are female and slower athletes who finish toward the back of the pack, although hyponatremia does occur in male athletes and appears to increase with the use of nonsteroidal anti-inflammatory drugs during competition. To avoid becoming hyponatremic, athletes should know their approximate sweat rate (see box 9.2) during all sports in which they participate and drink only enough to replace your losses. Drinking sodium-containing fluids such as higher-sodium fluid-replacement beverages or ingesting sodium-containing foods during events lasting more than two hours

Box
9.2

Estimating Individual Sweat Rate and Fluid Requirements During Exercise

› Determine nude body mass in kilograms (after using the restroom). Scale must be accurate to at least 0.1 kilogram or 0.2 pound.

› Perform regular exercise or training for one hour without consuming fluids. You can also exercise for 30 minutes and multiply the answer by two.

› Towel off and determine nude body mass.

› Subtract postexercise body mass from preexercise body mass.

› Body mass loss is directly proportional to fluid loss; one kilogram lost equals one liter of fluid, and one pound lost equals two cups of fluid.

Example:

An athlete weighs 90 kilograms before exercise and 88.6 kilograms after exercising for one hour.

› 90.0 – 88.6 = 1.4 kilogram

› 1.4 kilogram = 1.4 liters or 1,400 milliliters

› Sweat rate = 1,400 ml/hour

If this athlete replaces the fluid lost through sweat by consuming a 6 percent fluid-replacement beverage, he or she will consume 84 grams of carbohydrate per hour, which is greater than the current recommended intake of 30 to 60 grams per hour.

may also be prudent. Unfortunately, general symptoms of hyponatremia are nonspecific and include fatigue, nausea, and confusion. Severe cases can result in grand mal seizures, respiratory arrest, acute respiratory distress syndrome, coma, and death.

In addition to carbohydrate and fluid, several recent studies have also suggested that protein consumed along with carbohydrate and fluid may enhance aerobic endurance, reduce muscle damage, and improve fluid retention above that which occurs with carbohydrate alone or carbohydrate plus fluid.[12, 20, 22] The specific mechanisms for this effect of protein (given in a ratio of 4 grams carbohydrate to 1 gram protein) are not yet well understood and as such should be considered preliminary. In these studies, for example, the researchers tested aerobic endurance by having athletes exercise to exhaustion but did not determine if they would run or cycle faster with the protein-containing carbohydrate beverage compared to just the carbohydrate-containing beverage.

When and What to Eat During Training and Competition

The general guidelines for both fluid and carbohydrate intake during exercise are presented in table 9.1. As a general rule, carbohydrate ingestion should be a priority during competition and on days you train at a relatively intense effort for longer than 80 to 90 minutes. Remember, however, that carbohydrate may also be helpful for shorter, interval sessions or when you are unable to eat an adequate preevent meal. Currently, the recommendation is to aim for roughly 30 to 60 grams of carbohydrate per hour (approximately 0.7 g carbohydrate/kg body mass) with a focus on high-GI choices. For best results, you should consume carbohydrate at regular intervals (if allowed by the rules of your sport) and begin shortly after the onset of exercise.

Hot-off-the-press evidence, however, suggests that higher carbohydrate intakes—up to 100 grams per hour—may be beneficial during endurance and ultraendurance events such as marathon and ultramarathon runs, century and double century (160 and 320 km) bicycle races, and adventure racing. Athletes striving for higher hourly intakes of carbohydrate, however, need to ensure that the carbohydrate comes from several rather than a single sugar source. Although scientists used to think that muscle was able to take up and utilize a maximum of one gram of dietary carbohydrate per minute—regardless of body size—this exciting new research has suggested this is not true.[13, 32] The limiting factor apparently lies in the intestines, where different carrier proteins are responsible for escorting different sugars, such as glucose and fructose, across the intestinal wall. If only one type of simple sugar is consumed, we indeed can only absorb about 60 grams of sugar per hour, but if more than one type is consumed, we can recruit different carriers and absorb and oxidize up to 100 grams per hour. Fortunately, the carbohydrate found naturally in fruits and fruit juices is made up of a variety of sugar sources (see figures 9.1 and 9.2), as is the carbohydrate provided by many fluid-replacement products such as Gatorade.

Like carbohydrate intake, fluid intake during exercise should be closely monitored on days you train or compete for more than an hour. This of course is provided you are well hydrated at the start of exercise; otherwise, fluid intake is even more important. To prevent dehydration, the American College of Sports Medicine recommends that athletes drink enough fluid during exercise to replace what is lost through sweat.[2] A typical sweat rate is 800 to 1,500 milliliters per hour and is even higher during exercise in hot and humid environments, including the outdoors and non-air-conditioned gymnasiums. It is best, however, to have an idea of your own fluid requirements, which can change throughout your training season and in response to different types of exercise and different environments. See box 9.2 for information on calculating sweat rate and determining personal fluid requirements. Regularly obtaining your weight before and after exercise also helps you determine if you are under- or overdrinking. You should never gain weight during exercise because it means you are overhydrating and may be placing yourself at risk for hyponatremia.

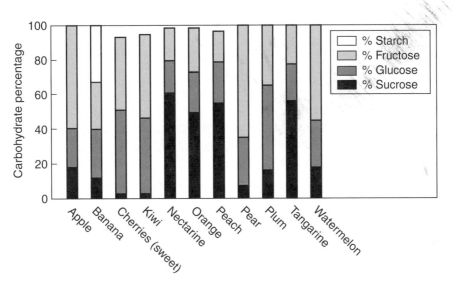

FIGURE 9.1 Type of sugar in selected fresh fruit.
Data from the United States Department of Agriculture (USDA).

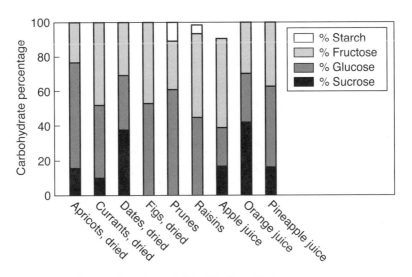

FIGURE 9.2 Type of sugar in selected dried fruit and juice.
Data from the United States Department of Agriculture (USDA).

Understanding your own fluid needs during exercise will help you establish a personal fluid intake plan according to the rules and rigors of your sport, and help ensure that you do not go overboard and consume too much fluid. For example, I typically aim to consume about one liter of fluid every hour, which is close to my sweat rate during moderately intense running. When I run a long race, I estimate how much fluid (in small cups) I need to drink at each water station based on the distance between stations and my estimated pace. If the stations are too far apart, such as in a marathon with water stations every five miles (8 km), I have to decide whether to ask a relative to supply water or to carry my own. During a training run, ride, or cross-country ski event, I might have the option of stashing water along a predetermined route or planning a route where I can get water at gas stations or from a friend's outdoor hose. If I played a team sport, I would estimate how much fluid I would need to consume during regularly scheduled breaks, bench time, and time-outs and balance that with my anticipated playing and bench time. This may sound like a bit of work, but improperly hydrating can impair performance and have life or death consequences.

Tips for Meeting Fluid and Carbohydrate Guidelines

Both water and sport drinks such as Gatorade and Powerade can replace fluid losses. In general, sport drinks that are labeled as a fluid-replacement beverage should contain 6 to 8 percent carbohydrate by volume along with a small amount of sodium and potassium (see box 9.3). They should not be carbonated, because carbonated beverages are more difficult to drink and less well tolerated while exercising. The advantage of sport drinks is that they are convenient and provide an easily absorbed source of carbohydrate and fluid that tastes good to most people during exercise. Alternatively, some of the newer sport gels pack 20 to 25 grams of carbohydrate in a small packet that can be carried easily. These are a good option if water is available along the route or on the sideline. Newer products, such as Clif Shot Bloks and Sport Beans, made by Jelly Belly, which taste somewhat like gummy bears, and regular jelly beans also provide carbohydrate, sodium, and potassium and must be consumed with water. Sport drinks and gels that contain protein along with carbohydrate are also available. The sport drink should be easily absorbed, and the gel should be consumed with water.

As a vegetarian, however, you may prefer natural or noncommercial sources of carbohydrate. In this case, diluted fruit juices (4 ounces [116 ml] of juice in 4 ounces of water produces a solution of approximately 6 percent), low-sodium vegetable juices such as carrot juice (7 percent solution), and solid foods such as fruit or bread ingested with water are appropriate. Honey, particularly in small packets, may also be of interest to some vegetarians for use instead of a sport gel. Research has shown that both honey and easily digested solid food are as effective as liquids in increasing blood glucose and enhancing performance, provided that they are ingested with water.[16, 19, 30] The guideline is to drink approximately 240 milliliters (8 oz) of water with every 15 grams of carbohydrate ingested to create a 6 percent solution. Be creative and create your own recipe for a homemade, fruit-based, fluid-replacement beverage. See box 9.4 for ideas.

A Special Note for Prolonged Endurance and Ultraendurance Events

If you participate in exercise events lasting more than five hours, you need to pay particular attention to your intake of carbohydrate and fluid, as well as sodium,

Box
9.3

What's Magic About 6 to 8 Percent?

The goal for athletes when drinking a carbohydrate-containing beverage is to get the fluid, sugars, and electrolytes into the body as quickly as possible without causing gastrointestinal upset. Therefore, it's important to know that the amount of sugar in a beverage strongly influences both how quickly the beverage empties from the stomach and also how rapidly it is absorbed by the intestines. Extensive research has shown that solutions containing 2 to 8 percent carbohydrate by volume from various sources (glucose, fructose, maltodextrins) are generally emptied quickly from the stomach and absorbed as well as or better than water. Their better absorption is attributed to the sugar and electrolyte content, which pulls water molecules beside them upon absorption in the intestines. Thus, beverages with 6 to 8 percent carbohydrate by volume do not compromise fluid replenishment during exercise and also provide an additional energy source. Some athletes may tolerate beverages with higher carbohydrate content by volume (up to 10 percent), but these beverages typically delay gastric absorption and may cause intestinal discomfort and diarrhea.

Although most fluid-replacement beverages such as Gatorade or Powerade fit the bill, most juices, fruit drinks, "energy drinks," and sodas are too concentrated to be rapidly absorbed without incident during exercise. You can determine the percent of carbohydrate by volume of carbohydrate-containing beverages as follows:

$$\frac{\text{Grams of carbohydrate per serving of beverage} \times 100}{\text{Total volume of serving}}$$

For example, 1 cup (236 ml) of apple juice contains 29 grams of carbohydrate.* The volume percent of carbohydrate in apple juice would be calculated as follows:

$$\frac{29 \text{ grams} \times 100}{236} = 12.3 \text{ percent}$$

Thus, apple juice needs to be diluted slightly to be well absorbed and utilized during exercise.

This calculation does not work properly in protein-containing beverages such as milk. Note, the volume percentage of carbohydrate is different from the percent of energy from carbohydrate.

*Values obtained from the USDA nutrient database at www.ars.usda.gov/main/site_main.htm?modecode=12354500.

potassium, other electrolytes, and maybe even protein. And remember that variety is key! An interesting phenomenon experienced by untraendurance athletes is that they get sick of carbohydrates—particularly sweet carbohydrates—right about the time they need them the most. Taking a variety of carbohydrate sources along

Box
9.4

Making Your Own
Fluid-Replacement Beverage

Use the following recipes to make a fluid-replacement beverage based on fruit juice that provides 6 to 7 percent carbohydrate by volume, 600 to 700 milligrams of potassium, and 291 milligrams of sodium (if 1/8 tsp salt is used) or 581 milligrams sodium (if 1/4 tsp salt is used). The beverage will be a natural mixture of glucose, fructose, and sucrose.

Recipe 1

> 3/4 cup (177 ml) of apple juice (preferably filtered)
>
> 1 1/2 cups (354 ml) of black cherry or grape juice
>
> Approximately 2 cups (472 ml) cold water to make 1 liter
>
> 1/8 to 1/4 tsp (0.75-1.5 g) table salt (not light, preferably iodized)

Recipe 2

> 2 1/4 cups (531 ml) of grape juice (preferably filtered)
>
> Approximately 2 cups (472 ml) cold water to make 1 liter
>
> 1/8 to 1/4 tsp (0.75-1.5 g) table salt (not light, preferably iodized)

in your jersey pocket, waist pack, or in your own cooler (if applicable) may help prevent the "sick of carbohydrate" trap. Things to bring along include different flavors of fluid-replacement beverages, whole and sliced fruit, trail mix, sport bars, baked potatoes with salt, pretzels, tortillas, peanut butter sandwiches, vegetarian burgers in buns, and, yes, soda and sour-tasting juices such as lemonade and grapefruit juice.

When it comes to drinking soda during an ultraendurance event, forget the carbonation rule. A bubbly cold soda or the taste of sour juice may be just what you need in the middle or end of the event. Just remember to follow it with an equal amount of water. Finally, tuck in a few packets of salt. Salt may be what you are craving and can enhance the palatability of your carbohydrate-rich foods. Believe me, this is the time you might want to put salt on your watermelon and even your peaches to help replenish sodium and possibly potassium lost during prolonged sweating.[9] Taking in sodium may also reduce the risk of hyponatremia, although this has not been completely backed up by research. A rough guideline is to strive for 230 to 460 milligrams of sodium and 119 to 195 milligrams of potassium per liter of fluids replaced.[9] If you prefer drinking plain water, the added sodium can come from salting your food or eating salty food. The important thing is to listen to your body. If you are craving salt, consume it, but not in the form of salt tablets, which generally are not recommended.[25] Finally, if a little protein in your sport drink or gel does indeed pan out (as discussed above), ultraendurance events are indeed the place to expect such benefit.

A Special Note for Team Sports

Team sports such as soccer, basketball, volleyball, and football also present a unique set of challenges. If you are on a team, you need to be prepared to play at all times but, unlike in endurance sports, may spend some time on the bench. Team athletes also must consume carbohydrate and fluids at times that are allowed by the rules of the game (e.g., half-time or time-outs). In many cases, team athletes are limited to specific sport drinks or products and may not be allowed to eat solid foods such as bananas or watermelon slices on the sideline. And you must remember that both your fluid and carbohydrate needs vary depending on how much of the actual game or match you play and then supplement accordingly. Going crazy on sport drinks and carbohydrate supplements, which is discussed in chapter 13, can lead to unwanted weight gain.

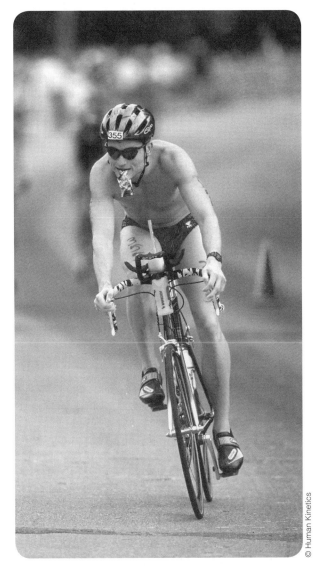

© Human Kinetics

Aim for variety in your during-exercise snacks, and determine a method and schedule of intake that works for you.

Keep a water bottle or two labeled with your name near at all times, and consider filling one with a sport drink for more intense or prolonged practices. In a study of elite Australian basketball, netball, and soccer players, researchers found that the factors influencing fluid replacement during exercise included providing each athlete a water bottle, proximity to water during training sessions, encouraging athletes to drink, and athlete awareness of his or her own sweat rate.[5] The duration and number of breaks or substitutions and the rules of the game are also influential, but you have no control over these influences.

Prioritizing the Postexercise Meal

The meal after exercise or competition is critical for providing the nutrients necessary for recovery and training adaptation. This meal, however, is often the one most neglected by athletes for reasons that are typically related to the lack of appetite that often occurs after grueling and long workouts and the desire to relax or celebrate—after all you have just worked hard! Not getting adequate nutrition after exercise, however, can negate your hard training efforts and also make training difficult in the following days.

It is currently recommended that athletes consume a mixed meal providing carbohydrate, protein, and fat soon after training, practice, or competition, and also strive to replace fluid lost during the session.[26] To replace lost body fluids, you should aim to consume about 150 percent of your body mass lost during exercise or about 1.5 liters of fluid for every kilogram of body mass lost (three cups for every pound lost), and include sodium and potassium in your recovery meals. This is important not only because both of these nutrients are lost through sweat and need to be replenished, but also because their replenishment helps restore fluid balance. Although the vegetarian diet is likely to contain ample potassium, which is abundant in fruits and vegetables, it may lack sodium-containing foods. Sodium intake can be a concern during periods of heavy training in athletes who avoid salt and processed foods. In fact, a more liberal intake of sodium is often appropriate for athletes, particularly if they notice salt residue on their dark-colored workout gear or find they have incredible cravings for salt.

Your specific postexercise nutrition priorities, however, will depend on the intensity of your training that particular day and your (or your coach's) training plans for the following days. For example, if you performed a two-hour run and have a fast-paced tempo run on your schedule tomorrow, your goal to replace muscle glycogen is a higher priority than if you have a rest day. Similarly, if you play most of a grueling volleyball match in the early morning, you need to aggressively replace as much carbohydrate as soon as you can if you hope to play your best in a match that evening or the following morning. In contrast, if you complete a tough 45-minute weightlifting or plyometrics workout, which is not likely to have depleted your glycogen stores, your focus will be on consuming protein along with carbohydrate to facilitate muscle growth and repair. In this case, neglecting postevent nutrition prevents you from optimizing the benefits of your resistance training.

Because muscle-glycogen stores can be completely depleted at the end of a hard practice or workout, carbohydrate consumption should always be a priority on harder training days. Consumption of carbohydrate 20 to 30 minutes after exercise is essential for replenishing muscle-glycogen stores and enhancing muscle recovery and muscle-protein synthesis. Research has consistently shown that muscle glycogen can be replenished within 24 hours, providing the postevent intake and overall diet is high in carbohydrate. Again, this is particularly important if training is to be resumed the following day because low muscle-glycogen stores can impair subsequent training and performance.

The current recommendation for replacing muscle glycogen and ensuring rapid recovery is to consume 1.5 grams of carbohydrate per kilogram of body mass within the first 30 minutes after exercise, and again every two hours for the next four to six hours.[26] A postexercise meal containing both protein and carbohydrate has been shown to be more effective for rapidly replacing muscle glycogen than ingesting carbohydrate only.[11] Researchers have shown benefits using a ratio of both three grams of carbohydrate to one gram of protein and four grams of carbohydrate to one gram of protein, but there is probably no magic to these ratios. Because hard exercise and competition often suppress your appetite—particularly during running events—it may be easier to consume a carbohydrate- and protein-containing beverage or snack immediately after exercise and then eat a mixed meal providing carbohydrate, protein, and fat a few hours later (see table 9.3 for snack suggestions that provide both carbohydrate and protein). This regimen allows you to begin replenishing muscle-glycogen stores while you shower, travel home, or find a restaurant for a postcompetition meal.

Efforts to consume a mixed meal that provides a high-quality source of plant or dairy protein, such as soy, other legumes, eggs, or milk, are probably sufficient for most vegetarian athletes. Consuming high-quality protein along with carbohydrate after endurance or resistance training supplies the needed amino acids to stimulate muscle-protein synthesis. Research has also found that consuming protein along with carbohydrate after endurance or resistance training stimulates

TABLE 9.3   Vegetarian Postexercise Snacks
That Provide Carbohydrate and Protein

Food	Carbohydrate-to-protein ratio
Small apple and 1 cup milk	27:8 (3.4 to 1)
Small apple and 1 slice soy cheese	15:6 (2.5 to 1)
Large banana and 2 Tbsp peanut butter	30:7 (4.3 to 1)
2 Tbsp raisins and 2 Tbsp almonds	15:7 (2.1 to 1)
4 graham cracker squares and 1 cup soy milk	34:10 (3.4 to 1)
1/2 large bagel with 1/4 cup cottage cheese	30:12 (2.5 to 1)
1/2 cup fruit with 1 cup plain yogurt	28:8 (3.5 to 1)
6-inch tortilla filled with 1/2 cup beans	30:7 (4.3 to 1)
1 cup low-fat chocolate milk	26:8 (3.2 to 1)

Refer to appendix E for guidance on converting English units to metric.

the building and repair of muscle and other tissue. Athletes who are trying to gain muscle should pay particular attention to their postexercise protein intake. As a final point, including fat in a recovery meal may also be important for replacing muscle fat stores following high-volume endurance training,[17] as discussed in chapter 4.

So there you have it! Consuming the right food and fluid before, during, and after exercise has great potential to improve—or at least optimize—your training and performance. In fact, prioritizing nutrition at these times has the potential to greatly affect your performance to a greater degree than any currently known dietary supplement or ergogenic aid, the topic of the next chapter.

Choosing Whether to Supplement

In the late 1990s, my colleagues and I conducted a study assessing the effect of creatine supplementation on off-season performance in female collegiate soccer players. My distinct memories from this study focus on one athlete, an extremely health-conscious semivegetarian player I had always enjoyed chatting with. She worked hard, loved tofu, and had been raised by parents who—it seemed—were a lot like me. When we approached her team about the creatine supplement study, she was very reluctant and told me privately that she was not comfortable taking anything "artificial" into her body. For some reason (probably related to peer pressure), however, she gave her consent to participate, which involved blindly receiving either creatine or a placebo mixed in a sport drink during the 13 weeks of spring training. Knowing what I knew, I was relieved to find out she had been randomized to the placebo rather than the creatine group. (Because I was the one in charge of dissolving the creatine or placebo in the sport drink and delivering it to the team after practice, I was privy to the randomization scheme.) What was interesting was that despite being given the placebo treatment (unbeknownst to her) she began experiencing side effects, which included nausea, headaches, shakiness, and weight gain. Two weeks before the end of the study she came to me—convinced she was in the creatine group—and dropped out of the study. She told me she couldn't take it any more but did agree to let us have access to her final performance data. Later, when we broke the code, she was extremely embarrassed and apologetic. Given the background events, however, it was understandable. She was so against taking the supplement—or any nonherbal supplement for that matter—that her mind allowed her to experience many of its side effects. As a consolation, we presented her with a bag of dried cranberries—a natural, albeit not very concentrated, vegetarian source of creatine.

Although it is probably stereotyping, I believe that vegetarian athletes think a little differently about supplements. Like most athletes, vegetarian athletes enjoy outrunning, outjumping, or outcompeting their competition, but as I see it, we tend to draw a different line between acceptable and unacceptable ways to gain a competitive edge. Vegetarian athletes don't necessarily want to win at all costs. They want to win by training hard, eating properly, and taking care of their health, rather than by taking a magic performance-enhancing formula (with unknown health risks). This does not mean, of course, that vegetarian athletes are not interested in herbal supplements to increase their immune function, allay the discomforts of menopause, or promote longevity. Vegetarian athletes may indeed be just as likely to use herbal or other natural supplements as nonvegetarian athletes, but not as likely to swallow the latest, most popular artificially synthesized performance-enhancing formula.

Because athletes are constantly bombarded with advertisements promoting new supplements, this chapter helps you understand the various types of supplements, their current level of regulation, and when or if you may want to consider their use. In view of the fact that several ergogenic aids may enhance performance in certain situations, and that quite a few herbal supplements have promise as health enhancers or natural remedies, the chapter also provides information on how you can evaluate each supplement that appears on the shelf. After reading this chapter, you should feel confident in your choice to supplement or not supplement and will be armed to make informed decisions in the future. Although the purpose of this chapter is not to review the most popular supplements—because many enter and exit the market quickly—the chapter ends with a summary of selected supplements that may be of interest to vegetarian athletes.

Supplement Primer

Athletes spend millions of dollars on dietary supplements each year for the purpose of improving performance or health. Athletes' attraction to supplements can probably be explained by their competitive instincts. Ancient warriors used various concoctions believed to possess magical properties to help them outfight their enemies just like ancient and even current-day Olympians use them to gain an edge over their opponents.

Supplements that promise even a small advantage are appealing in the athletic arena because events can be won or lost by the slimmest of margins: less than a second during a sprint to possess the ball or a sprint to the finish line. The breathtakingly close finish at the 2005 New York City Marathon is just one example. After running 26 miles (41.8 km), Paul Tergat of Kenya and Hendrick Ramaala of South Africa ended up neck and neck for the final 385 yards (352 m) with Tergat eventually winning by just a step. Other events are often won by an even closer margin. In the 1996 Olympic Games in Atlanta, for example, the United States' Gail Devers won the women's 100-meter track event. Her time of 10.95 seconds was 0.01 seconds faster than the third-place winner. No matter what your philosophy, the temptation to take a supplement that may offer you a split-second of an advantage is always there, challenging your desire to perform better, feel better, or live longer.

Before we continue, it is important to understand the definitions of supplements and ergogenic aids, particularly because athletes and coaches often use these terms interchangeably. In the United States, the Dietary Supplement Health and Education Act (DSHEA) defines a *dietary supplement* as a food product added to the total diet that contains at least one of the following ingredients: a vitamin, mineral, herb, botanical, or amino acid metabolite; it could also be a constituent, extract, or a combination of any of these ingredients.[29] An *ergogenic aid,* on the other hand, is typically defined as a substance or strategy that improves athletic performance by improving work production. The word's roots are *ergo,* which means work, and *genic,* which means generation.

Before DSHEA, which was passed in 1994, botanicals and herbals were considered neither food nor drugs. Now, supplements that promote improved athletic performance are regulated by DSHEA; whereas, ergogenic aids that are not supplements, including carbohydrate-loading strategies, aerodynamic handlebars, and leg shaving, are not regulated by the DSHEA.

Can Supplements Be Trusted?

Although the practice of medicine is, for the most part, grounded in science, the same cannot necessarily be said for supplements. For a medical treatment to become an accepted practice or standard of therapy, there must be evidence, supplied by human clinical trials, that the treatment is likely to benefit rather than harm the people who receive it.[1] If a treatment shows no benefit, it will not make it into the standards of care manual or to the shelves of your local pharmacy.

For a prescription or over-the-counter drug, the U.S. Food and Drug Administration (FDA) requires that pharmaceutical companies conduct clinical trials in adults before seeking approval.[1] During these trials, the participants' response, side effects, and established doses are monitored and documented. The study results are then reported to the FDA and likely submitted for publication in peer-reviewed scientific journals. Although not perfect, this process, lasting approximately 15 years from discovery to consumer use, reduces the likelihood that ineffective and unsafe drugs reach the market. Once a drug is released, the FDA mandates that information pertaining to the drug's active ingredients, safety, dosage, and expected reactions be available and also expects physicians to report any ill effects experienced by patients taking the drugs. The drug may then later be removed from the market. This recently happened with the weight-loss drug Redux.

Supplements, on the other hand, require much less regulation before they are available to the consumer. Clinical trials documenting efficacy, safety, and dosage are not required and are exempted from evaluation by the FDA by the 1994 DSHEA act.[29] As a result, supplements are released on the market sooner.

The manufacturers are required to supply only a single scientific report as supporting evidence and that report need not even pertain to that specific product.[1] For example, if Supplement X is a caffeine herbal cocktail and one report documenting the possible effects of generic caffeine is available, Supplement X can be released even if its mixture is ineffective or produces side effects. Once a supplement reaches the shelves, the FDA can remove the product only if it can be proven unsafe when taken as directed. Furthermore, whereas the FDA has the authority to inspect the facilities of any drug manufacturer and to verify that the ingredients are pure, this safeguard does not apply to supplements. In the past, contaminated supplements have produced adverse reactions that were difficult to treat because the source of the contaminant was not easily identified. One such example occurred a few years ago when an herbal "cleansing system" was found to be contaminated with the heart medication digitalis. This caused life-threatening cardiovascular reactions in two women.[1]

That said, however, it is also important to mention that the seemingly lax regulation of dietary supplements by the FDA does not mean that all supplements are unsafe or that their effects are poorly documented. Herbs are in fact regulated by Germany's Commission E, the equivalent of the FDA.[1] Any herb that is widely used in Germany or other parts of Europe, where herbal remedies are an accepted part of medical practice rather than being considered "alternative medicine," is likely to be accompanied by reports from studies concerning its effectiveness and safety. These reports are typically published in German medical journals, and summaries of specific herbs are available to the public (see table 10.1). Some are translated and available through scientific databases such as Medline. As a result of growing interest, it is becoming easier to find herbal remedies in the United States from reputable companies in standardized extracts that are equivalent to those used in Germany and to be reasonably certain of their effects. Unfortunately, there is much less supporting evidence for nonherbal supplements and ergogenic aids, including enzymes, prohormones, hormones, and amino acids.

Evaluating a Supplement for Potential Benefits and Risks

To decide whether a dietary supplement is right for you, you must keep both an open mind and a watchful eye. Keeping an open mind, nonetheless, may be a bit easier for some athletes than for others. I must admit, I still struggle with the concept of using supplements, particularly ergogenic aids, even though I have read hundreds of scientific reports and even noted improvements in performance from using creatine, both in my studies and in my own experience. What I have finally come to terms with—by keeping an open mind—is that some supplements have the potential to enhance the health and performance of some athletes, particularly when used over the short term. But regular use of these supplements should be considered only after an athlete—vegetarian or not—ensures that he

TABLE 10.1 Sources for Information About Dietary Supplements

Organization	Information
SupplementWatch www.supplementwatch.com	Operated by a privately held corporation consisting of a network of scientists, physiologists, nutritionists, and other health professionals dedicated to educating people about the pros and cons of dietary supplementation. Updated monthly by staff who review scientific papers, research abstracts, and medical journals in order to provide comprehensive and up-to-date information. Contains information on more than 300 vitamins, minerals, and herbs, explaining the theory behind the health-benefit claims associated with each supplement. Specific subsections include "what is it," health-benefit claims, theory, scientific support, safety, and dosage. A significant portion of the Web site is provided free.
U.S. Food and Drug Administration Dietary Supplement Site http://vm.cfsan.fda.gov/~dms/supplmnt.html	Provides information on the regulation of supplements and the Dietary Supplement Health and Education Act (DSHEA). Provides limited information on supplements.
HealthWorld Online www.healthy.net/nutrit/nutinfo/dietsup	Site includes information on a wide range of vitamin and dietary supplements including vitamins, minerals, amino acids, supplemental oils, bioflavonoids, and antioxidants. It is written by medical doctors, and descriptions have a scientific tone. Sections in each entry include description, sources, functions, uses, requirements, deficiency, and toxicity. Entries also provide information on research studies.
HerbMed www.herbmed.org	This interactive, electronic herbal database provides hyperlinked access to the scientific data underlying the use of herbs for health. It is an evidence-based information resource provided by the nonprofit Alternative Medicine Foundation. Information on 54 herbs is available free, and information on more than 100 other herbs is available to subscribers. In addition to reports on clinical research, case studies, and descriptions of traditional use, listings also link to further information on contraindications, toxicity, adverse effects, and drug interactions, as well as an herb's chemical constituents and biochemical mechanisms of action.
American Botanical Council (ABC) www.herbalgram.org	This online resource for herbal news and information is presented by the ABC, a leading independent, nonprofit, international member-based organization that provides education using science-based and traditional information to promote the responsible use of herbal medicine. Provides information on Commission E. Nonmembers have access to some of ABC's general resources and samples from the databases. Full access is available to members who pay a yearly fee.
Dietary Supplement Quality Initiative (DSQI) www.supplementquality.com	This site provides information and a method for sharing information on supplement quality and supplement manufacturers.
PubMed Central http://www.pubmedcentral.nih.gov	The U.S. National Institutes of Health's free digital archive of biomedical and life sciences journal literature. The user can search the site using text or key words to gain access to published research on supplements. All abstracts and some papers are available electronically.
American Herbal Pharmacopoeia (AHP) www.herbal-ahp.org/index.html	AHP's mission is to promote the responsible use of herbal medicines and ensure that they are used with the highest degree of safety and efficacy achievable. AHP has developed standards for identity, purity, and analysis for botanicals, as well as a set of monographs on specific herbal supplements, some of which are free on the Web site.
United States Pharmacopeia (USP) www.usp.org	USP is an independent, science-based public health organization. The pharmacopeia is the official public standards-setting authority for all prescription and over-the-counter medicines, dietary supplements, and other healthcare products manufactured and sold in the United States. The USP may be available at libraries.

or she follows a good sports diet (see box 10.1) and evaluates each supplement for its potential risks and benefits.

In my case, I tried creatine for several months as we prepared to conduct our supplementation study on the female soccer players and noted an amazing improvement in my bench press performance, which had not budged for years. I did not continue using creatine for very long, however, because I felt that as a recreational athlete who was planning to start a family, any small benefit to my already acceptable strength performance was not worth the unknown risks of long-term supplementation. Maybe I would have decided differently if I were a close contender for the Olympic Trials.

Keeping a watchful eye then becomes important for athletes at all levels who are interested in either performance- or health-enhancing dietary supplements. Keeping a watchful eye involves carefully evaluating the supplement of interest, its research, safety, and cost so that you can decide whether the potential benefits outweigh the known and unknown risks and deciding if taking the supplement fits

---

Box 10.1

Do You Really Need to Supplement?

Before taking a supplement, ask yourself the following questions:

1. Do I eat breakfast regularly?
2. Do I eat at least three meals a day at regularly scheduled times?
3. Am I consuming enough, but not too much, energy to support my level of physical activity?
4. Do the bulk of my calories come from carbohydrate? Alternatively, am I taking in the recommended amount of carbohydrate for my sport and level of training?
5. Do I watch my fat intake, making sure my choices are smart and that I am getting enough but not too much of the right kinds of fat?
6. Do I eat a variety of foods from each of the major food groups?
7. Do I eat at least three servings of fruit a day?
8. Do I eat at least two servings of vegetables a day?
9. Do I consume adequate carbohydrate and fluids when training and during competition?
10. Do I drink enough water to maintain normal hydration?

If you cannot answer yes to each of these questions, why take a supplement? Don't expect supplements to replace a daily balanced diet.

USA Today, 1996.

with your personal value system. These steps are discussed in detail and can be used to evaluate all types of dietary supplements.

Evaluate the Product and Its Claims

The first step in evaluating a supplement is to first carefully evaluate the product and the claims being made. This includes taking a look at who is making the claims and whether the claims seem possible. Many times, products are sold by testimonials from other athletes, fitness buffs, self-proclaimed nutritionists, or medical doctors, all of whom can be very convincing. If the product sounds too good to be true, it probably is. Also, consider whether the product claims that it contains secret ingredients or special formulas. Under an amendment to the DSHEA, companies are now required to list all of the ingredients but are not required to tell which ones are likely to be beneficial. Just as a comparison, creatine and caffeine have known chemical structures with known actions but are not heavily advertised by themselves. Instead, cocktails containing "magic or special formulas" of these and other special ingredients are advertised. Although it is probably more profitable and exciting to offer a special concoction, such formulas require that you—the athlete—look up each ingredient to determine its possible efficacy and safety. Furthermore, it is less likely that good research supporting the benefit of a formula compared to a pure herb or compound is available, and more likely the formula may contain contaminants along with shady ingredients.

Determine Whether Research Exists to Back Up the Claim

The next step is to determine whether adequate and scientifically sound research is available to back up the supplement's claims or support its efficacy. The research should, of course, be done on humans, preferably active ones, and not on mice, rats, chickens, or overweight TV watchers. Also, you don't need to have a PhD in nutrition to figure out whether the research is sound. This step entails checking the supplement company's Web site (which typically lists supporting studies), calling the company to get further details, and most important, searching for the product and published product research on PubMed Central and other reputable Web sites including SupplementWatch (see table 10.1). In your search, remember that one study does not justify research. Neither does an abstract or two from a meeting or an unpublished study described only on a supplement company's Web site. The studies conducted should also be randomly assigned, placebo controlled, and double or single blinded. Randomly assigned, placebo controlled means that about half the athletes are randomly assigned to take the supplement and the other half are assigned to take the look-alike placebo. Double blinded means that neither the athlete nor the investigators conducting the test know who is taking what. This helps eliminate bias on the part of the athlete and the investigator. Single blinded means that just one party, for example, the athlete, is unaware of who is taking what. Although not as scientifically sound, this protocol is used when it is impossible to "blind" a party. For example, it would be difficult to blind athletes randomly assigned to a vegetarian compared to a mixed diet or a high-carbohydrate compared to a low-carbohydrate diet. Studies should also, if possible, include a crossover design in which study participants take one treatment—supplement or placebo—and later cross over to the other treatment. Crossover studies, however, are difficult to use with athletes because of training influences and are almost impossible to conduct when supplements are stored in the body for longer than a week or so (as is true with creatine and carnitine). Studies in which all participants knowingly take a supplement are for the most part worthless because of the placebo effect. This well-documented phenomenon holds that about one-third of the people given a sugar pill, or placebo, will experience benefits or side effects simply because they are told that they will.

Determine Whether the Supplement Is Safe, Vegetarian, and Legal

If, after your research, the product still seems promising, the next steps are to determine whether there are possible safety or toxicity issues associated with it, whether it is vegetarian (or vegan), and whether it is indeed legal, and not necessarily in that order. A first step in this process may be to look up information on the noted and possible side effects from the published research or from one of the Web sites listed in table 10.1. If the product seems relatively safe and you feel compelled to try it, the next step may be to seek a reputable brand. Although there are no guarantees, house brands from large grocery or drug stores might be your safest bet. These brands—because of their visibility and economic clout—are more likely to impose high standards on their suppliers. Once you have selected a brand or two, call the company or manufacturer to obtain specifics on how the product is manufactured and if animal derivatives are included as ingredients or in processing. This step is not necessary for an herbal supplement, which is of course vegan, or bovine colostrums, which are not vegetarian, no matter how you look at it, but it is a necessity for many nonherbal supplements, such as creatine. The final step is to ensure that the supplement of interest is legal. It is easy to determine if a substance is banned or restricted for use in a sport by checking with the national body governing that sport (if, of course, one exists). For example, the National College Athletic Association (NCAA) Web site lists all substances banned or restricted for athletes competing under the NCAA guidelines and currently includes anabolic agents such as dehydroepiandrosterone (DHEA), androstenediol, androstenedione, and a list of popular stimulants including ephedra.[2] Caffeine is also a limited substance.

Determine the Potential Risks and Costs of Supplementing

The final step in this process is to determine whether supplementing is worth it. Taking a supplement—including an herbal one—has potential health, ethical, and financial risks. Remember that because the FDA does not strictly regulate the supplement industry, any given supplement may contain pesticides, banned substances, and other contaminants and may lead to long-term health complications or disqualification from an athletic event. Knowing how long people have been taking a certain substance may also help you determine its risks. Ginseng, for example, has been used as an herbal therapy for years (although not in the United States) and its safety, when not mixed with other products, is well documented. In contrast, creatine has been on the market for a little more than 10 years. Although it appears to be safe over the short term, its long-term effects—particularly when taken regularly for years—simply are not known.

Also, as a vegetarian athlete, you need to ensure that supplementation fits your value system and your budget. Do you define natural as what you get from food and herbs or does it also include an artificially synthesized ergogenic aid? If it is OK to supplement with a commercially produced carbohydrate electrolyte beverage, is it also OK to mix in a little creatine, or is that somehow cheating? Although your response may depend on your competitive level and whether your opponents are taking supplements, the question is one that only you can answer.

The final important question comes down to economics. Can you afford the cost of the supplement? You should consider this in the context of how much the supplement costs as well as how much healthy food you could purchase if you were not spending that money on supplements. For example, if you believe that fresh blueberries or whole-grain sourdough bread from the local bakery is too expensive, you should think twice about buying supplements.

Supplements of Interest to the Vegetarian Athlete

Although there are a zillion supplements out there, only a handful may be of interest to vegetarian athletes. These supplements, along with several health-enhancing herbal supplements, are briefly discussed in the following section. This discussion is by no means an endorsement of their use but is an effort to provide information about their potential benefits and to expose hype, whichever the case may be, and the list is not exhaustive. However, if you decide to try a supplement, you should first ensure that you are eating well (see box 10.1). And remember, you should never substitute supplements for a good sports diet.

Creatine

Most of the creatine in the body is found in skeletal muscle where it exists primarily as creatine phosphate, which is an important storage form of energy that buffers ATP (see chapter 2). Many studies conducted since the early 1990s have found that oral creatine supplementation is effective at increasing body mass by one to two kilograms (2.2-4.4 lbs) and performance during high-intensity, short-duration exercise tasks such as strength training and repetitive high-intensity cycling or sprinting intervals.[5, 14, 15, 26] Supplementation, however, does not appear to enhance performance during swimming or endurance running.[5, 14, 15, 26]

The average dietary intake of creatine is about two grams per day in meat eaters[4] and is negligible in vegetarians. This makes sense because creatine is found primarily in muscle tissue. Even though creatine can be made in the body from the amino acids glycine, arginine, and methionine,[4] low concentrations of creatine in the blood[10, 24] and skeletal muscle[6, 13, 18] have been noted in vegetarians, as well as nonvegetarians placed on a vegetarian diet. Several studies have also found that vegetarians respond better to oral creatine supplementation than nonvegetarians.[6, 24] In these studies, vegetarians were found to experience greater increases in skeletal muscle creatine phosphate, lean tissue mass, and work performance during weight training[6] and anaerobic bicycle exercises[24] than nonvegetarians did. One study, however, did not find these benefits.[7] Thus, it is often suggested that vegetarian athletes may benefit from regular or periodic supplementation with creatine.

Creatine supplementation has not been associated with short-term safety issues, but its long-term safety is not known. Creatine comes in several forms. The pure powder form can be dissolved in warm water and mixed into carbohydrate-containing beverages. Evidence suggests that carbohydrate, mainly glucose,[12] enhances creatine absorption. According to several well-known manufacturers, creatine is not synthesized using animal derivatives. If you

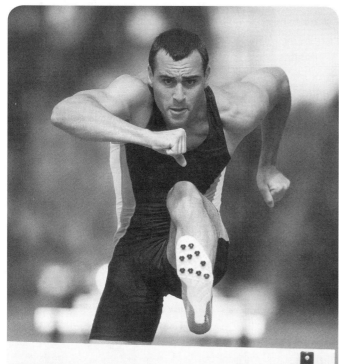

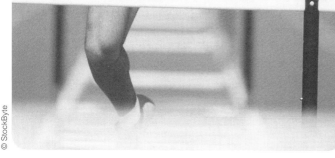

Creatine may help increase body mass and performance during high-intensity, short-duration activity, so it's a supplement to consider for vegetarians, since they often don't obtain much from their diets.

decide to try creatine, however, take pure creatine monohydrate, not creatine mixed with a cocktail of other ingredients, and contact the manufacturer to verify that your brand is vegetarian. The usual dose is three to five grams per day. Although many research studies have used loading protocols of 15 to 20 grams per day for five to seven days followed by a lower maintenance dose, this loading phase is not necessary as a regular dose of three grams per day will achieve the same increase in muscle creatine.[26]

Carnitine

Carnitine plays a central role in the metabolism of fat. Its role is to transport fatty acids into the body's energy-generating powerhouse—the mitochondria—to be burned for energy. Carnitine is found in meats and dairy products but not in plant foods. Like blood concentrations of creatine, blood concentrations of carnitine have been found to be lower in vegetarians[10] despite the liver's ability to produce it from the amino acids lysine and methionine.[23] In addition, blood carnitine concentrations have been found to be lower in obese people following a diet that is very low in calories,[9] which suggests that carnitine levels could be low in anyone who restricts calories.

Not surprisingly, carnitine has been targeted as a potential "fat burner" and endurance-performance enhancer. Studies addressing the ergogenic potential of carnitine, however, have been ambiguous, with several suggesting a beneficial effect of carnitine supplementation and others indicating no effect at all. Several previous studies suggested that carnitine supplementation of two to six grams per day increased fat utilization during endurance exercise, but others failed to find that supplementation spared glycogen or enhanced endurance when taken in doses of up to six grams per day.[25] It has also been noted that although carnitine concentration in blood goes up with supplementation, the enzyme system responsible for transporting fatty acids into the mitochondria is not increased.[25] This suggests that supplementation is unlikely to enhance what capacity the body already has. Although carnitine supplements are generally not considered an effective ergogenic aid for athletes, some sources—including SupplementWatch—suggest that supplements be considered for vegetarians who may not consume adequate carnitine or its precursor amino acids in their diets.[25] However, clinical evidence is not available to support or refute this suggestion. Carnitine is available in pill and liquid forms and many companies offer a vegetarian version. Adverse side effects have not been found from taking two to six grams per day for up to six months.[25]

Caffeine

Caffeine is probably the most casually and widely used sport-enhancing supplement because of its availability and social acceptance. Caffeine and its sister derivatives theophylline or theobromine occur naturally in certain plant-based foods including coffee, tea, and chocolate, and caffeine is also added to soda, sport bars and gels and some medications (see table 10.2). Caffeine is thought to improve performance by both stimulating the central nervous system (CNS) and facilitating force production in the muscle. As a CNS stimulant, caffeine specifically affects perception of effort, wards off drowsiness, and increases alertness. Well-controlled laboratory studies have found that caffeine (3-13 mg/kg body mass) taken one hour before or during exercise improves endurance performance, most notably by improving performance time in a racelike setting.[8] Studies demonstrating a benefit of caffeine on shorter, more-intense events are less abundant but also suggest an ergogenic potential.[21]

Vegetarian athletes who enjoy coffee, tea, or other caffeinated beverages may find it beneficial to consume a cup or two (236-472 ml) of strong coffee or tea about an hour before exercise, although some suggest that caffeine from supplements may be more effective.[11] Contrary to previous ideas about caffeine consumption,[11, 21] habitual caffeine intake does not appear to diminish caffeine's ergogenic properties. Nor does it lead to dehydration or electrolyte imbalance during exercise.[3] High levels of caffeine are banned by the NCAA, but only at levels possible from supplementation. For example, an athlete would have to drink approximately six cups (1,416 ml) of strong coffee before exercise to exceed

TABLE 10.2   Caffeine and Theobromine Content of Selected Beverages and Foods

Food or beverage	Portion	Caffeine (mg)	Theobromine (mg)
Coffee, brewed from grounds	6 fl oz	71	—
Coffee, instant	1 tsp	28	—
Espresso, restaurant brewed	1 fl oz	64	—
Tea, black	6 fl oz	36	4
Hot cocoa	12 fl oz	4	115
Cola	12 fl oz	29-99	
Lemon lime soda with caffeine	12 fl oz	55	
Rockstar energy drink	8 fl oz	75	
Red Bull energy drink	8 fl oz	80	
Milk chocolate	1 bar (1.55 oz)	9	90
Clif Bar (cool mint chocolate and peanut toffee buzz)	1 bar	50	

Values obtained from the USDA National Nutrient Database for Standard Reference (http://www.ars.usda.gov/nutrientdata), and selected manufacturers. Information on green tea is not currently available. Many energy bars and gels contain caffeine. Check the product information for your favorite brands (caffeine content is not typically listed on the label). Use these values to convert English measurements to metric: 1 fl oz = 29.6 ml = 28.4 g; 1 tsp = 4.7 g.

the urinary caffeine allowable level of 15 micrograms per milliliter. Caffeine has also been prohibited by the International Olympic Committee, but in 2004 it was moved to its Monitoring Program.

Beta-Hydroxy-Beta-Methylbutyrate (HMB)

Beta-hydroxy-beta-methylbutyrate, or HMB, is a metabolite of leucine, a branched-chain amino acid that plays a role in regulating protein metabolism. It is found in small amounts in some protein-rich foods, including fish and milk, but the body can produce it if total protein and leucine intake is sufficient.[25] You should be set if your diet is adequate in protein as discussed in chapter 5 and provides about 0.25 to 1 gram of leucine per day.[25] This is easily accomplished on a plant-based diet because just one cup of regular tofu or one cup of legumes alone provide over 1 gram of leucine.

Of interest to athletes is the evidence that HMB reduces muscle breakdown and may protect against muscle damage. For example, creatine kinase, an indicator of muscle damage, is reduced following exercise in subjects consuming HMB.[19] Research in humans as well as cattle, pigs, and poultry suggests that HMB can increase muscle mass in all species and increase strength[25] in humans. In fact, leucine is commonly added to chicken feed for the purpose of improving the muscle tissue and providing bigger chicken breasts (perhaps another reason most of us are vegetarian). In humans, a recent meta-analysis of hundreds of supplements showed that HMB, along with creatine, was one of the few that augmented lean mass and increased strength when combined with a program of resistance training.[20] Thus, HMB is sometimes recommended to athletes trying to minimize protein losses and muscle breakdown, particularly when initiating training[16] or during very high-intensity training.[25] Not all studies, however, support the benefits of HMB supplementation, which may suggest that training status and stages of training are important. One study conducted in well-trained resistance athletes found that HMB supplementation did not improve strength or alter body composition.[16]

The recommended dose of HMB depends on training intensity: one gram per day on rest and easy days and about three grams on heavy training days.[25] No side effects have been reported in animal studies, which have used large doses of HMB for several weeks, or in human studies giving as much as four grams per day,[25] although I question the researcher's ability to truly monitor side effects in animals. Supplemental forms of HMB often contain magnesium stearate derived from an animal source and are commonly packaged in capsules made with animal-based gelatin. At least one company, however, offers a version for vegetarians.

Conjugated Linoleic Acid

Conjugated linoleic acid (CLA) is an isomer of the essential fatty acid linoleic acid (discussed in chapter 4). Specifically as an isomer, the molecular structure is slightly rearranged with a conjugated double bond occurring at carbons 10 and 12 or carbons 9 and 11.[22] The significance of this rearrangement is that it results in a different fatty acid with altered chemical functions. Whereas the essential fatty acid linoleic acid is found in the diet in vegetable oils, CLA is found primarily in meat and dairy products.

CLA may be of interest to vegetarian athletes because it is purported to increase lean tissue by suppressing catabolic hormones, increase energy expenditure, reduce body fat, and fight cancer.[22] The majority of research on CLA supplementation, however, has been conducted on animals. Livestock studies have found that supplemental CLA, somewhat like HMB, promotes growth and prevents muscle wasting but also suppresses body fat accumulation.[25] Studies in humans, for the most part, have noted that CLA supplementation does not appear to have the impact noted in animal studies.[22, 27] In exercising people, one study reported a decrease in body fat in healthy men and women exercising 90 minutes, three days a week for 12 weeks,[28] and another reported no effect during 28 days of resistance training in resistance-trained men.[17]

Nonetheless, CLA is a supplement that may be touted for vegans because they obtain very little in their diets, and also for health-conscious people because of its purported anticancer potential (found in animal studies). CLA may be a supplement to continue watching. CLA is typically delivered in a gelcap, and the typical recommended dosage is three to five grams per day taken in three doses with meals. Although the form of CLA most commonly used in dietary supplements is manufactured from vegetable oils such as sunflower oil,[25] the gelcaps themselves are usually made from animal-based gelatin. No side effects have been reported with CLA supplementation; however, caution is advised because the majority of the work has been done on animals.

Herbal and Other Supplements

Depending on your objective, there are probably a handful of herbal and other types of supplements likely to provide health benefits. Although Commission E and SupplementWatch are the best sources of information for these supplements, table 10.3 lists products that are considered safe and effective for their reported uses. If you are interested in these or other supplements, evaluate the supplement—herbal or otherwise—using the tools discussed earlier, paying particular attention to data obtained from the reputable Web sites listed in table 10.1.

I hope this chapter has given you an overview of dietary supplements and also taught you how to evaluate supplements and their place in your diet as a vegetarian athlete. The next chapter focuses on how diet may influence two common athletic maladies: muscle cramps and muscle injury and inflammation.

TABLE 10.3 Selected Herbal and Other Supplements That May Offer Health Benefits

Supplement	Use	Reported value and effect
Echinacea	Stimulates immune system function Prevents upper-respiratory-tract infections	May be beneficial in reducing the severity and duration of symptoms associated with the common cold and flu. Echinacea preparations should not be viewed as a cure for the common cold.
Ginkgo biloba	Improves memory and mental sharpness Alleviates symptoms of Alzheimer's disease Acts as an antidepressant Improves circulation Thins blood Acts as an antioxidant	Research suggests it may be valuable for an array of health concerns related to problems with microcirculation in the brain, legs, or sex organs. Ginkgo biloba's neuroprotective effects are well established, and its benefits in improving mental function and memory in healthy subjects looks promising.
Ginseng	Relieves stress Enhances athletic performance Promotes well-being Enhances immune system Acts as a stimulant Lowers blood sugar Improves cognitive function	Scientific evidence of the benefits is considered inconclusive. The adaptogenic role of ginseng has proven beneficial for many thousands of years so ginseng may, therefore, prove valuable for normalizing substances during stressful conditions.
St. John's wort	Alleviates mild depression	May be effective as a low-dose tricyclic antidepressant in treating mild depression.
Melatonin	Promotes sleep Reduces symptoms of jet lag Slows the aging process Increases secretion of sex hormone Acts as an antioxidant	Serves as a nonaddictive alternative to over-the-counter chemical sleep aids. Particularly useful as a short-term regulator of sleep/wake cycles, e.g., resetting your body clock after crossing several time zones. Melatonin can induce or deepen depression in susceptible people. Melatonin supplements may also be dangerous for people with cardiovascular risks.

Adapted from information summarized by Supplement Watch. Available: http://www.supplementwatch.com. Please refer to this and other sites for updates as well as information about safety concerns and recommended dosages. All supplements listed are thought to be safe for generally healthy people.

11

Reducing Muscle Cramps and Inflammation

M y neighbor e-mailed me the day after the Marine Corps Marathon and wanted to meet right away. His e-mail did not say much except that he had developed severe leg cramps about 10 miles (16 km) into the race and had a terrible time finishing. I was disappointed because I knew he had trained hard—diligently following one of Runner's World *magazine's marathon training plans. I knew because I saw him running in the neighborhood most mornings and he was now passing me in races.*

When we met, we chatted about the marathon and days leading up to it. He said he consumed adequate fluids the morning of the race and had drunk fluids at all the water stations until 10 miles (16 km). But when I asked about the days before the race, it seemed that travel had interfered with his typical fluid-intake patterns. He admitted that he might have started the race somewhat dehydrated. Nothing else about his diet or training seemed off-kilter; he had tapered and reported that he paid attention to his carbohydrate intake. He wanted to know, of course, if prerace dehydration had caused his cramps, but given their nature, I could only say that I believed it had contributed. Indeed, I reminded him that before the next marathon—which he was already planning—he must consume adequate fluid with the carbohydrate and the other components of his diet, and we would then hope for the best.

Both muscle cramps and overuse inflammatory injuries are common, painful physiological disturbances that regularly frustrate athletes. Because both can be caused by a change in your training routine—for example, you run faster and farther than you are accustomed to—your diet can potentially assist in controlling or reducing these maladies. Although no conclusive evidence is available, muscle cramps are thought to occur during severe dehydration and as a result of fluid and electrolyte imbalances[37]—which suggests that dietary factors may be involved. Recent research in people with arthritis also suggests that dietary factors—mainly omega-3 fatty acids and vitamin D—can help control inflammation and may help athletes control nagging overuse and inflammatory injuries. This chapter reviews the basics of both muscle cramps and inflammation and discusses the dietary factors that can potentially—but not necessarily—help prevent or control muscle cramps and musculoskeletal inflammation. Unlike the information in the other chapters, however, the information presented here is provocative and somewhat speculative.

Inside a Muscle Cramp

If you have ever had a muscle cramp, you understand well that cramps are, by definition, painful, spasmodic, involuntary contractions. Typically, they are of little medical consequence but pose an inconvenience for athletes. Cramps tend to occur at night (nocturnal cramps) or during or after unusually prolonged exercise (exercise-associated cramps), but they can occur during apparently typical exercise conditions, either early or late in the session. It is still not known why they occur because—believe it or not—little scientific research has been done on the subject.[6] This has resulted in a perpetuation of myths about the cause and treatment of cramps.[6]

Fortunately, there has been interest recently in investigating both why muscles cramp and what specifically occurs during a cramp. Collectively, research suggests that skeletal muscle cramps can occur during a diverse range of conditions[6] and result when the sensitivity of the reflexes between the muscles and tendons and the spinal cord are altered.[30] Researchers from the University of Cape Town Medical School in South Africa have found evidence that muscles cramp because of both sustained firing by the nerves in the spinal cord to the muscle and limited protective reflex function by the Golgi tendon organ governor.[30] Normally, excitatory impulses from the spinal cord are fired in an intermittent rather than sustained pattern, and protective impulses from the Golgi tendon organ (by way of the spinal cord) cause muscles to relax under excess tension. Researchers at the University of Cape Town also argue that these changes occur in association with fatigue and are particularly notable in the muscle groups that contract in a shortened position for prolonged periods.[30] Examples include the hamstrings and the quadriceps muscles in cycling and running, the calf muscles in swimming or when sleeping, and the diaphragm muscles in most physical endeavors. Accordingly, only muscles that undergo frequent lengthening during prolonged exercise are prevented from cramping because stretching the muscle activates the protective stretch reflex via the Golgi tendon organ.

In agreement with the findings from the Cape Town group, the accepted treatment of cramps is passive stretching.[6, 30] Passive stretching also reduces the electrical conductivity of the muscle, which in one study was found to be elevated in endurance athletes actively experiencing muscle cramping.[34] Although there are no proven strategies for preventing exercise-induced muscle cramping, regularly stretching may be beneficial along with attaining conditioning adequate for the sport activity, correcting muscle balance and posture problems, muscle relaxation therapy, and sport psychology therapy aimed at mental preparation for competition. The benefit of other strategies, such as incorporating plyometrics or eccentric muscle strengthening into training regimens, treating myofascial trigger points, and maintaining adequate carbohydrate reserves[6] and adequate mineral electrolyte status through diet, is speculative and requires further research.

Causes of Muscle Cramps

Even less is known about what causes or triggers a muscle cramp. Causes of muscle cramps proposed in the past include extreme environmental conditions of heat or cold, inherited abnormalities of carbohydrate or fat metabolism, and exercise-induced imbalances in fluid or the major electrolyte concentrations in the body, which include sodium, potassium, calcium, and magnesium.[6] An imbalance of the major electrolytes is suspected because these electrolytes are involved in generating electrical currents in the body and occur during muscle contraction and when sending a nerve impulse.

More recently, however, researchers have suggested that cramping is simply caused by fatigue. A recent analysis of published scientific findings on the triggers of muscle cramps found that few studies support the idea that any of these disturbances—other than possibly fatigue—are the underlying cause of the typical cramping that occurs during endurance and ultraendurance events. It is nevertheless important to mention that the cause of muscle cramps may be different for each athlete and that muscle cramping is not necessarily associated with fatigue that is more pronounced than it was at times that muscle cramping did not occur. Thus, studies that compare athletes who cramp during a race or event to those who do not might be missing valuable information if only average group rather than individual data are compared and food and fluid intake are ignored.

In addition, because the body defends its concentrations of certain electrolytes in the blood—mainly those of sodium, potassium, calcium, and magnesium[36]—serum electrolyte concentrations may not reflect muscle electrolyte concentrations. Hence, it is possible that the concentration of certain electrolytes may be low within the muscle cell, but appear normal or just slightly lower in the blood. Of course, as you can imagine, gathering such data in muscle and blood is precluded for practical reasons because the only way to measure muscle-electrolyte concentrations is by taking a muscle biopsy. As dedicated as I am to science, I cannot imagine undergoing a muscle biopsy during or following an exercise-associated cramp. Muscle biopsies can themselves induce cramps, making this a very difficult area to investigate.

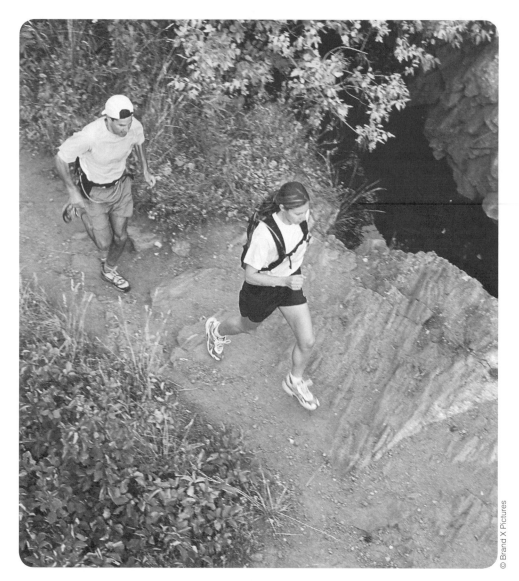

© Brand X Pictures

Readily available fluid sources, such as hydration packs, during prolonged activity help prevent dehydration and painful muscle cramps. Use caution, however, since over-drinking may lead to hyponatremia.

Diet and Muscle Cramping

If you look at the information presented in most exercise physiology and sports nutrition books, you will notice an obvious omission of discussions of muscle cramps. This is probably because little is known about muscle cramps. Nonetheless, I am a true believer that imbalances of fluid or the mineral electrolytes— sodium, potassium, calcium, and magnesium—in the diet should be ruled out as contributors to all nocturnal and exercise-associated cramps.

Fluid Imbalances and Dehydration

Whether fluid imbalances and mild dehydration can trigger muscle cramping is open to debate. Although we know that muscle cramps can and do occur with severe dehydration and heat injury, there is no conclusive evidence that consuming adequate fluid with or without electrolytes will prevent typical nocturnal or exercise-associated cramping. In fact, studies have found that runners, cyclists, and triathletes who develop cramps during an endurance event are no more likely to be dehydrated or to have lost greater amounts of bodily water than are those who do not develop cramps during the same race.[31, 34, 38] In my practice, however, I have noted anecdotally that maintaining a proper fluid balance indeed helps many endurance and team athletes avoid cramps, particularly those that occur after exercise or when sleeping at night. In one case, I worked with a male tennis player from Switzerland who had a history of severe cramping and fatigue after practice that was relieved by a regular and diligent fluid-consumption schedule. In her book, well-known sport nutritionist Nancy Clark tells an amusing story about a runner who eliminated his painful muscle cramps by following the simple postexercise advice to first drink water for fluid replacement and then have a beer for social fun.[10]

Sodium

Sodium is one of the main positively charged mineral ions or electrolytes in body fluid. The body needs it to help maintain normal body-fluid balance and blood pressure, and in conjunction with several other electrolytes, it is critical for nerve impulse generation and muscle contraction. Sodium is distributed widely in nature but is found in rather small amounts in most unprocessed foods. In most developed countries, however, a significant amount of sodium is added from the salt shaker (1 teaspoon [6 g] contains 2,325 milligrams of sodium) or by food manufacturers in processing (as listed on the food label). Because sodium intake can vary, the typical Western diet contains 10 to 12 grams of salt (3.9 to 4.7 g of sodium) per day.

Because sodium plays an important role in regulating blood pressure and fluid and electrolyte balance, the body has an effective mechanism to help regulate the levels of sodium in the blood on a variety of sodium intakes. If the sodium concentration in the blood starts to drop, a series of complex events leads to the secretion of a hormone called aldosterone, which signals the kidneys to retain sodium. If sodium levels are too high, aldosterone secretion is inhibited, which allows the kidneys to eliminate some sodium through urination. Another hormone, called *antidiuretic hormone (ADH),* also helps maintain normal sodium levels in body fluids by signaling the kidney to retain water and sodium. Typically, levels of both aldosterone and ADH increase during exercise, which helps conserve the body's water and sodium stores.

Actual sodium-deficient states caused by inadequate dietary sodium are not common because the body's regulatory mechanisms are typically very effective.

Humans even have a natural appetite for salt, which helps assure that they take in enough sodium to maintain sodium balance. Indeed, I have great memories of eating salty tortilla chips wet with a little water—so more salt would stick—after long cycling races in Arizona. Thankfully, these sodium-conserving mechanisms are activated in athletes who lose excessive sodium and other electrolytes during prolonged sweating (see box 11.1).

Although muscle cramps are reported to occur during the sodium-deficient state, some researchers believe that alterations in sodium balance are not involved in exercise-associated cramps.[31, 34] This is despite the fact that significantly lower postexercise serum sodium concentrations have been found in endurance athletes who experienced cramps during a race compared to those who did not develop cramps.[31, 38] One of the reasons this is downplayed may be because serum sodium concentrations remain within the normal range, despite being significantly lower in the athletes with muscle cramps.

Nevertheless, it is important for athletes to consume enough sodium to replace what is lost through sweat (see box 11.1). Despite the regulatory mechanisms discussed earlier, it is possible for vegetarian athletes to be at risk for muscle cramps and other problems because of low sodium intake. The reason is most likely because they ignore their salt craving cues—eating mostly unprocessed and unsalted foods—while continuing to lose considerable salt through sweating. The recommendation set by the USDA's Dietary Guidelines for Americans to keep sodium intake to 2.3 grams or less per day is not appropriate for most athletes because of their higher sodium losses. Thus, while it is not likely that low sodium intake is the cause of cramps in most athletes, it is certainly possible that a vegetarian athlete prudently following a low-sodium diet for health reasons might experience muscle cramps that would be relieved with more liberal use of the salt shaker.

Box
11.1

Composition of Sweat

Sweat is about 99 percent water but does contain several major electrolytes and other nutrients. The major electrolytes found in sweat are sodium and chloride. Although it varies, an average of about 2.6 grams of salt, or 1.01 grams of sodium, are lost with each liter of sweat produced during exercise. A typical sweat rate is between 800 and 1,500 milliliters per hour and may be even higher during exercise in hot and humid environments, including the outdoors and non-air-conditioned gymnasiums. Other minerals lost in small amounts include potassium, calcium, magnesium, iron, copper, and zinc. Certain athletes—particularly those who lose large amounts of sweat—may need to increase their dietary intake of these nutrients to replace the loss.

Potassium

Potassium is the major electrolyte found inside all body cells, including muscle and nerve cells. It works in close association with sodium and chloride in the generation of electrical impulses in the nerves and the muscles, including the heart muscle. Potassium is found in most foods, but is especially abundant in fresh vegetables, potatoes, certain fruits (melon, bananas, berries, citrus fruit), milk, meat, and fish. Table 11.1 lists the 20 best vegetarian sources of potassium.

TABLE 11.1 Top 20 Plant-Based Sources of Potassium

Food	Portion	Value
Beet greens, cooked	1 cup cooked	1,309
White beans, canned	1 oz	1,189
Baked potato, flesh and skin	1 medium	1,081
Green soybeans, cooked	1 cup cooked	970
Lima beans	1 cup cooked	955
Marinara sauce, already prepared	1 cup	940
Hash browned potatoes, home prepared	1 cup cooked	899
Winter squash, all types	1 cup cooked	896
Soybeans, cooked	1 cup cooked	886
Spinach, cooked	1 cup cooked	839
Tomato sauce	1 cup	811
Plums, dried or stewed	1 cup	796
Sweet potato, canned	1 cup cooked	796
Pinto beans	1 cup cooked	746
Lentils	1 cup cooked	731
Plantains	1 cup cooked	716
Kidney beans	1 cup cooked	713
Split peas	1 cup cooked	710
Navy beans	1 cup cooked	708
Prune juice	1 cup	707

Refer to appendix E for guidance on converting English units to metric.

Data from "Reports by Single Nutrients," *USDA National Nutrient Database for Standard Reference, Release 18*. Available: http://www.ars.usda.gov/Services/docs.htm?docid=4451.

Potassium balance, like sodium balance, is regulated by the hormone aldosterone. A high serum potassium level stimulates the release of the hormone aldosterone, which leads to increased potassium excretion by the kidneys into the urine. A decrease in serum potassium concentration elicits a drop in aldosterone secretion and hence less potassium loss in the urine. As with sodium and calcium, potassium is typically precisely regulated, and deficiencies or excessive accumulation are rare. Potassium deficiencies, however, can occur with conditions such as fasting, diarrhea, and regular diuretic use. In such cases, low blood–potassium concentrations, called *hypokalemia,* can lead to muscle cramps and weakness, and even cardiac arrest caused by impairment in the generation of nerve impulses. Similarly, high blood–potassium concentrations, or *hyperkalemia,* are also not common but can occur in people who take potassium supplements far exceeding the recommended daily allowance. High blood–potassium concentrations can also disturb electrical impulses and induce cardiac arrhythmia.

Even though little evidence is available to support a link between potassium intake and muscle cramps, it is quite interesting that most athletes—and nonathletes alike—think that the banana is the first line of defense in preventing muscle cramps. If only it were that simple. Furthermore, athletes following vegetarian diets are not likely to experience muscle cramping as a result of low potassium intake because the vegetarian diet provides an abundance of potassium. An athlete who is recovering from an intestinal illness, restricting calories, or taking diuretics or laxatives should, nevertheless, make an effort to consume potassium-rich foods (see table 11.1), particularly if he or she is experiencing muscle cramping. Because of the dangers of hyperkalemia, potassium supplements are not recommended unless closely monitored by a physician. The recommended daily intake for potassium is 4,700 milligrams per day for adults.

Calcium

As discussed in chapter 6, the vast majority of calcium found in the body is found in the skeleton where it lends strength to bone. Calcium, however, is involved in muscle contractions, including that of the heart, skeletal muscles, and smooth muscle found in blood vessels and intestines, as well as the generation of nerve impulses. Blood calcium is tightly controlled and regulated by several hormones, including parathyroid hormone and vitamin D.

Although impaired muscle contraction and muscle cramps are commonly listed as symptoms of calcium deficiency, many exercise scientists feel that low calcium intake is not likely to play a role in most muscle cramps. This is because if dietary calcium intake were low, calcium would be released from the bones to maintain blood concentrations and theoretically provide what would be needed for muscle contraction. This thinking, however, does not completely rule out the possibility that muscle cramping could be caused by a temporary imbalance of calcium in the muscle during exercise. Certainly, we know that people with inborn errors in calcium metabolism in skeletal muscle (which will be discussed later) are prone to muscle cramping.

Despite so little being known about low calcium intake and muscle cramps, calcium is one of the nutritional factors people most associate with relieving cramps, second only to the potassium-rich banana. Although to my knowledge studies have not assessed whether dietary or supplemental calcium affects exercise cramps in athletes, a recent report found that calcium supplementation was not effective in treating leg cramps associated with pregnancy.[39] On the other hand, anecdotal reports from athletes are common. Nancy Clark tells of a hiker who resolved muscle cramps by taking calcium-rich Tums and of a ballet dancer whose cramping disappeared after adding milk and yogurt to her diet.[10] Because calcium intake can be low in the diet of some vegans and vegetarians, inadequate calcium should also be ruled out in vegetarians experiencing muscle cramps.

Magnesium

In addition to its role in bone health, magnesium plays an important role in stabilizing adenosine triphosphate (ATP), the energy source for muscle contraction, and also serves as an electrolyte in body fluids. Muscle weakness, muscle twitching, and muscle cramps are common symptoms of magnesium deficiency.

Limited data have suggested that magnesium status is indirectly related to the incidence of muscle cramps.[11] In these studies of endurance athletes, the athletes who developed muscle cramps were found to have serum magnesium concentrations that were different from their competitors who did not cramp.[31, 38] The research, however, presents a confusing story because serum magnesium was significantly lower in cyclists who cramped during a 100-mile (160 km) bike ride [38] and significantly higher in runners who cramped during an ultradistance race.[31] In both studies, serum magnesium remained within the normal range but was low-normal in the cyclists who cramped and high-normal in the runners. Interestingly, studies in pregnant women have found that supplementation with magnesium (taken as magnesium lactate or magnesium citrate in doses of 5 millimoles in the morning and 10 millimoles in the evening) show promise for treating pregnancy-associated leg cramps. Research, however, has not addressed whether dietary or supplemental magnesium can prevent or reduce muscle cramps in athletes.

Vegetarian athletes are not likely to experience muscle cramping as a result of low magnesium intake because the typical vegetarian diet is abundant in magnesium. Low magnesium intake, however, is possible for people restricting calories or eating a diet high in processed foods. Low magnesium intake should be ruled out in cramp-prone athletes. Table 11.2 lists the 20 best vegetarian sources of magnesium. A more extensive list is found in table 6.1 on page 70.

Carbohydrate

Inadequate carbohydrate stores have also been implicated as a potential cause of muscle cramps. Theoretically, it makes sense that hard-working muscles might

TABLE 11.2 **Top 20 Plant-Based Sources of Magnesium**

Food	Portion	Value
Spinach, frozen	1 cup cooked	156
Pumpkin seeds	1 oz	151
Soybeans	1 cup cooked	148
White beans	1 cup cooked	134
All-Bran cereal (Kellogg's)	1/2 cup	109
Green soybeans	1 cup cooked	108
Brazil nuts	1 cup cooked	107
Lima beans, frozen	1 cup cooked	101
Beet greens	1 cup cooked	98
Navy beans	1 cup cooked	96
Okra, sliced	1 cup cooked	94
Baking chocolate, unsweetened	1 square (28 g)	93
Southern peas, black-eyed and crowder	1 cup cooked	91
Oat bran muffin	1 medium (57 g)	89
Pinto and great northern beans	1 cup cooked	86
Buckwheat grouts, toasted	1 cup cooked	86
Brown rice	1 cup cooked	84
Raisin Bran cereal (Kellogg's)	1 cup cooked	80
Kidney beans	1 cup cooked	80
Almonds and cashews	1 oz	78-79

Refer to appendix E for guidance on converting English units to metric.

Data from "Reports by Single Nutrients," *USDA National Nutrient Database for Standard Reference, Release 18*. Available: http://www.ars.usda.gov/Services/docs.htm?docid=4451.

experience cramping in association with the depletion of its power source—carbohydrate. While all athletes should consider the recommendations presented earlier to optimize performance, athletes with a history of cramping during prolonged exercise should ensure that they consume adequate carbohydrate during exercise and in the days before and days following an endurance event.

Checking Your Diet

If you have a history of muscle cramps—either nocturnal or exercise induced—the first step may be a nutrition check to ensure that your diet is not contributing to the cramps (see box 11.2). As mentioned earlier, cramps tend to occur in some athletes who work their muscles to exhaustion, but in my experience also occur in well-conditioned athletes for no apparent reason. Paying attention to the timing and pattern of cramping can also be helpful. Cramps associated with dehydration, for example, typically occur in the latter parts of prolonged exercise but may

---

Box 11.2

Ruling Out Nutritional Causes of Cramps

Nutrition may be involved in nocturnal or exercise-associated muscle cramps. Although the following nutrition tips are not guaranteed to resolve this malady, they should help ensure that a poor diet does not contribute to the underlying cause of cramping. Keep in mind that dietary change may not immediately resolve cramps.

> Follow the guidelines for fluid intake before, during, and after exercise (see chapter 9). Both too little and too much fluid can potentially induce muscle cramps.

> Consume enough sodium in your diet to replace that lost through sweat. Vegetarian athletes eating mostly whole and unprocessed foods and who do not salt their food may risk low sodium intake.

> Eat an abundant amount of fresh fruits and vegetables—not just bananas. The vegetarian diet is typically rich in potassium, but vegetarians who eat poorly or who take laxatives or diuretics may have poor potassium status.

> Obtain calcium from a variety of plant sources and, if appropriate, dairy sources. Plant foods that are rich in easily absorbed calcium include low-oxalate, green, leafy vegetables (collard, mustard, and turnip greens), tofu set with calcium, fortified soy and rice milks, textured vegetable protein, tahini, certain legumes, fortified orange juice, almonds, and blackstrap molasses.

> Eat a diet full of whole grains, nuts, seeds, and legumes. Although vegetarian athletes may be at an advantage when it comes to dietary magnesium intake, athletes who eat diets high in refined foods should watch their intake of magnesium. Plant foods that are rich in magnesium include seeds, nuts, legumes, unmilled cereal grains, dark-green vegetables, and dark chocolate. Refined foods and dairy products tend to be low in magnesium.

> Consume ample carbohydrate both in your overall diet and in association with exercise (as discussed in chapters 3 and 9). Muscles depleted of their carbohydrate stores may be more likely to cramp.

> Consume adequate energy. Insufficient energy consumption can compromise your intake of important electrolytes, including potassium, calcium, and magnesium.

indeed be present at the beginning of the event if you started exercise partially dehydrated. Technically, cramps caused by a deficiency of sodium, calcium, or magnesium could occur any time but also might not manifest until later as compromised stores of these minerals are lost through prolonged sweating or are diluted by drinking water only without electrolytes.

Although making improvements in your diet will never hurt—and may in the long run help you improve your overall health and performance—making these improvements is not guaranteed to prevent muscle cramping. I worked with a former training partner who began to experience severe calf cramps during running but not cycling. The cramps started suddenly sometime in her early thirties and did not appear to be related to poor conditioning or a change in her training. Despite trying everything imaginable—nutritionally or otherwise—she finally gave up running and is now placing in master's cycling events. Oddly, she has never experienced a cramp during cycling.

My colleagues and I also worked with an indoor-fitness enthusiast who taught the toughest spinning class I have ever taken. Despite being in awesome shape, he could not exercise outdoors without his quadriceps locking up. Many times he had to hobble home because his cramps would not let up. After assessing him in the lab, we finally came to the conclusion that his cramping was related to malignant hyperthermia (MH), a rare genetic condition characterized by an abnormal release of calcium from its storage site in muscle, the sarcoplasmic reticulum. Although his sister had been diagnosed with MH, discovering that the condition was the cause of his cramping was beneficial because people with MH can experience severe reactions during anesthesia, including muscle rigidity, increased body temperature, metabolic acidosis, and even death.[20] Nothing could be done to his diet to improve his condition. In addition to MH, other genetic and metabolic disorders that can result in exercise-associated cramping in seemingly fit athletes include a deficiency of muscle carnitine palmitoyl transferase (the enzyme that helps escort fat into the mitochondria for oxidation[8]) and myotonia.[14, 35]

Inflammation and Injury 101

Inflammation is something every athlete knows as redness, pain, and swelling but probably does not quite understand. That goes double for many nutritionists, coaches, and exercise physiologists. Although often a nuisance, inflammation is necessary for your body to protect itself from infection, to regrow damaged tissue, and to begin healing. The immune system responds to both infection and signs of injury, which include broken cell parts and spilled cell constituents, by directing the inflammatory response. This results in the accumulation of both fluid and special immune cells. Once the cause is resolved, the inflammation usually subsides. In cases such as joint stress in osteoarthritis or the autoimmune response with rheumatoid arthritis, the inflammation reaction continues out of control and can cause tissue damage rather than repair.

Tissue damage that results from a sport injury typically involves local and short-lived inflammation, which in some cases can become long term, or chronic.

Tissue damaged in response to injury recruits white blood cells traveling through blood to the scene of the injury (see figure 11.1). The immune system then activates various types of immune cells during the inflammatory and healing process. Many of these cells contain and secrete tissue-remodeling agents that play a role in healing. Some of these substances stimulate blood clotting to halt bleeding, and other molecules gently pry open the tissue so it can begin to sew itself back together and close up the wounded area. Acute inflammatory reactions can be painful because swollen tissue compresses nerves and because chemical messengers activate nerve cells and communicate to the brain that the injury hurts. The purpose of pain, of course, is to get you to pamper your injured area a bit so it can heal, but we all know how well that works in athletes.

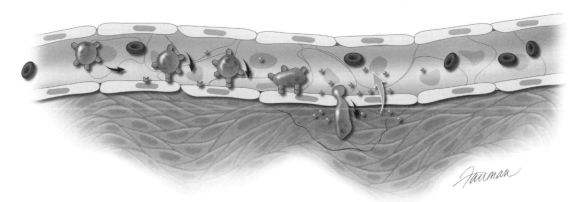

FIGURE 11.1 **Tissue damaged in response to any type of injury (including a sport-related injury) recruits white blood cells traveling through blood to the scene of the injury. Illustrated here is the activation of a type of white blood cells called neutrophils that then move into the injured tissue in response to chemical signals. This process is important for tissue healing.**
Illustration © Fairman Studios, LLC.

We understand very little about whether overuse injuries are caused by a chronic or overreactive inflammatory response. Scientists, however, are just beginning to understand the role that chronic, unchecked, inflammation can play in the development of many chronic diseases including multiple sclerosis, arthritis, heart disease, and cancer. What this means to an otherwise healthy athlete is unknown, but read on to see how diet may play a role in the inflammatory response.

Diet and Inflammation

Given what we know about inflammation, the question that should come to mind is whether your diet can prevent or contribute to the minor inflammatory injuries that occur in muscles, joints, and tendons or can influence how your body reacts to acute inflammation from a sport injury. Although no one would expect good nutrition to prevent an ankle sprain, nutrition could potentially control the inflammatory response that occurs after the ankle is sprained, perhaps allowing injured tissues to heal faster or more completely. Nutrients that might be involved and deserve a nutrition check include the omega-3 fatty acids (or the ratio of omega-3 to omega-6 fatty acids), vitamin D, and the antioxidant and anti-inflammatory phytochemicals found in plant foods and seasonings (see box 11.3).

Box 11.3

Nutrition Tips for Reducing Inflammation

> ➤ Strive to improve the ratio of omega-3 to omega-6 fatty acids in your diet by consuming at least two servings of foods that supply omega-3 fats every day and eliminating—as much as possible—your intake of omega-6-rich corn, safflower, sunflower, and cottonseed oils. Omega-3 rich foods are listed in table 11.3 and include flaxseed oil, ground flaxseed, canola oil, hemp oil, walnuts, and commercially available products with added flax.

> ➤ Maintain adequate levels of vitamin D, either by spending time outside in the sun or through supplementation (see box 6.1). Vitamin D supplementation of 2,000 IU per day[9] might be worth trying if you experience bone, joint, or tendon problems, including swelling and stiffness.

> ➤ Consume a diet rich in fruits, vegetables, and fresh herbs. When experiencing inflammation from a nagging sport injury, try green tea, ginger tea, pesto, pomegranate juice, or other foods naturally high in anti-inflammatory compounds.

> ➤ Stay tuned for more research!

Omega-3 Fatty Acids

As discussed in chapter 4, both omega-3 and omega-6 fatty acids are used to create a family of signaling molecules called *eicosanoids* (and include prostaglandins). The eicosanoids are important and potent controllers of many body functions including inflammation and immune function. The signaling molecules created from omega-3 fatty acids, however, behave differently than those created from the omega-6 fatty acids. Those created from the omega-3s direct blood vessels to dilate, encourage blood to stay fluid, and reduce the inflammation response, whereas those created from the omega-6s (particularly arachidonic acid found in eggs, meat, and dairy) promote blood clotting, constrict blood vessels, and encourage inflammation. Overall, the type of inflammatory response is determined by the type of fat consumed in the diet. Research has shown that increasing the omega-3 fatty acids in the diet, particularly the longer chain eicosapentaenoic and docosahexaenoic acids, reduces the production of and tissue response to aggressive inflammatory-response cellular signals, called cytokines.[15] These cytokines control the wide range of symptoms associated with trauma and infection and are thought to promote the inflammation associated with a variety of ailments including arthritis, inflammatory bowel disease, and asthma.

Although omega-3s are thought to reduce inflammation and lower the risk for many age-related diseases, it is not known whether they affect nagging athletic injuries. Studies in people with rheumatoid arthritis, however, have shown that regularly consuming two to three grams of omega-3 fats helps decrease joint tenderness and swelling.[4, 16] As is reviewed in box 11.4, rheumatoid arthritis is rooted in the immune and inflammatory responses.

Although we all know that nonblinded experiments of one can be biased and misleading, I nonetheless performed such a study on myself to determine if upping the omega-3s in my diet would improve the swelling I had been experiencing in my left knee after strenuous or prolonged running. My strategy was to eliminate the oils high in omega-6s from my diet, eat a large handful of walnuts, which are rich in omega-3s, and drink a smoothie made with one tablespoon of flaxseed oil almost daily (although daily ended up being three to four times a week). The verdict was indeed favorable. After a month or so, I noted only minimal swelling, which nearly a year later is nonexistent. Is it worth a try? You bet! Even if bumping up the omega-3s in your diet at the expense of the omega-6s has no effect on your nagging injuries, it may provide other health benefits. It is hard to predict where you might feel the effects of increased omega-3 intake, but it could have an impact anywhere you experience inflammation, including your joints, muscles, or tendons.

Practically speaking, the easiest way to improve your ratio of omega-3 to omega-6 fatty acids is to strive to include two or more servings every day of foods that supply omega-3 fats and limiting—as much as possible—foods high in omega-6 fats: oils made from corn, safflower, sunflower, and cottonseed and dairy products and eggs, which are high in arachidonic acid. A serving of omega-3 fats according to the Vegetarian Food Guide Pyramid is one teaspoon of flaxseed oil, two teaspoons of canola oil or soybean oil, one tablespoon of ground flaxseed, or a quarter cup of walnuts.[1] Other good sources of omega-3 fatty acids can be found in table 11.3. If you decide to bump up those omega-3s at the expense of the omega-6s, keep in mind that dietary changes may not produce immediate results because it takes time to significantly alter the fatty-acid composition of your cells' membrane through diet, which is the fat storage source used to make inflammatory markers.

Vitamin D

Recent research reveals that vitamin D, in addition to its major influence on bone, also plays a role in modulating the body's inflammatory and immune responses.[17] Vitamin D, however, appears to exert its anti-inflammatory effect by blocking

Box
11.4

Arthritis and the Athlete

Arthritis is one of the most prevalent chronic disease conditions in the United States and other countries and is the leading cause of disability in the United States. The two most common types of arthritis are osteoarthritis and rheumatoid arthritis. The major differences between the two types are that osteoarthritis is not systemic (bodywide) or autoimmune in origin but involves cartilage destruction with asymmetrical inflammation and is caused by joint overuse. Rheumatoid arthritis is a systemic autoimmune disorder that results in symmetrical joint inflammation. Understanding arthritis and its prevention may be important for athletes striving to stay injury free.

Osteoarthritis is formally known as degenerative arthritis or degenerative joint disease and is the most prevalent form of arthritis. It is developed through a chronic process characterized by softening of the joint cartilage. It typically affects the joints of the knees, hips, ankles, and spine, which bear the bulk of the body's weight. The elbow, wrist, and ankle are less often affected. The early stage of osteoarthritis is marked by stiffness after standing and when rising from a chair. Inflammation occurs at times, but it is not a primary symptom of this condition. Although some research has found that sports or strenuous activities that subject joints to repetitive high impact and loading increase the risk of degeneration of the joint cartilage,[33] this appears to be somewhat controversial.

Rheumatoid arthritis is a debilitating and frequently crippling disease that is less common but often more severe than osteoarthritis. It occurs more frequently in women than in men, with the peak onset commonly occurring between 20 and 45 years.[19] It typically affects cartilage, bone, tendons, and ligaments as well as the synovial membranes and blood vessels. Although the etiology of rheumatoid arthritis is unclear, it is known to be a chronic systemic autoimmune disorder and may be provoked by a virus or by constant stress, from obesity or inappropriate strenuous exercise, that initiates the inflammatory process. The inflammatory process, which involves cytokines, is also thought to play a role.[13] Chronic inflammation appears to begin in the synovial membrane and then progress to subsequent damage in the joint cartilage. Epidemiological studies have documented that development of the disease in the northern hemisphere is more common in winter than in summer, as are exacerbations of the disease.

production of the inflammatory cytokines (at the gene level), and regulating the function of certain inflammatory cells.[25] Because of this, vitamin D may also be important in maintaining healthy muscles and joints over the long haul and aiding in controlling chronic joint inflammation. Like in the case of the omega-3s, studies have not yet addressed the importance of vitamin D in acute or chronic sport

TABLE 11.3 **Plant Sources Rich in Omega-3 Fatty Acids**

Food	Portion	Total fat (g)	Omega-6 (g)	Omega-3 (g)
Canola oil	1 Tbsp	14	2.8	1.3
Flaxseed	2 Tbsp	8.2	1.0	4.3
Flaxseed oil	1 Tbsp	13.6	1.7	7.3
Hemp seed oil[§]	1 Tbsp	14	2.5	7.0
Soybean oil	1 Tbsp	13.6	6.9	0.9
Walnuts, English*	7 halves (14 g)	9.2	5.4	1.3
Walnut oil*	1 Tbsp	13.6	7.2	1.4
COMMERCIAL PRODUCTS**				
FlaxPlus Multibran Cereal (Nature's Path)	3/4 cup	1.5	na	0.5
FlaxPlus Waffles (Nature's Path)	2 waffles (78 g)	9		1.0
Flax and soy granola cereal, (Zoe's)	1/2 cup	5	na	2.2

[§]Obtained from product label, information not contained on USDA nutrient database.

*English walnuts, but not black walnuts, are a good source of omega-3 fatty acids.

**Commercial products with added flax or hemp are becoming available in local, national, and international markets.

Use these values to convert English measurements to metric: 1 Tbsp = 14.2 g; 1 cup = ~230 g (see appendix E).

Data from "Reports by Single Nutrients," *USDA National Nutrient Database for Standard Reference, Release 18.* Available: http://www.ars.usda.gov/Services/docs.htm?docid=4451

injuries. Several large-scale studies, however, have found that vitamin D protects against cartilage loss and disease progression in people with knee osteoarthritis[21] and favorably reduces symptoms[40] and risk of disease in people with rheumatoid arthritis.[24] Although the mechanism of action of vitamin D is likely to be different in the two types of arthritis, the findings illustrate the potential impact of vitamin D status on joint health and inflammation. In osteoarthritis, vitamin D most likely acts to prevent the softening of the joint cartilage, whereas in rheumatoid arthritis it most likely acts to reduce immune response and inflammation.

It is not known how much vitamin D is needed for healthy joints. The Vitamin D Council recommends that blood concentrations of 25-hydroxyvitamin D be maintained above 80 nanomoles per liter (approximately 30 ng/mL), which can be accomplished by sensible sun exposure (usually 5 to 10 minutes of exposure to the arms and legs or the hands, arms, and face two or three times a week) or regular intake of foods fortified with vitamin D or supplements[18] (see chapter 6). Vitamin D supplementation at the level of 2,000 international units (IU) per day[9] might be worth trying if you are experiencing bone, joint, or tendon problems, including swelling and stiffness.

Antioxidants and Anti-Inflammatory Agents

Many plant products—including fruits, vegetables, plant oils, and herbs—contain specific nutrients or phytochemicals that may have antioxidant or anti-inflammatory properties. Antioxidants—including vitamins C and E—protect body tissues, which include muscles and joints, against free-radical damage and possibly also age-related degeneration. Anti-inflammatory agents, on the other hand, block or reduce the inflammatory response, acting in a manner that is either similar to or different from the action of nonsteroidal anti-inflammatory agents, aspirin, and ibuprofen[2] (see box 11.5). It is not known whether dietary antioxidants or anti-inflammatory agents can help prevent or reduce symptoms associated with sport or overuse injuries. Several studies, however, have found that high intakes of antioxidant vitamins, especially vitamin C, protect against cartilage loss and disease progression in people with osteoarthritis of the knee.[22] Vitamin D has the same effect. Smaller studies also suggest that many plant products, most notably pomegranate fruit extracts,[2] may slow cartilage deterioration and reduce inflammation associated with both osteoarthritis and rheumatoid arthritis. Because trials to establish the efficacy and optimum dosage of these compounds for treating human inflammation are currently needed,[2] your best bet is to ensure that your diet is rich in a variety of fruits and vegetables, including tomato products, and contains olive

---

Box 11.5

Herbs and Plant Products With Proposed Anti-Inflammatory Properties

➤ Basil

➤ Olive oil, which contains oleocanthal in newly pressed extra virgin versions

➤ Willow bark, which contains salicin, the chemical in aspirin

➤ Pomegranate fruit

➤ Green tea (epigallocatechin-3-gallate)

➤ Cat's claw

➤ Thunder god vine

➤ Turmeric (curcumin)

➤ Ginger

➤ Tomatoes and tomato-based drinks (Lyc-O-Mato)

Selected list of plant and herb products that may have anti-inflammatory properties. This list is not meant to be inclusive or be an endorsement for product use. It was compiled from various sources.[2, 3, 5, 27, 29]

oil and fresh herbs and spices. Giving green tea, ginger tea, pomegranate juice, and dishes with basil and olive oil a try may not hurt. Beyond that, stay tuned for this research to evolve.

Considering Supplements

If you have recurring painful or swollen joints or have been diagnosed with arthritis (see box 11.4), chances are you have heard about or even considered taking the dietary supplements glucosamine or chondroitin sulfate or both. Both are sold to reduce joint pain and improve joint function and are even thought to stimulate cartilage synthesis or perhaps inhibit its breakdown. Although their mechanism of action is unknown, both play a role in joint function. Glucosamine is an amino sugar that may help form and repair cartilage, whereas chondroitin is part of a protein that aids in the elasticity of cartilage. Chondroitin also attracts water, providing a cushioning effect within joints.

Whether these supplements are beneficial for the long-term treatment of non-specific joint pain or arthritis, however, is still open to debate. For the most part, studies have found that the combination of glucosamine and chondroitin may produce positive effects for many people with joint pain.[23] One study found that 12 weeks of supplementation with glucosamine alone provided pain relief and improved function in patients with prior cartilage injury or osteoarthritis or both.[7] Another large-scale government-funded study in people with knee arthritis found that supplementation with a combination of both substances for 24 weeks reduced pain only in those with the most severe pain.[12] While both glucosamine and chondroitin are not commonly vegetarian—glucosamine is commonly derived from shrimp shells, and chondroitin sulfate is extracted from shark cartilage—vegan and vegetarian versions are available from several companies (type in vegan glucosamine and vegan chondroitin on your web browser). I, however, am still holding out for a study that compares the effects of omega-3 fatty acids, vitamin D, and plant antioxidants to those of glucosamine and chondroitin. I won't even tell you which I think will be more beneficial.

If you are prone to muscle cramps or muscle or joint inflammation, my hope is that this chapter provided you with ideas on how diet may help prevent or alleviate these maladies. We next discuss how you can incorporate all the information we have covered thus far into a healthy vegetarian meal plan.

12

Creating a Customized Meal Plan

The women's athletic trainer asked me to see a 22-year-old tennis player to determine whether her weakness, fatigue, and history of frequent infections were related to her diet. Like several of the vegetarian athletes I had worked with, she was from Germany—apparently a good place to live if you are a vegetarian athlete. She had a hearty appetite and reported eating a diet that consisted mostly of bagels with European cheese, potatoes, rice, pasta, cereal, dense crusty bread (if she could get it), and lots of vegetables. She said she consumed at least two servings of dairy products a day but typically ate fruit only in the morning. She was also a coffee drinker and admitted to recently adding a little fish to her diet to see if it would help her fatigue. She was not interested in taking a multivitamin (as recommended by her coach). Despite her fatigue and regular infections, she denied any real detriment to her playing record.

Although her eating habits were not too bad, her meal plan needed revising. Without a doubt she was getting ample carbohydrate, but I was a little concerned about her protein, iron, and zinc intake. Because results from a routine blood analysis were pending—and would have provided only a basic screening for anemia—I could not directly determine whether her diet was the cause of her frequent infections. I could, however, work with her to customize a meal plan that would better provide all of the essential nutrients. I felt that the overall nutritional quality of her diet could be improved by including legumes, nuts, fruit, and power house vegetables, such as leafy greens and orange and red vegetables, and limiting coffee to one or two cups (236-472 ml) daily. I recorded in my nutrition note that we reviewed pyramid-style eating (vegetarian-style), emphasizing easy ways to add fruit and plant-protein foods to her current plan.

The task of eating well can be daunting for many athletes. There are indeed a zillion nutrients to consider—or at least it may seem that way—along with the additional nutrition guidelines for athletes. You need enough carbohydrate to fuel high-intensity activity, enough protein to build body tissue, including muscle, and enough but not too much energy in the form of calories. You also need the right balance of dietary fat and an adequate intake of calcium, iron, iodine, zinc, riboflavin, vitamin C, vitamin K, and many other vitamins and trace minerals. On top of that you need to think about all those phytochemicals. Or do you?

Quite honestly, what you need is a game plan: a meal plan upon which to build a healthy diet to ensure that you get enough of the right kinds of macronutrients (carbohydrate, fat, and protein), micronutrients (vitamins and minerals), and phytochemicals. The meal plan should set the framework and help you develop an eating pattern for a busy vegetarian athlete and then set you free to eventually eat well intuitively. Indeed, the purpose of this chapter is to help you put together all the pieces discussed in this book to come up with a customized eating plan. The remaining step, which will be covered in chapter 14, is learning how to whip up quick meals and snacks that fit into your customized game plan.

Pieces of a Healthy Diet

Various eating plans have been developed to teach people how to meet nutrient needs through good food choices. These food guidance systems have been available in the United States since before the 1930s and have included the basic four food groups and the original USDA Food Guide Pyramid.[3] Although the design of the earlier food guidance systems made it difficult to personalize a nutrition plan—particularly for a vegetarian—the new tipped-over USDA pyramid, now called MyPyramid, emphasizes that one size does not fit all. Although most food guidance systems developed by the government or private entities were designed for an average citizen, not an athlete, we can borrow and easily customize a plan for vegetarian athletes using MyPyramid or any of the vegetarian pyramids. Before we begin, however, it is important to first understand the pieces that contribute to a healthy diet: food groups and variety.

Why Food Groups?

In my earlier days as a nutritionist I failed to recognize the importance of food groups. In fact, I was disturbed by some of the categories: the meat group for obvious reasons and the fruit and vegetable groups, which incorrectly categorize many fruits—including tomatoes, squash, and pumpkin—as vegetables. It was not until I taught my first college-level sports nutrition course to exercise science and health promotion students that it hit me—during my own lecture—just how ingenious this system is. Maybe you are a faster learner than I am, but foods are grouped into major categories based on the key nutrients that those foods contribute to the diet (see table 12.1). Although some variability exists among the different foods in each category, this system *guides* people to select a variety of foods from each group to meet their nutrient needs so that they can enjoy eating food rather than trying to remember which foods provide B vitamins, protein, or iron. The estimated number of servings from each category was determined by nutritionists based on how much food from each food group people need to consume to meet daily nutrient needs. Indeed, although fruit is a great source of many nutrients, if fruits alone made up the bulk of your diet (or your calories) instead of grains, you might lack B vitamins, iron, and zinc even though you would get ample carbohydrate, fiber, and vitamin C. Therefore, what you need to do is choose foods from each category and use them to create individual meals and snacks.

Admittedly, I am not always enthralled with the category names and mandatory inclusion of the dairy group—because they are somewhat limited for vegans and vegetarians—but I do find that the food categories in general make considerable sense. Basically, the grain group includes cereals, bread, pasta, rice, and all other whole- or milled-grain products, which provide carbohydrate, some protein, iron, potassium, zinc, copper, thiamin, niacin, riboflavin, folate, vitamin B_6, biotin, and vitamin E. The meat and bean group (which is called the beans [legume] and meat analogue group from this point forward) provides protein, iron, zinc, thiamin, niacin, and vitamins B_6 and B_{12}. The fruit group is divided from the vegetable group based on their carbohydrate and general nutrient profile, which are slightly different. The only group arguable is the milk and dairy group because certain foods from each of the other categories, with the exception of fruit and oil, can contribute significantly to calcium intake (see figure 12.1). Dairy foods do however provide a source of riboflavin and vitamin B_{12} for vegetarians. The final group is the discretionary calorie group, which includes sweets, fats, and even sport supplements. Unfortunately, lumped within the same category in MyPyramid are nuts and healthy oils, which should be included in higher levels in an athlete's diet, along with added processed sugars, trans fats, and other "junk" items that should be limited in the diet.

Why Variety?

Although the concept of variety has been discussed in other parts of this book, I mention it here briefly to emphasize that the additional piece of a plan for healthy eating includes the selection of a variety of foods from each major food category. Because there are no perfect foods, the variety of components increases an athlete's chance of taking in adequate vitamins, minerals, and phytochemicals. For example, although walnuts are the only nuts high in omega-3 fatty acids, the other nuts provide different oils and alpha- and gamma-tocopherols (vitamin E derivatives) that also contribute to a healthy diet. Spinach—which is not an absorbable source of calcium—is one of the top sources of folate, vitamin B_6, beta-carotene, lutein, vitamin E, and magnesium. In addition, fruits and vegetables lacking in

TABLE 12.1 Key Nutrients Provided by the Food Categories Used in Most Food Guidance Systems

Category	Nutrients provided by group	Food and typical servings
Grains	Carbohydrate Protein (some) Minerals: iron, potassium, zinc, copper, selenium,* iodine* Vitamins: thiamin, niacin, riboflavin, folate, B_6, biotin, E Phytonutrients Whole grains also provide fiber, magnesium, chromium, vitamin E.	**1 equivalent =** 1 slice bread 1/2 cup cooked grain, rice, or pasta 1 oz ready-to-eat cereal
Vegetables	Carbohydrate (starchy vegetables) Fiber Minerals: iron, potassium, zinc, selenium,* iodine* Vitamins: A and carotenoids, C, folate, and K Phytonutrients Dark-green leafy vegetables also provide riboflavin, vitamin B_6, magnesium.	**By MyPyramid** **1/2 cup vegetables =** 1/2 cup raw or cooked vegetable or juice 1 cup raw leafy greens **By Vegetarian Food Guide Pyramid** 1/2 cup cooked = 1 cup raw
Fruits	Carbohydrate Fiber Vitamins: A and carotenoids, B_6, C, folate (selected fruits) Phytonutrients	**1/2 cup fruit =** 1 medium fruit 1/2 cup cut fruit or fruit juice 1/4 cup dried fruit
Milk	Protein Minerals: calcium, iodine, potassium Vitamins: Riboflavin, B_{12}, biotin, A, and D (fortified)	1 cup milk or yogurt 1 1/2 oz natural cheese
Meat (for comparison)	Protein Minerals: iron, zinc Vitamins: thiamin, niacin, B_6, B_{12}	1 oz any type of meat
Beans (legumes) and meat analogues	Protein Minerals: calcium, iron, magnesium, potassium, zinc, copper, molybdenum Vitamins: folate, thiamin, niacin, riboflavin, B_6, biotin	**1 protein equivalent =** 1/2 cup legumes 1/2 cup tofu or tempeh 2 Tbsp nut or seed butter 1/4 cup nuts 1 oz meat analogue 1 cup soy milk 1 egg 1 oz cheese
Nuts	Protein Fiber (some) Minerals: iron, calcium, magnesium, zinc, copper, chromium, selenium* Vitamins: folic acid, vitamin E, other tocopherols Essential fatty acids: linoleic acid, linolenic acid	**1 protein equivalent =** 1/4 cup nuts
Healthy oils	Essential fatty acids: linoleic acid, linolenic acid Vitamin E	1 tsp

*Content of selenium and iodine vary significantly depending on the content of the soil.
Serving sizes obtained from MyPyramid and the Vegetarian Food Guide Pyramid.[2]
Refer to appendix E for guidance on converting English units to metric.

one type of anti-inflammatory phytochemical are high in a phytochemical that enhances the body's ability to detoxify cancer-causing agents. Thus, the more variety, the better!

Helpful Models for Vegetarian Athletes

Teaching vegetarian athletes what their meal plan should look like can be a bit more challenging than educating nonvegetarian athletes. First, for vegetarians in general, the framework of what makes up a nutritious meal is not always there—particularly for those who grew up in a meat-centered household where the response to "what's for dinner?" was answered based on the meat being served. "Chicken" was for dinner rather than "chicken, rice pilaf, garden salad, and whole-grain bread." This way of thinking often leaves new vegetarians with the idea that they need to have a meat analogue for dinner and that rice pilaf with almonds and leafy greens cannot stand alone as a meal. My husband is still known to say, "We did not have any protein tonight," and then have to listen as I recall the content of all the protein-rich plant foods in the meal along with the nuts and occasional egg and cheese in the seemingly "no protein" dishes.

Second and third, few food guidance systems for vegetarian athletes exist, and those that do exist are of limited use to vegans and vegetarians who consume little dairy. For example, the vegetarian version of one food plan for endurance athletes recommends that vegetarian athletes consume 5 to 10 one-cup (236 ml) servings of milk products per day, depending on their energy intake.[1] This is a little more milk than most vegetarian athletes desire or tolerate. The other limitation in existing systems is that they are not flexible enough to allow athletes to tailor their intake of carbohydrate, protein, and fat to their training requirements. For example, as a 52-kilogram (115 lb) female endurance athlete, my carbohydrate and protein needs on a 3,000-calorie diet are different than those of a 65-kilogram (143 lb) softball player during her strength-building season. Although we're both consuming 3,000 calories, I might need more carbohydrate, and the softball player might need a bit more protein.

That said, however, I have successfully used many of the food guidance systems—including the USDA Food Guide Pyramid and the food plate, used in the United Kingdom and a few other countries—to help vegetarian athletes develop a custom plan or to simply fine-tune their current eating plan. Although my personal favorite is the food plate model, I have found that both models serve a purpose and depend on the athlete's background, sex, and ability to eat intuitively. In looking over many of the nutrition notes I kept on the college and local athletes I've counseled over the years, I found that I most often used the food pyramid model with athletes who needed structure or who needed to lose weight. In contrast, I used the food plate more with people who were intuitive eaters—meaning they were able to maintain a healthy weight without much thought—but just needed some education on what their plates should look like. It also looked as if I discussed the food pyramid more with women and the food plate more with men. Although I never used a specific vegetarian version of the pyramid or plate (because I didn't like any that were available at the time), I admittedly would have found much benefit in the Vegetarian Food Guide Pyramid published in 2003 by Messina, Melina, and Mangels (see figure 12.1).[2]

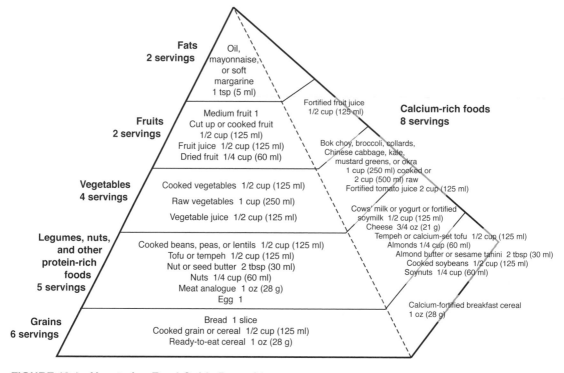

FIGURE 12.1 Vegetarian Food Guide Pyramid.

Customizing Your Meal Plan

Although MyPyramid, the Vegetarian Food Guide Pyramid, and the food plate model each present limitations to vegetarian athletes, they can guide you in customizing your meal plan and learning to eat intuitively. This section discusses how you can use either MyPyramid or the Vegetarian Food Guide Pyramid to put together a custom meal plan. Then we will discuss how the food plate model can be adapted for a more intuitive eating approach.

Your first step for customizing a meal plan is to estimate your energy needs using one of the methods discussed in chapter 2 and to round your estimate to the nearest 200 calories. It is also helpful to estimate your carbohydrate and protein needs as discussed in chapters 3 and 5. The next step is to consult table 12.2 to obtain the recommended number of servings you need to consume from each of the major groups if using MyPyramid (top of table) or the Vegetarian

TABLE 12.2   Creating a Meal Plan Using the USDA Food Guide Pyramid or the Vegetarian Food Guide Pyramid

Amount of food from each major food group, based on MyPyramid, required to satisfy various caloric needs for active vegetarians.

Calories per day	1,800	2,000	2,200	2,400	2,600	2,800	3,000
Bread	6 eq (oz)	6 eq (oz)	7 eq (oz)	8 eq (oz)	9 eq (oz)	10 eq (oz)	10 eq (oz)
Vegetables	2 1/2 cups	2 1/2 cups	3 cups	3 cups	3 1/2 cups	3 1/2 cups	4 cups
Fruits	1 1/2 cups	2 cups	2 cups	2 cups	2 cups	2 1/2 cups	2 1/2 cups
Milk	3 cups	3 cups	3 cups	3 cups	3 cups	3 cups	3 cups
Beans and analogues	5 eq	5 1/2 eq	6 eq	6 1/2 eq	6 1/2 eq	7 eq	7 eq
Tabulation							
Carbohydrate range (g)*	256	271	288	311	332	352	386
Protein range (g)**	78-97	81.5-101	87-108	92.5-115	98.5-124	104-131	106-134
Discretionary calories	195-290	265-310	265-310	265-310	360-510	360-510	360-510

Amount of food from each major food group, based on Vegetarian Food Guide Pyramid, required to satisfy various caloric needs for active vegetarians.

Bread	6 eq (oz)§	6 eq (oz)	7 eq (oz)	8 eq (oz)	9 eq (oz)	10 eq (oz)	10 eq (oz)
Vegetables	2 cups	2 1/2 cups	3 cups	3 cups	3 1/2 cups	3 1/2 cups	4 cups
Fruits	2 cups	2 cups	2 cups	2 cups	2 cups	2 1/2 cups	2 1/2 cups
Beans, nuts, and analogues	5 eq	6 eq	6 eq	7 eq	7 eq	8 eq	8 eq
Fat§	2	2	2	2	2	2	2
Tabulation							
Carbohydrate range (g)*	227.5	247.5	270	292.5	318	355	365
Protein range (g)**	63-82	70-90	74-96	83-107	87-113	96-124	99-127

Servings sizes for MyPyramid obtained from USDA MyPyramid (www.mypyramid.gov). Serving sizes for the Vegetarian Food Guide Pyramid were modified from the original source by V. Messina, V. Melina, and A Mangels[2] (figure 12.1) by adding additional servings of various food groups as energy needs increase.

§Values in this column for each group are the minimum amounts, according to the Vegetarian Food Guide Pyramid, necessary to meet nutrient needs for nonathlete vegetarians. Vegetarian Food Guide Pyramid fat servings do not increase as calories increase because it is a minimum requirement.

*Carbohydrate content is estimated using the methods described in chapter 3, assuming half of the vegetable servings are starchy and half are not, half of the protein servings are from legumes, and half the milk (if appropriate) is from carbohydrate-rich milk or plain yogurt (rather than from cheese). Carbohydrate content under each energy level can be increased by selecting mostly starchy (carbohydrate-rich) vegetables and adding discretionary carbohydrate sources, including simple sugars and sport drinks, bars, and gels.

**Protein content is estimated using the methods described in chapter 5 where each protein and milk equivalent provides 7-8 g protein and each grain and starchy vegetable provides 2-3 g protein.

Refer to appendix E for guidance on converting English units to metric.

Food Guide Pyramid (bottom of table). If your energy needs are greater than 3,000 calories per day you can use the 3,000-calorie recommendations as a starting point because, as we will discuss later, these servings are an estimate of the *minimum* number of servings needed in each group for a healthy diet. Thus, you will simply follow a 3,000-calorie diet but eat larger portions at each meal. You can also consult table 12.3 if you need ideas for which food groups could be added to extend calories.

In deciding which pyramid to consult, I recommend using MyPyramid if you regularly consume two to three servings of milk, yogurt, or cheese daily and the vegetarian version if you are vegan or consume few milk products. Just as an aside, one advantage to using MyPyramid is that it has an interactive online version (www.mypyramid.gov) that allows you to print out custom worksheets and use MyPyramid Tracker to perform an in-depth assessment of your diet quality. In fact, if you decide to use MyPyramid as your framework, using the downloadable worksheets for a few weeks may be all you need to get you on the track of intuitive eating.

Once you have an idea of your estimated daily servings from each category, the next step is to begin customizing your plan on paper. An example of a 3,000-calorie diet based on MyPyramid is shown in table 12.4, and table 12.5 shows a

TABLE 12.3 Food Combinations That Provide 250 Additional Calories

Combination	Example	Actual nutrients in example
Bean (protein)—1 equivalent (eq) Fruit—1 cup Healthy oil—1 tsp	1/2 cup black beans 1 cup pineapple 1 tsp hemp seed oil	228 kcal 8 g protein, 5 g fat, 40 g carbohydrate
Bean (protein)—1 eq Healthy oil—1/2 tsp	1 cup pinto beans 1/2 tsp canola oil	165 kcal 15 g protein, 2.5 g fat, 44 carbohydrate
Grain—2 eq Nuts—1 oz	1 cup white rice 1 oz walnuts	287 kcal 6 g protein, 18 g fat, 26 g carbohydrate
Grain—2 eq Healthy oil—1 tsp	2 slices whole-grain bread 2 tsp trans-fat-free margarine	222 kcal 6 g protein, 11 g fat, 26 g carbohydrate
Starchy vegetable—1 cup Healthy oil—1 tsp	1 large sweet potato 1 tsp hazelnut oil	222 kcal 9 g protein, 9 g fat, 37 g carbohydrate
Fruit—1 cup Dairy or soy milk—1 cup Healthy oil—1 tsp	1 cup peaches in own juice 1 cup yogurt 1 tsp flaxseed oil	250 kcal 11 g protein, 5 g fat, 40 g carbohydrate
Healthy oil—2 Tbsp	1 Tbsp flaxseed oil 2 Tbsp ground flax seeds	230 kcal 23 g fat

The energy and macronutrient values are approximate and will vary depending on actual food choices. They will also vary depending on the accuracy of portion sizes. Refer to appendix E for guidance on converting English units to metric.

3,000-calorie diet based on the Vegetarian Food Guide Pyramid. The easiest way to start customizing your plan is to start with each group, such as the grain group, and divide the suggested number of servings into meals and snacks, remembering to include nutrition you'll take in during exercise, if appropriate. Keep in mind that there will also be room for added fats and discretionary calories depending on your energy needs. In the sample plan in table 12.4, 3 of the 10 grain equivalents were placed in the breakfast meal, 3 in the lunch meal, and 4 in the dinner meal.

TABLE 12.4 3,000-Calorie Vegetarian Meal Plan Using MyPyramid

Meal	Categories and suggested servings	Sample plan 1	Sample plan 2
Breakfast	Grain—3 equivalents (eq) Fruit—1/2 cup Milk—1 serving	2 slices whole-wheat toast 1 Tbsp no-trans-fat margarine* 1 oz cornflakes 1 cup skim milk 1 medium orange	3 (5-inch) pancakes 1 Tbsp no-trans-fat margarine* 2 Tbsp maple syrup* 1/2 cup blueberries 1 cup vanilla nonfat yogurt
Morning snack	Fruit—1 cup Protein—1 eq	1/2 cup raisins 1 oz almonds	1 large apple 2 Tbsp peanut butter
Lunch	Protein—2 eq Grain—3 eq Milk—1 serving Vegetable—1 cup	Vegetarian burger (60 g) on a large poppy seed bagel 1 1/2 oz cheddar cheese 2 cups mixed greens 2 Tbsp Italian dressing*	1 cup marinated and baked tofu with 1 tsp sesame oil* 1 1/2 cups wild rice 1 cup steamed yellow squash 8 oz skim or soy milk
Afternoon snack	Vegetable—1 cup	1 cup baby carrots 1 Tbsp ranch dressing*	1 baked potato topped with 2 Tbsp light sour cream*
Dinner	Protein—3 eq Grain—4 eq Milk—1 serving Vegetable—2 cups	1 1/2 cups black beans with 1/2 cup onions 2 cups long-grain rice with 1 Tbsp olive oil* and topped with 1/2 cup tomato 1 cup steamed spinach 1 cup skim milk	1 1/2 cup lentil taco mix with 1/2 cup onion 4 (6 in) tortillas 1 oz cheddar cheese 1/2 cup each tomato, red bell pepper, green bell pepper, and lettuce
Evening snack	Fruit—1 cup Protein—1 eq	1 cup sliced bananas 1 oz walnuts 1/2 cup frozen yogurt*	Large baked pear 1 oz pecans Brown sugar*

*Discretionary calorie items

Sample meal plan 1 provides ~3,066 kcal (56% carbohydrate, 30% fat, 14% protein), 442 g carbohydrate, 114 g protein, 105 g fat (7% saturated), 4.6 grams omega-3 fats, 1,348 mcg folate, 141 mg vitamin C, 27 IU vitamin E, 1,728 mg calcium, 32 mg iron, 15 mg zinc, and 797 mg magnesium. It also provides more than the RDA for men and women athletes for riboflavin (3.7 mg), vitamin B_6 (3.9 mg), and vitamin K (1,190%) and adequate levels of other trace minerals.

Sample meal plan 2 provides ~3,065 kcal (55% carbohydrate, 29% fat, 16% protein), 442 g carbohydrate, 125 g protein, 110 g fat (7% saturated), 2.4 grams omega-3 fats, 1,062 mcg folate, 299 mg vitamin C, 12 IU vitamin E, 2,118 mg calcium, 31 mg iron, 18 mg zinc, and 624 mg magnesium. It also provides more than the RDA for men and women athletes for riboflavin (2.5 mg), vitamin B_6 (2.9 mg), and vitamin K (94.7%) and adequate levels of other trace minerals. Refer to appendix E for guidance on converting English units to metric.

TABLE 12.5 3,000-Calorie Vegan Meal Plan Using the Vegetarian Food Guide Pyramid

Meal	Categories and suggested servings	Sample plan 1	Sample plan 2
Breakfast	Grain—3 equivalents (eq) Fruit—1/2 cup Protein—1 eq	2 slices whole-wheat toast 1 Tbsp no-trans-fat margarine* 1 oz cornflakes 1 cup fortified soy milk 1 medium orange	3 (5 in) pancakes 1 Tbsp no-trans-fat margarine* 2 Tbsp maple syrup* 1 oz vegetarian sausage 1/2 cup calcium-fortified orange juice
Morning snack	Fruit—1 cup Protein—1 eq	1/2 cup raisins 1 oz almonds	1 large apple 2 Tbsp peanut butter
Lunch	Protein—2 eq Grain—3 eq Vegetable—1 cup	Vegetarian burger (60 g) on a large poppy seed bagel 2 cups mixed greens 2 Tbsp Italian dressing*	1 cup marinated and baked tofu with 1 tsp sesame oil* 1 1/2 cups wild rice 1 cup steamed yellow squash
Afternoon snack	Vegetable—1 cup	1 cup baby carrots 2 Tbsp tofu-based dip*	1 baked potato topped with 2 Tbsp soy sour cream*
Dinner	Protein—3 eq Grain—4 eq Vegetable—2 cups	1 1/2 cups black beans 2 cups long-grain rice with 1/2 cup onions and 1 Tbsp olive oil* and topped with 1/2 cup tomato 1 cup collard greens	1 1/2 cups lentil taco mix with 1/2 cup onion 4 (6 in) tortillas 1/2 cup each tomato, red bell pepper, green bell pepper, and lettuce
Evening snack	Fruit—1 cup Protein—1 eq	1 cup sliced bananas 1 oz walnuts 1/2 cup Soy Dream dessert*	Large baked pear 1 oz pecans 1 Tbsp brown sugar*
Training snack	Other	2 cups fluid-replacement beverage*	1 cup fluid-replacement beverage*

*Discretionary calorie items

Sample menu 1 provides ~2,972 kcal (60% carbohydrate, 28% fat, 12% protein), 461 g carbohydrate, 91 g protein, 98.9 g fat (4% saturated), 4.2 grams omega-3 fats, 1,258 mcg folate, 151 mg vitamin C, 29 IU vitamin E, 1,125 mg calcium, 29 mg iron, 12 mg zinc, and 630 mg magnesium. It also provides more than the RDA for men and women athletes for riboflavin (1.9 mg), vitamin B$_6$ (3.1 mg), and vitamin K (1,114%) and adequate levels of other trace minerals.

Sample menu 2 provides ~3,055 kcal (55% carbohydrate, 31% fat, 13% protein), 434 g carbohydrate, 104 g protein, 112 g fat (5.5% saturated), 3.6 grams omega-3 fats, 991 mcg folate, 320 mg vitamin C, 16.5 IU vitamin E, 1,630 mg calcium, 30 mg iron, 14 mg zinc, and 516 mg magnesium. It also provides more than the RDA for men and women athletes for riboflavin (2.9 mg), vitamin B$_6$ (3.8 mg), and vitamin K (114%) and adequate levels of other trace minerals. Refer to appendix E for guidance on converting English units to metric.

Once you have placed all of the groups, list several ideas for foods and mixed dishes for each group. I admit that this is easier to do when lunch consists of a cheese sandwich made with two slices of bread and one and a half ounces (42 g) of cheese instead of vegetable and cheese pizza or stir-fry. Because combinations of foods from two or more food groups are common in our diet, you will need to estimate how much of each of the different food types is in the dish to determine how it fits into a pyramid-style meal plan. For example, a slice of vegetable and cheese pizza contains a serving of grain in the crust, a half to a full serving of protein in the cheese and an eighth cup or so of vegetables, depending on how loaded with vegetables it is. It is also likely to be fairly high in fat and thus contain some discretionary calories. Learning to properly count mixed foods is easiest if you prepare the foods yourself and can then estimate what went into the recipe and how much of that recipe you had for dinner. And while making your estimates, it is hoped that you will also recognize, based on your food plan, that if you have pizza, it is best served as a part of a meal consisting of a huge green salad and an additional source of carbohydrate, such as French bread, fruit, or fruit juice.

In coming up with sample menu ideas, you should also evaluate whether the plan seems reasonable for you—based on your preferences and training schedule—and whether it is too structured. Although most plans specify a greater number of servings of vegetables than fruits because of the higher nutrient density and phytochemical content of vegetables compared with fruit,[2] the sample 3,000-calorie plans have too many vegetables and not enough fruit for my lifestyle. With three kids, I find it is much easier to grab several colorful pieces of fruit than to prepare and eat the recommended vegetable servings. I also feel that the argument in favor of more vegetables than fruit is a moot point if you regularly include legumes in your diet. So I swap a few fruits for a few vegetables. Furthermore, if this sample plan calls for more dairy products than you would like, you could drop one or two and simply include calcium-rich greens—as part of your vegetables—on the days you don't consume much dairy. Indeed if this plan appears too restrictive—because, for example, you don't want to be stuck with a vegetable every day for a snack—you can either grin and bear it for a few weeks or try the checklist approach (see figure 12.2). I say grin and bear it because this meal plan is something you should try to stick to for several weeks or months as you learn to incorporate this healthy eating pattern into your lifestyle. Over the weeks, you will learn to intuitively select a variety of different foods at meals and throughout the day.

The checklist approach, on the other hand, is a more flexible method of ensuring that you get adequate servings from each group. I counseled both a female volleyball player and a male mountain bike police officer who found it helpful to use a daily checklist. Although both of these athletes were checking off foods to ensure that they made good choices and did not overeat, all athletes can use the checklist to ensure that they eat foods that will meet their nutrient needs. The checklist is something you use for just a short time and reinstate later if your eating habits begin to stray off-track. Within a short period you will most likely find—as I do—that you can keep the checklist in your head to help you make healthy choices throughout the day.

The last piece of the plan is to pencil in how you will meet specific personal nutritional goals that are not included in the pyramid plan (see box 12.1). Examples include meeting your vitamin D needs by spending a little time in the sun or increasing your intake of omega-3 fatty acids.

Daily Target

Grains _____ **servings (1 oz, 1 slice, 1/2 cup)**

Vegetables _____ **cups (raw or cooked)**

*1 cup leafy greens = 1/2 cup

Fruit _____ **cups (1/2 cup = 1 medium fruit)**

Milk and dairy _____ **1 cup milk or 1/1/2 oz cheese**

Omega-3 fats _____ **g**

DAY OF WEEK _____					
Grains					
Vegetables					
Fruit					
Milk and dairy					
Protein					
Healthy oils					

Instructions: Carry in pocket or purse or post on refrigerator. Check box after eating a snack or meal. Strive to meet daily target (at a minimum). Refer to appendix E for guidance on converting English units to metric.

FIGURE 12.2 **Sample checklist for recording food intake.**

From _Vegetarian Sports Nutrition_ by D. Enette Larson-Meyer, 2007, Champaign, IL: Human Kinetics.

Box
12.1

Tips for Meal Planning

> See table 12.2 for a list of the estimated number of servings from each major food group required to satisfy various calorie needs for active vegetarians. Choose additional foods from any of the groups or from the discretionary calorie group as needed to meet energy needs.

> Choose a variety of foods from the major food groups.

> If you do not consume dairy products, choose five to eight servings per day of calcium-rich foods. Those conveniently listed in the third dimension of the Vegetarian Food Guide Pyramid provide approximately 10 percent of an adult's daily requirements. A more extensive list of calcium-containing plant foods is in chapter 6.

> To meet iron needs, follow the pyramid plan and select a variety of iron-rich grains and legumes. Aim to consume a fruit or vegetable that contains vitamin C along with most meals to boost absorption. See chapter 7 for more information.

> Incorporate healthy fats in cooking and in dressing up foods and limit foods that are high in saturated and trans fats (as suggested in chapter 4).

> Include foods rich in omega-3 fatty acids as discussed in chapter 4 and shown in figure 4.4.

> Although not mandatory, a daily serving or two of nuts is a good idea, unless you have nut allergies. Nuts add additional energy, healthy fats, and an abundance of other nutrients (see table 12.1). Servings of nuts and seeds can also serve as a source of protein and be used in place of servings from the fats group for people limiting energy requirements.

> If you are vegan, include at least three good sources of vitamin B_{12} in your diet every day. These include one tablespoon (15 ml) of Red Star T6635 nutritional yeast, one cup (236 ml) of fortified soy milk, one ounce (28 g) of fortified cereal, and 1.5 ounces (42 g) of fortified meat analogue. Servings for vegetarians include half a cup (118 ml) of cows' milk, three-quarter cup (172 g) yogurt, and one egg.

> Use iodized salt when cooking and in salting foods, particularly if you live in an area where the concentration of iodine in the soil is low.

> Get adequate vitamin D from daily sun exposure or through fortified foods or supplements. Use of vegetarian vitamin D is controversial (see chapter 6).

> Get most of your daily calories from the foods in the Vegetarian Food Guide Pyramid. One-third to one-half should come from whole food sources. Limit consumption of overly processed foods, which contain added sugars, high-fructose corn syrup, and unhealthy fats.

It is important to reemphasize that the plan is just a plan. It estimates what you need, and around this framework you will strive to make good food choices that will include mixed dishes and possibly also alcohol (see box 12.2). You will add or subtract foods and servings based on your training and your hunger level. As an athlete, your energy needs fluctuate daily with your training schedule and your nonsport activities. Attempting to follow a rigid meal plan would be crazy. This is one of the difficulties experienced by researchers doing controlled studies on athletes. For instance, in one of my studies I used myself as a subject and placed

---

Box 12.2

How Do Coffee, Tea, and Alcohol Fit In?

There is nothing wrong with a little coffee, tea, wine, or beer. Consumed in moderation, all can be included in a healthy sport diet and may even provide health benefits. Although most people are aware of the abundance of antioxidants found in both green and black tea, some people may not yet know that several healthful phytochemicals have also been isolated from coffee. I suppose we should not be surprised, because most plant foods seem to deliver their own set of unique phytochemicals. Similarly, although most people know about the health benefits of wine, which are at least partially linked to a certain class of antioxidant called flavinoids and found in grapes, others may not yet know that higher-quality microbrewery or European-style beer (not the watered-down versions produced by the major U.S. breweries) is also chock full of nutrients and nonnutrients originally found in the hops or malted barley.

So how should these fit into your meal plan? Quite simply, they provide mostly discretionary calories. Although coffee and tea are basically calorie free, the sugar or cream added should be included in the discretionary group. For the latte or cappuccino fan, the amount of milk or soy milk mixed with your espresso is nearly equal to one milk serving. Wine and beer offer calories from alcohol (7 kcal/g) as well as some carbohydrate.

When you should consume these beverages is another story. Because many of the components in tea and coffee potently inhibit iron absorption, they should not accompany a meal. Wine and beer do not appear to interfere with nutrient absorption, but you should limit them as suggested by the *Dietary Guidelines for Americans:* up to one drink per day for women and up to two drinks per day for men. Typically, 12 ounces (348 ml) of regular beer, 5 ounces (145 ml) of wine, or 1.5 ounces (43.5 ml) of 80-proof distilled spirits count as a drink. Although there are no hard-and-fast guidelines for tea and coffee, limiting intake to one or two cups (236-472 ml) per day is also a good idea. Athletes should also recognize that the postexercise meal period is not the best time to consume alcohol or caffeine-containing beverages because the body needs to rehydrate. Coffee and tea, however, may provide an ergogenic benefit when consumed before an event (see chapter 10).

myself on a 2,800-calorie diet. Indeed, 2,800 calories met my needs the first two days—when I was sitting at my desk—but on the third day, when I spent a little time gardening, it was not nearly enough. By 5:00 I had consumed all of the food in my research bag and was starved the rest of the evening. Therefore, the final step in the planning process is to begin following your custom meal plan while remembering that this plan provides a framework and does not list everything you are supposed to eat. At times you will need to supplement your diet with healthy oils and additional carbohydrate-rich foods, including sport products and healthy desserts to meet your training needs. Additional or larger servings of the foods listed are, of course, also appropriate.

The tabulation of the estimated carbohydrate and protein content provided for each calorie level (table 12.2) should help you determine whether you need to add more carbohydrate, protein, or fat. For the sample 3,000-calorie plans shown in tables 12.4 and 12.5, healthy oils, healthy desserts, and fluid-replacement beverages were added to increase calories and carbohydrate. It is interesting to note, however, how much more room there is for these foods when milk is eliminated from the diet and that you can eliminate milk and still meet or exceed calcium recommendations. The additional milk and dairy, however, help increase the protein content of the vegetarian meal.

This brings us to a final question of whether athletes should develop customized meal plans for rest days. My answer is to play it by ear. In my experience, many athletes with high energy needs actually eat more, not less, on their regularly scheduled rest days. A rest day allows them to catch up because it can be a struggle to maintain neutral energy and carbohydrate balance on vigorous training days. Athletes with varied training or work schedules, and therefore varied energy needs, might develop a maintenance plan based on an energy level that includes regular physical activities but not training and then simply increase portions or add sport supplements and healthy desserts according to their hunger on training days.

Learning to Eat Intuitively

If you feel that the pyramid method takes too much planning or is simply not your style, you might find that the food plate model is just what you need to learn to eat well intuitively. What I like about the food plate is that it seems less burdensome than the pyramid and some athletes, notably football players and cyclists, seem to accept it more readily. To begin using the food plate, you need to be familiar with the food group categories discussed and be able to visualize your lunch or dinner plate divided in thirds (see appendix B). On a healthy athlete's plate, grains are piled on one-third, or slightly more, of the plate, and fruits and vegetables together are piled on another third. The remaining third contains a combination of protein-rich sources, dairy, healthy oil, dessert, and even additional grains. The problem, of course, is that this takes visual imagination and makes it more difficult to specify calorie level or to emphasize or limit particular foods in each category.

Nevertheless, I have found that visualizing a healthy plate or cereal bowl helps athletes pack healthier lunches, cook healthy dinners, and make better selections at restaurants or buffet meals. As a quick example, if I were serving black-bean chili for dinner, which is a source of protein and is also a vegetable, visualizing the plate might remind me to serve the chili over rice or with corn bread, to add grains, and with a leafy green salad or fruit salad or a healthy dessert.

Further Assistance with Meal Planning

You are lucky to live in a day and age where most of the foods you select at the grocery store "wear" nutrition labels and where accurate nutrition information is at your fingertips. Both resources can help you figure out how specific foods— particularly mixed and unusual foods—fit into your meal plans.

Using Food Labels

Food labels—as you are aware—provide information on the nutrient content as well as the ingredients in most food products available in supermarkets. Most consumers are familiar with the nutrition facts label that lists the serving size by weight or volume; the number of servings in the container; the calorie content and grams of protein, carbohydrate, and fat and milligrams of sodium in a serving; and the percentage of Recommended Daily Allowances for at least eight nutrients. Although the nutrition facts are somewhat intuitive, it is important for athletes to remember to check serving sizes because the size of a serving is often small and to keep in mind that many of the percentages given are for a reference individual on a 2,000-calorie diet. You can, however, use the grams of carbohydrate, protein, saturated fat, trans fat, and total fat to help determine how the product fits in with the rest of your daily requirements and whether the food is a good source of a particular nutrient, such as calcium, iron, or zinc. These nutrients are listed only as a percentage of the daily value (%DV), but the actual amount in milligrams or micrograms can be calculated using the information listed in table 12.6. As an example, the cereal in figure 12.3 provides 17%DV for calcium. Because the DV for calcium is 1,000 milligrams, the cereal provides 170 milligrams of calcium (0.17 × 1,000 mg = 170 mg). Also, without performing calculations, you can tell from the %DV that this product is a decent source of calcium. A good nutrient source provides 10% to 19%DV, and a high source provides more than 20%DV.

The ingredient list is the other component of a food label. It lists the ingredients in the food product in descending order by weight. Hence, ingredients listed first are present in the largest amounts in the food, and those listed last in the smallest amounts. The labels, however, do not indicate how much of any ingredient is included in the food. Although the average consumer often ignores the ingredients list, it can be helpful in many instances. For example, the ingredients list can help vegetarian athletes get an idea of how much of a multigrain product contains whole grains, determine if a product labeled trans free is truly trans free (as dis-

TABLE 12.6 Reference Values for Nutrition Labeling

Nutrient	Daily value (DV)
Saturated fatty acids	20 g
Cholesterol	300 mg
Sodium	2,400 mg
Potassium	3,500 mg
Total carbohydrate	300 g
Fiber	25 g
Protein	50 g
Vitamin A	5,000 IU
Vitamin C	60 mg
Calcium	1,000 mg
Iron	18 mg
Vitamin D	400 IU
Vitamin E	30 IU
Vitamin K	80 mcg
Thiamin	1.5 mg
Riboflavin	1.7 mg
Niacin	20 mg
Vitamin B_6	2.0 mg
Folate	400 mcg
Vitamin B_{12}	6.0 mcg
Biotin	300 mcg
Pantothenic acid	10 mg
Phosphorus	1,000 mg
Iodine	150 mcg
Magnesium	400 mg
Zinc	15 mg
Selenium	70 mcg
Copper	2.0 mg
Manganese	2.0 mg
Chromium	120 mcg
Molybdenum	75 mcg
Chloride	3,400 mg

Food labeling is based on a 2,000 kcal intake for adults and children at least 4 years old. From the US Food and Drug Administration. Available: http://www.cfsan.fda.gov/~dms/flg-7a.html.

cussed in chapter 4), and see if a food product contains animal products. If you are interested in learning more about the vegetarian purity of specific common ingredients, the Vegetarian Resource Group offers a *Guide to Food Ingredients* for a nominal fee (www.vrg.org). Food ingredient lists are also important for athletes

Nutrition Facts
Serving Size: 1 oz (about ▢ cup) healthy grain flakes alone and in combination with ▢ cup vitamin D fortified skim milk
Servings Per Container: about 12

Amount Per Serving	Cereal	Healthy Flakes with 1/2 cup skim milk
Calories	100	140
Calories from Fat	15	20
	% Daily Value**	
Total Fat 1.5g*	2%	2%
Saturated Fat 0g	0%	0%
Trans Fat 0g	0%	0%
Polyunsaturated Fat 1.1g		
Monounsaturated Fat 0.5g		
Cholesterol 0mg	0%	0%
Sodium 190mg	8%	11%
Total Carbohydrate 22g	7%	9%
Dietary Fiber 7g	28%	28%
Sugars 6g		
Protein 4g		
Vitamin A	0%	6%
Vitamin C	0%	0%
Calcium	2%	17%
Iron	15%	15%

*Amount in cereal. One-half cup of skim milk contributes an additional 40 calories, 65mg sodium, 6g total carbohydrate (6g sugar), and 4g protein.
**Percent Daily Values are based on a 2,000 calorie diet. Your daily values may be higher or lower depending on your calorie needs:

		Calories	2,000	2,500
Total Fat	Less than		65g	80g
Sat Fat	Less than		20g	25g
Cholesterol	Less than		300mg	300mg
Sodium	Less than		2400mg	2400mg
Total Carbohydrate			300g	275g
Dietary Fiber			25g	30g

Calories per gram
Fat 9   Carbohydrate 4   Protein 4

Ingredients: Organic whole-wheat flour, organic corn, organic wheat bran, organic evaporated cane juice, organic flaxseed, organic oat bran, organic barley malt extract, rice extract, sea salt, tocopherols (natural vitamin E).

FIGURE 12.3   **Sample nutrition facts label and ingredient list.**

with allergies or intolerances to food products or preservatives such as monosodium glutamate.

Using the USDA or Other Nutrient Databases

The USDA National Nutrient Database for Standard Reference is one of the best sources for looking up accurate information on food products. It is available free online and allows athletes to quickly look up the nutrient profile for specific foods. It is a great source for looking up produce or for checking the nutrient profile of a common oil (before you mail order it). For example, if you wonder if it is worth it to give up your iceberg lettuce and switch to darker greens, you could do a quick comparison of iceberg and see that among other things, iceberg has 10 times less vitamin A per serving than red-leaf or other darker greens. The database, however, is not perfect. It is missing several common vegetarian foods (or has them listed in unusual ways) as well as international foods such as hemp seed oil and vegemite. Information on the nutrition content of many products can also be found at food company Web sites or by contacting the company.

After finishing this chapter you should feel equipped to customize a vegetarian meal plan to support your current training. Although the remaining step—covered in chapter 14—is learning how to whip up quick meals and snacks, you should first consult chapter 13 if you are unhappy with your current body weight.

13

Adapting the Plan to Manage Weight

She came to see me for weight loss in early January of her freshman year. She had gained a little more than 30 pounds (14 kg) during the fall season, and it was difficult to hide even on her 5-foot, 11-inch (180 cm) frame. She was under the impression—based on something her parents had said over the holiday break—that her weight gain was "caused by the carbohydrate." Because I had worked closely with the team in the preseason and during the season, I had an idea that there was more to the story. I knew it was not because of carbohydrate, unless there had been an abundance of the nutrient.

As we spoke further about her first semester on the volleyball team, it came out that she—like the majority of freshman players—traveled frequently with the team but spent more time sitting on the bench than playing. When the team went for their postgame meal, she feasted as much, if not more, than her upperclassmen teammates who had played most of the game. And yes, even though her choices had been fairly healthy, she simply ate more calories than she was expending. Part of it, she admitted, was eating because everyone else was eating. The other part, however, was eating out of frustration and boredom. It is never easy sitting on the sidelines when you really want to play.

Weight struggles and issues with body weight in athletes are not unusual. Nearly three-fourths of the athletes I saw as a nutritionist for a college team came to me for concerns about weight loss or weight gain. Of course, this is a biased sample because I did not see all athletes, but it illustrates that many athletes, despite hours of hard training, are not immune to weight-related issues. Vegetarian athletes are no exception. Although some athletes struggle with real issues that may be caused by poor eating habits or a particular genetic makeup different from their desires, other athletes struggle with issues related to unrealistic expectations—either their own or those of their coaches or parents. Although it is true that excess weight can hinder performance in some athletic activities, athletes do not and should not feel that they need to fit a specific mold or body type in order to be a good athlete. This section focuses on how a vegetarian meal plan can be adapted when necessary to promote weight loss or weight gain and ultimately assist in lifelong weight management. It also briefly addresses the relationship between body weight and performance and discusses conditions in which weight-loss or weight-gain efforts may not be appropriate.

Physics of Weight Management

Simply put, weight maintenance is a matter of balancing the energy consumed with the energy spent. Body weight changes when there is a long-term imbalance between energy consumed from foods, beverages, and supplements and calories expended during training and the activities of daily living. Losing one pound (0.45 kg) of body fat requires an energy, or caloric, deficit of 3,500 calories. To lose this much in one week, there must be a negative balance of 500 calories each day. This is accomplished by eating less, being more active, or a combination of the two. To gain this much as body fat, there must be a positive balance of at least 3,500 calories.

That said, however, some people can overeat a bit on occasion and manage to avoid gaining weight, whereas others gain weight every time they eat an excess calorie. The difference in these people is mainly related to their ability to waste, or burn off, some of the excess energy consumed. The person who gains weight puts nearly every excess calorie into his or her body fat stores. The resistant gainer, on the other hand, increases his or her metabolism enough that a smaller proportion of the excess calories is stored as body fat. The average person wastes about 12 percent of the excess energy consumed and thus banks about 78 percent of the excess calories.[12, 13] The other important factor is that the resistant gainer may—without even thinking about it—increase physical activity or fidgeting after overeating, thereby spontaneously increasing energy expenditure. The opposite is true to some extent with regard to weight loss. The resistant reducer loses a bit less than predicted because metabolism slows somewhat to fend off weight loss, and he or she may even subconsciously decrease physical activity level. These reactions do not occur in the person who loses weight easily. What causes these differences in metabolism in response to overeating or calorie restriction is not well understood but is likely related to variations in enzymes and hormones that regulate metabolism, including skeletal muscle energy-generating enzymes, thyroid hormone, and sympathetic nervous activity.

It should be stressed, however, that although these differences in metabolism exist in response to energy restriction or energy excess, they are small relative to the big picture and do not support the contention that a person can achieve a 3,500-calorie deficit with no effect to his or her weight. Instead, these differences in metabolism explain why two college athletes with similar energy needs who splurge on 500-calorie ice cream sundaes every night for two weeks (in excess of their energy requirements, of course) gain different amounts of weight, or why a person who eats 500 calories less than needed every day for a week loses three-quarters of a pound instead of the predicted pound. And if you are wondering if your sex makes a difference—it does. Women are more likely to gain weight easily and have a difficult time losing it. But that is a generality. Some men have what we call a conservative metabolism that makes it easier for them to gain weight, and some women have a wasteful metabolism that makes it easier for them to lose it. If truth be told, I have worked with male athletes who struggle to keep weight off and female athletes who are able to eat *everything* they want but cannot gain an ounce. Indeed, in our weight-conscious, food-abundant society, these women are considered lucky; however, during a famine, their faster metabolisms wouldn't serve them so well.

Overweight Issues for Vegetarian Athletes

Beyond the basic concept of energy balance, the prevention of weight gain and the promotion of weight loss are not simple issues, even for athletes. Although it is true that athletes typically expend a lot of energy, they are still subject to both overeating and a sedentary lifestyle when they are not training. One or a combination of both can promote a positive energy balance that either leads to weight gain or prohibits body fat reduction. As mentioned earlier, some athletes are more destined to weight gain because of their genetic makeup, which can include the tendency to overeat, move less, or efficiently bank excess energy. As a group, athletes appear to be particularly prone to weight gain during their freshman year of college and after experiencing a major injury, undergoing surgery, taking a new job, getting married, having children, or going through menopause. Although the reasons for weight gain are different for each athlete, typically stress, boredom, and the habit of eating a lot are somehow involved. My father, a former football player, for example, is overweight because he still eats as if he is training for the Fiesta Bowl.

Although it is true that a small percentage of athletes may experience problems with the thyroid—the gland that produces the important energy hormone thyroxin—in association with weight change, most people gain weight simply because they eat more than they move. For example, freshmen athletes commonly gain weight during their first year because they play less during games or matches yet eat as much as their junior and senior teammates. Adult athletes often gain weight because real-life responsibilities either decrease the time they have to exercise or provide an environment that encourages overeating. From personal experience, I can testify that vegetarian athletes are also destined to gain weight if they shift uninformed to a vegetarian eating pattern. As you can imagine, weight gain is inevitable when you sprinkle sunflower seeds and cheese on everything just to ensure that you get enough protein.

Deciding Whether You Need a Weight-Loss Plan

Weight reduction is a different ballgame for athletes than it is for nonathletes. If you or your coach believe that you need to lose weight, it is important that you first seriously consider whether your weight-loss goals are necessary or realistic. I have worked with too many athletes who believe that they need to weigh a little less to run faster or look better in their team uniform. These athletes are not really candidates for a weight-loss diet, but for one that directs their focus toward better eating habits. Although studies have found a negative relationship between body fat and athletic performance that requires the body to be moved in space, the relationship is actually weak, explaining 9 to 49 percent of the variation in performance during various running and jumping activities.[15] Also because studies were typically conducted in cross-sectional groups of active people,[15] not competitive athletes, the results should not be taken to mean that you will perform better if you go on a "diet" to lose a few pounds of fat. You may instead lose lean tissue along with fat tissue. And loss of lean mass, if it is muscle that is important to acceleration, power, or other aspects of sports performance, could decrease performance. Loss of body fat can also be detrimental. Body fat serves as padding in contact sports and loss of too much fat may increase your injury rate and, in combination with a negative energy balance, alter the circulatory pattern of hormones including estrogen and testosterone.

Thus, the bottom line is that you should consider reducing your weight only if you have recently gained weight (not associated with puberty) and you are not performing as you did before. You may also consider modifying your diet according to a weight-loss plan if you have been slightly overweight your whole life, providing you are persistent in your efforts to improve your eating habits so that you can achieve a healthy body weight over the long haul. In that case, you are probably someone who gains easily and has a difficult time losing, so you will need to overcome your body's desire to store excessive calories by learning to eat just what you need. If you are an athlete with a stable body weight within the normal range and you perform decently, however, you should not embark on weight-loss efforts with the idea that you will perform or look better if you just drop a little weight. Part of being a strong and successful athlete is learning to accept your body for what it is and making the most of it through participation in athletics. Athletes come in all sizes and shapes!

Pieces of the Weight-Reduction Plan

The meal plan for an athlete trying to lose weight is similar to the meal plan for any athlete, but it contains slightly fewer calories than are necessary to maintain weight. Exactly how many fewer depends on your body size or total energy requirements and training and performance goals. I firmly believe that athletes should not restrict calories during the regular season or peak season, unless of course they have been benched, are sitting out that season, or are not expecting a peak performance that season. Restricting calories is a goal for the preseason and off-season. During this time, athletes on a weight-reduction plan should strive to eat 300 to 500 calories per day less than their required energy needs, which would promote a weight loss of about half a pound to a pound (0.22-0.45 kg) per week. Athletes weighing more than 200 or 250 pounds (90-112 kg) can get by restricting up to—but no more than—1,000 calories a day, which should promote a reduction of one to two pounds (0.45-0.9 kg) per week. An athlete wanting to cut weight or body fat during the season should instead strive to improve his or her eating habits, and

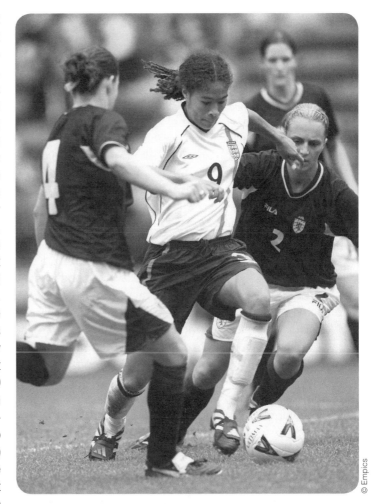

© Empics

Weight loss does not necessarily ensure improved performance. Many factors go into the decision to try to lose or gain weight.

then embark on weight-loss efforts during the off-season. Although it is common for athletes in certain sports to restrict calories to make weight or cut body fat, this practice is not healthy and may result in poorer-than-expected performance.

The biggest mistake an athlete can make during his or her efforts to reduce body weight or body fat is to choose a diet that excludes one or more of these vital nutrients: carbohydrate, protein, vitamins, minerals, and, yes, even fat. Another mistake is to follow a diet that excessively restricts calories. The next sections discuss why a balanced diet is vital to your performance and why weight loss should occur slowly.

Get Your Carbs   Carbohydrate is the only fuel that can sustain the moderate to high level of activity that is required in most sport and athletic endeavors and is the one preferred by the brain and central nervous system. Excessively restricting carbohydrate diminishes your ability to train long and hard, which most likely will come back to haunt you. For example, if you go out for an hour run with low glycogen reserves caused by a low-carbohydrate weight-loss plan, chances are you will run at a lower percent effort and cover fewer miles. This, of course, will burn fewer calories and, unless it is your easy day, induce less of a training effect. If you have enough energy to make it through the run, you most likely will finish the workout more tired than usual and seek the comforts of your couch or cozy office chair and be less likely to expend effort (calories) getting out of the chair to walk down the hall, up the stairs, or into the kitchen. If you somehow make it into the kitchen, your carbohydrate-craving liver and muscles will most likely strain your willpower and . . . well, you get the idea—suddenly you are eating ravenously.

How much carbohydrate you need on your weight-loss plan depends on your body weight and level and type of training, but a good general rule is to eat about one or maybe two grams of carbohydrate per kilogram of body weight *less* than you should be striving for (see table 3.1 on page 27). For example, a 242-pound (110 kg) baseball player would most likely require six to seven grams of carbohydrate per kilogram body weight (660 to 770 g of carbohydrate) during preseason training. If this athlete wants to reduce his body weight, he should strive to consume five to six grams of carbohydrate per kilogram of body weight (550 to 660 g of carbohydrate). This would reduce his caloric intake by 440 calories (4 kcal per g × 110 g of carbohydrate) and be close to the 500-calorie deficit recommended to lose about a pound (0.45 kg) a week. You will know you have restricted carbohydrate intake too much if you experience early fatigue during your training or note a rapid change in your body weight. Typically, losing a pound or two over the course of a day or two can be attributed to the lost water weight that occurs when glycogen stores in the liver and muscle are low. This happens because every gram of glycogen in the muscle and liver is stored along with three to four grams of water. So if you reduced your body's glycogen stores by 500 grams, you would notice a 1.5- to 2-kilogram (3.3 to 4.4 lb) weight loss almost overnight.

Get Your Protein   Although the obvious goal of a weight-reduction plan is to restrict the intake of energy and energy-producing nutrients, this does not hold true for protein. During active weight loss, when your energy balance is negative, you may need to increase the percentage of calories you take in as protein to help reduce the loss of muscle tissue and to prevent your resting metabolic rate from slowing. This is because more dietary protein is "burned" for energy when the body has a negative energy balance, resulting in less protein available for building and repairing lean body tissue. Thus, extra dietary protein during weight loss spares body protein. In addition, some researchers believe that protein, compared to fat and carbohydrate, may help you feel fuller sooner, produce alertness, and requires that your body expend more energy to digest and metabolize a meal (called the thermic effect of food).[4] Hence, a little extra protein may be advantageous during weight loss.

Unfortunately, although most experts agree that there may be an advantage to including more protein in an energy-restricted diet, it is not known just how much protein is beneficial for a typical dieter, let alone an athlete. Nevertheless, it has been my experience that athletes fare well when they strive for a protein intake in the upper range recommended for endurance or strength athletes (see chapter 5) and emphasize protein from higher-quality sources. What this means is that vegetarian athletes may want to consider eating complementary proteins at most meals during active weight loss. Although this is not necessary when energy is balanced because the limiting amino acids consumed from a single plant source are buffered by the body's amino acid pools, it may be beneficial during weight loss when these amino acid pools are not as plentiful because of the lower energy intake combined with the body's increased use of protein for energy. Although no research currently supports this suggestion, it does not take much effort to complement or eat higher-quality proteins because these foods are a natural part of our culture (see chapter 5 for further detail).

Include Fat Judiciously   Although it is true that we should reduce dietary fat during weight loss, particularly to ensure that we get enough carbohydrate and protein, athletes should by no means attempt to follow a diet that is nearly fat free. The main reason is because humans like fat. It tastes good and allows us to enjoy eating, even when we are trying to drop a few pounds. If we deprive ourselves of fat by eating the bread without the olive oil or having the raisins without the walnuts, we may be setting ourselves up for an "I can't stand the deprivation any longer" binge. That said, however, athletes also need to recognize that a substantial amount of research suggests that it is easier to overeat fat-containing foods.[17]

Therefore, you should continue to include small amounts of smart fat choices—nuts, seeds, flavorful oils, full-fat soy products, and strongly flavored cheeses—in your daily diet, but cut back on fat-containing foods, such as chips, crackers, fried tofu, or any food that triggers the "I have to eat the whole thing" effect. In fact, if you have a binge food, such as ice cream, chocolate, or cashews, avoid bringing them into your house or keeping them in your desk drawer, or purchase them only in very small packages.

Include Fruits, Vegetables, Vitamins, Minerals, and Energy-Dense Foods   When you restrict your energy intake, you increase your chance of taking in inadequate amounts of vitamins, minerals, and phytochemicals. You can avoid the low-vitamin-and-mineral trap if you continue to eat nutrient-dense fresh and frozen fruits and vegetables—without limits. These foods are also high in soluble and insoluble fibers, which may promote satiety. Athletes who struggle in their decision about which foods to eliminate or reduce to create a calorie deficit may want to emphasize low-sugar, low-starch vegetables such as carrots, cooked and fresh leafy greens, onions, tomatoes, and parsnips and cut back on fruit juice and starchier vegetables. Athletes who restrict energy may also want to consider taking a multivitamin and mineral supplement even though it is typically only imperative for those consuming less than 1,200 calories a day.

Drink Plenty of Fluids and Cut Back on Supplements   As mentioned in chapter 9, it is important to drink enough fluids daily to keep well hydrated. This is additionally important during weight loss because the body's need for fluid is often misinterpreted as a desire to eat. During weight reduction, drink plenty of water throughout the day and avoid high-calorie fluids, such as regular soda, sweetened tea, and full-fat milk. Also drink fluid-replacement beverages only when needed, for example, during a long training session. These and other sport supplements add calories and may even suppress fat oxidation during and after exercise. When you are actively seeking weight loss, it is better to drink water and snack on carbohydrate- and protein-rich snacks such as a banana with peanut butter and dairy or soy yogurt with fresh fruit. Save the supplements for when you need them.

Watch Portion Sizes   As mentioned earlier, an eating plan that promotes healthy weight loss should look like the meal plan in chapter 12 but contain slightly fewer calories than required to maintain weight. Thus, if you already eat well, you may simply want to watch your portion sizes. If you don't eat well, you should go ahead and create a meal plan for weight reduction. It is interesting to note that the amount of food considered to be a normal portion has escalated over the past 20 or 30 years. Research from the Department of Nutrition, Food Studies, and Public Health at New York University has found that portion sizes in eating establishments are now two to eight times greater than recommended serving sizes.[26] This has also influenced what we consider to be normal at home. Because you consume more calories when more food is on your plate, you can reduce energy intake simply by putting less on your plate and focusing on smaller portions. Although this may be difficult in certain social situations, for example, when eating with your running buddies or when celebrating with the team at the postgame meal, remember that everyone has a different metabolism. Either find a vegetarian buddy to split a healthy meal with or take half of it home for the next day. Another option is to choose a healthy soup and salad or a small entree with steamed vegetables. And by all means, avoid all-you-can-eat buffets, even if their options for vegetarians are limited.

Go Slowly   If you are an overweight athlete, losing slowly is not necessarily the message you want to hear. College athletes and students in my sports nutrition course have often asked me why an athlete shouldn't simply go on a more extreme low-calorie diet for six to eight weeks during the off-season and be done with it. Why prolong this "dieting thing"? Although there are probably a zillion reasons to go slowly, the first and most important reason not to rush things is that these extreme diets do not typically contain real foods and thus do not teach athletes how to make the appropriate changes to their eating and lifestyle habits necessary for long-term success. Second, rapid weight loss tends to promote greater loss of valuable lean tissue or muscle than does slower weight loss and also does not allow for much training apart from moderate walking. No athlete wants to lose muscle and also experience a six-to-eight-week detraining effect. Chances are they may never perform the same again. Third, athletes are typically overachievers. If you placed one on a 1,000-calorie diet, he or she would strive for 500, which could endanger his or her life. I saw an extreme case in which a football player placed himself on an extremely low-calorie diet after being called "fatty" by his coach. By the time the team physician referred him to me, he had been consuming just a six-inch (15 cm) sub sandwich and a liter of soda daily for eight weeks. He had dangerously elevated concentrations of creatine phosphate, an enzyme that dwells in skeletal and cardiac tissue and is released with tissue damage. Indeed, he dropped 30 pounds, but he had been experiencing such an amazing breakdown of muscle tissue that he could have ended up with acute renal failure. The final reason is simply that lowest-energy diets do not always bring about the best weight-loss results because they reduce lean mass, resting energy needs, and spontaneous physical activity. They are rarely successful.

Creating or Modifying a Plan for Weight Loss

A meal plan customized for weight reduction helps athletes determine an energy level that promotes healthy weight loss (see box 13.1). To customize your meal plan for weight reduction, estimate your energy needs using one of the methods discussed in chapter 2, subtract 500 to 1,000 calories (according to the information discussed on page 198), and round your estimate to the nearest 200 calories. Use this target energy level to obtain the recommended number of servings you need to consume from each of the major food groups as shown in table 12.2 (page 177) and to develop a pyramid-style meal plan designed specifically for weight loss. For example, if the estimated daily energy needs of a female synchronized swimmer were approximately 2,550 calories per day during her off-season, she would subtract 500 calories from her daily needs to promote weight loss and then round 2,050 to the nearest 200 calories to come up with a 2,000-calorie target. Her plan should contain six grain equivalents, 2.5 cups (575 g) of vegetables, two cups (460 g) of fruit, three cups (708 ml) of milk, and 5.5 to 6 servings of protein (if using MyPyramid). A sample menu showing both a vegetarian and vegan 2,000-calorie-per-day weight-loss plan is shown in table 13.1. Remember that with any plan, you may need to adjust the carbohydrate or protein foods a bit to meet your training needs and may also add additional servings of leafy greens and other nonstarchy vegetables, which contain only 10 to 20 calories per half cup (115 g) serving. If you find you are starving on the plan, feeling fatigued, or dropping weight too quickly, you may have underestimated your daily energy needs and should adjust up by adding an additional serving or two of carbohydrate or protein depending on your training needs.

Other Tricks to Promote
Weight Loss or Maintenance

In addition to understanding the basic principles of weight loss and having a meal plan, a handful of other "tricks" or ideas may aid in weight loss or in weight maintenance following weight reduction. These are briefly reviewed in the following sections.

Box
13.1

Tips for Adopting a Plan
to Promote Weight Loss

➤ To promote a weight loss of about half to one pound (0.22-0.45 kg) per week, eat a well-balanced vegetarian diet that contains 300 to 500 calories per day less than you need. Larger athletes with higher energy expenditures can eat about 500 to no more than 1,000 calories per day less than needed. This will promote a reduction of one to two (0.45-0.9 kg) pounds per week. Customize the meal plan for weight reduction by estimating energy needs (using one of the methods discussed in chapter 2), subtracting 500 to 1,000 calories, and rounding to the nearest 200 calories. This calorie target can then be used to develop a pyramid-style meal plan as discussed in chapter 12.

➤ Eat plenty of fresh fruits and vegetables, which are packed with water, fiber, vitamins, minerals, and much more. You can add as many nonstarchy vegetables to the plan as you want because they add few calories.

➤ Learn to take smaller portions of food.

➤ Avoid the all-you-care-to-eat buffets.

➤ Drink plenty of water and other low-calorie beverages.

➤ Limit your intake of alcohol and sugar-containing beverages, including sport drinks.

➤ Spread food intake throughout the day and don't skip breakfast—or for that matter, lunch or dinner. Three meals and three snacks as shown in the sample meal plans may be appropriate for spreading out food intake.

➤ Keep a food log recording when and why you eat. The worksheets downloaded from the MyPyramid Web site (www.mypyramid.gov) may be useful for logging your daily progress in relation to your pyramid plan.

➤ Assess your nontraining physical activity. If needed, get off the couch!

➤ Watch emotional eating. If you feel like snacking, take a walk or have a cup of coffee or tea instead.

➤ Fix an enjoyable vegetarian meal, and splash on the flavored vinegar if desired.

➤ Watch your calcium. Although it is not a magic bullet, it ensures good bone health.

➤ Learn lifelong healthy habits that will help you maintain a healthy body weight. You will have greater success if you think you are following a healthy meal plan rather than a diet.

➤ Go slowly and don't look for magic.

TABLE 13.1 2,000-Calorie Vegetarian Meal Plan for Weight Loss

Meal	Categories and suggested servings	Vegetarian meal (using MyPyramid)	Vegan meal (using the Vegetarian Food Guide Pyramid)
Breakfast	Grain—2 equivalents (eq) Fruit—1/2 cup Milk—1 serving	1 slice (1 oz) whole-wheat toast 1 cup (1 oz) shredded wheat 1 tsp no-trans-fat margarine* 1 cup skim milk 1/2 cup sliced strawberries	1 multigrain English muffin (2 oz) 2 tsp no-trans-fat margarine* 1 Tbsp apricot preserves* 1/2 cup fortified orange juice
Morning snack	Fruit—1/2 cup Protein—1 eq	1/4 cup raisins 1 oz almonds	1 small apple 2 Tbsp peanut butter
Lunch	Protein—2 eq Grain—2 eq Milk—1 serving Vegetable—1/2 cup	1 cup mixed greens 1 Tbsp red-wine vinegar and 1 Tbsp olive oil* Vegetarian burger (60 g) on a French roll (2 oz) 1 cup milk	1/2 cup baby carrots Tofu-salad sandwich made with 1 cup firm tofu, 1 Tbsp soy mayonnaise, 1 Tbsp mustard* 2 slices whole-wheat bread
Afternoon snack	Fruit—1/2 cup	1 medium orange	1/2 cup unsweetened apple sauce 1 cup hot tea
Dinner	Protein—2 eq Grain—2 eq Vegetable—1 1/2 cups	1 cup vegetable soup 1 cup black beans with 1/4 cup onions 1 cup long-grain rice with 1 tsp canola oil* and topped with 1/2 cup tomato 1/2 cup steamed spinach drizzled with red-wine vinegar	1 cup black-eyed peas topped with 1/2 cup green onions 1 cup brown rice 1 piece homemade corn bread made with canola oil* 1 cup steamed collard greens
Evening snack	Fruit—1/2 cup Milk—1 serving	1/2 cup sliced bananas 1 cup nonfat yogurt 1 Tbsp honey*	1 small Asian pear 1 cup fortified soy milk* 1 ounce walnuts*

*Discretionary calorie items

Refer to appendix E for guidance on converting English units to metric.

Don't Skip Breakfast   You have been told this before, but now there is research to support it. Successful dieters report eating breakfast every day.[24] Eating a morning meal helps reduce later consumption of fat and minimizes impulsive snacking during the day. It is common for people who don't eat breakfast to make up the missed calories later in the day and even consume more calories than they would if they had eaten breakfast. And as an athlete, you need the additional energy and carbohydrate to help you perform your best. Be sure to include breakfast in your custom meal plan.

Start With a Low-Calorie, High-Volume Appetizer   Interesting research by Barbara Rolls—who has spent her career studying eating behavior and weight management—at Pennsylvania State University has found that consuming food or meals with a low energy density, measured in calories per gram of food, aids in weight control.[20] Our bodies, it seems, do not have calorie meters but rather volume meters, meaning that our hunger is satisfied by a certain volume of food, not a certain number of calories. Consuming foods with low energy density, such as certain fresh fruits and vegetables, whole-milled cereals and grains, legumes, and broth-based soups, helps us feel more satisfied with fewer calories than if we had eaten more dense foods, such as meats, cheese, pizza, ice cream, and candy. To incorporate this plan, try eating broth-based soup, yogurt, a leafy salad, or vegetable before or with each meal and make it a point to select more foods with a low energy density. Choosing foods with fewer calories per volume allows more satisfying food portions and—if you make good choices—more vitamins, minerals, and phytochemicals per gram of food. Note, however, that drinking a calorie-free beverage such as water or diet soda with a meal does not count toward the volume of food it takes to satisfy the appetite, as is commonly believed.[5] And consuming a calorie-containing beverage adds to the total calories of the meal. It seems our bodies are simply unaware of the volume that comes from a beverage.

Limit Alcohol   Conventional wisdom states that the cause of a "beer belly" may be just that: the alcohol in beer. Recent advertisements for low-carbohydrate beer, however, would like us to believe it is really the calories from carbohydrate and not the alcohol that increases our girth. Although it is true that excess calories cause weight gain, it is also true that alcohol intake can slow fat metabolism. In the early 1990s, a group of well-known energy metabolism researchers from Switzerland found that when alcohol was either added to the diet or substituted for other foods, 24-hour fat utilization decreased by nearly 33 percent in both cases.[21] Carbohydrate and protein metabolism were not affected. Energy expenditure was slightly increased (by 7 and 4 percent) but was not elevated enough to offset the effect of alcohol on fat balance. Although the researchers concluded that habitual consumption of ethanol in excess of energy needs favors fat storage and weight gain, the amount of alcohol used in the study (96 grams) was quite a bit higher than one would consume in a five-ounce (145 ml) glass of wine with dinner (16 grams). The effects of just one glass of wine or a microbrew, however, are not known. Nonetheless, other reasons to limit alcohol are that it may promote snacking[22] and reduce your body's ability to store muscle glycogen.[2]

Try Vinegar   Research is preliminary, but given that vinegar can enhance the flavor of many vegetables and vegetarian dishes, adding it to your diet may be worth a try. Swedish researchers recently found that consuming vinegar as part of a meal reduces the body's insulin response to carbohydrate and increases feelings of satiety following that meal.[14, 16] In this study, researchers had volunteers consume three different amounts of vinegar on different days in random order, the highest amount being two to three tablespoons (30-45 ml) along with 50 grams of high-glycemic carbohydrate from white bread. The researchers found that the higher the vinegar intake the greater the effects on dose response. Although these findings deserve follow-up, they suggest that adding vinegar to your meals may help you eat less and reduce cravings brought on by sugar peaks after meals. Try a vinegar and olive oil dressing on fresh greens. Drizzle it on top of cooked greens, legumes, or legume-based soups, or use it in pasta salads and rice dishes. Also, create a beverage by mixing a few tablespoons of a flavorful vinegar, such as raspberry, with plain or seltzer water. Vinegar-based drinks have recently taken off in Japan, owing to beliefs in their medicinal properties. Although vinegar is not likely to be the be-all and end-all for promoting weight loss, adding a bit to your meals may keep you on track and may also help boost iron absorption.

Wear a Pedometer   Sure, you spend a lot of energy training for your sport, but what do you do when you are not training? Wearing a pedometer to get an idea of how physically active you are during your nontraining time may benefit your weight-loss program. I have found in working with athletes that many are sedentary when not training. Quite a few drive everywhere, circle the parking lot to get the closest spot, and spend a lot of time sitting at a desk or on the couch. If you exert little physical effort except during training, a pedometer may help you learn to be more physically active. Your goal? First measure what you do now and then increase the value by 10 to 15 percent each week until you approach 10,000 steps. In addition to helping you control your weight, increasing your movement, particularly through walking, may also assist with active recovery because it increases blood flow to your hard-worked muscles. This helps provide a fresh supply of oxygen and other nutrients and removes lingering postexercise metabolites. As an athlete, however, keep in mind that you should increase your daily steps by walking more in your daily activities, including to and from practice, and not by engaging in racewalking. I don't want a call from your coach!

Write It Down   Research shows that monitoring the type of food you eat plays an important role in successful weight loss and maintenance. Writing down all the drinks and food you consume in a day, at least for a while, helps make you aware of the food you consume and why you consume it. Many weight-conscious people also feel that keeping food records keeps them accountable and helps them avoid binge foods because they don't want to have to write it down. As an athlete, writing it down also allows you to check the adequacy of your carbohydrate and protein intake.

Don't Count on the Calcium—Just Yet   Chances are you have seen the yogurt ads promising that three servings a day will help you squeeze into an "itsy bitsy, teenie weenie, yellow polka dot bikini." If not, maybe you have heard the news that a researcher from the University of Tennesee, Michael Zemel, has patented the idea that dairy products promote weight loss. Or maybe you've heard that the Physicians Committee for Responsible Medicine, a provegan medical group, is petitioning the federal government, saying the claims that dairy consumption promotes weight loss are false and misleading. What, then, does this mean to you as a weight-conscious vegetarian athlete? Right now it simply means don't count on the calcium, or maybe I should say *milk*.

Indeed, evidence is emerging of a link between dairy consumption and weight loss if you are fairly overweight or obese. Several recent clinical trials have found that consuming three or more dairy products markedly accelerates weight and body fat loss during caloric restriction.[27] In one study of 34 otherwise healthy obese adults, those who consumed three servings of light yogurt (for a total of 1,100 mg of calcium) daily lost 22 percent more weight and 61 percent more body fat than those on a similarly restricted low-dairy (500 mg of calcium) diet. Take caution, however, because the majority of evidence linking increased dairy and weight loss comes from animal or observational studies[27] and is not noted in all investigations.[6]

How calcium might affect weight loss is a good question. The theory is that a high-calcium diet—1,200 milligrams per day—inhibits the production of calcitriol, a hormone that tells cells to generate more fat. Conversely, on a low-calcium diet more calcitriol is released resulting in bigger, plumper fat cells. But supplements alone won't suffice. According to Zemel, you need to consume dairy foods because bioactive compounds in milk, yogurt, and cheese supposedly work with calcium to nearly double the effectiveness of fat burning and weight loss. Research studies, however, have never compared the weight loss effects of plant sources of calcium to dairy calcium and also have not looked at athletes who need to trim just a little weight. Stay tuned, I am sure there is more on the horizon.

Don't Think About the D Word   Believe it or not, one of the best ways you can achieve success is to forget the D word—diet, that is. Many people are done in by their "diets." They are overzealous, restrict too much, including their favorite foods, and suddenly begin cheating and maybe binging, and soon they are off the diet. Many even gain weight. Instead, stick to a healthy plan as suggested in this chapter that realistically restricts energy by no more than 500 or 1,000 calories per day. This promotes a slow weight loss and allows you to incorporate some of your favorite foods. If you crave ice cream, have a small dish. In the big picture, you are trying to improve your eating habits over the long term, which includes learning to make better choices more often and overeat less often—if ever.

Don't Look for Magic   Every week something new is thought to aid in weight loss or help you achieve a healthy body weight. Although some of these aids are harmless foods or products you may already be using, others have the potential to be costly or dangerous, even if they are natural. Take oolong tea,[7] green tea, coffee,[23] or hop extract for example. A recent study found that supplementing the diet of rodents with isomerized hop extract (containing isohumulones)—normally found in pale ales and other styles of beer—prevented weight gain in rodents.[25] In humans, a study conducted in the Netherlands found that people who consumed large amounts of caffeine (more than 300 mg) had greater success at reducing body weight, fat mass, and waist circumference (as well as maintaining resting energy expenditure) than did those who consumed little or no caffeine.[23] Certainly, if you already enjoy a glass of hoppy beer or cup of tea or coffee, relax and know it may help just a wee bit. If you don't, consider that the evidence is not strong enough for you to start taking hop, green tea, or caffeine pills. Furthermore, always use caution when considering new weight-loss information (just as you do with ergogenic aids and herbal supplements). A seemingly innocent weight-loss aid that has been in the news lately is bitter orange peel. This product, which is touted as an ephedra-free weight-loss agent elevates heart rate and blood pressure, especially when taken with caffeine, and may be nearly as dangerous as ephedra. The bottom line is to simply eat a well-balanced plant-based diet and know that there may be a bit of magic simply in some of what you're already doing.

Physics of Weight Gain

Unfortunately, it is safe to say that scientists know a lot less about the energy demands of muscle gain than they do about fat loss. We know that if you were to overeat 3,500 calories you should gain close to a pound (0.45 kg) of body fat, but most athletes are not looking to gain body fat. Furthermore, as mentioned earlier, there is considerable variation in the amount of weight that would be gained by consuming the extra 3,500 calories. Some would gain almost exactly one pound (0.45 kg) , and others, because they can "waste" a higher percent of the excess energy they consume, would gain a bit less. Gaining muscle, however, is somewhat more complex. One pound of muscle contains quite a bit less energy than fat—about 2,500 calories compared to 3,500 calories—but additional energy costs are required to promote gains in lean tissue. These include the cost to run the body's protein-making machinery, to arrange the amino acids consumed in the diet into the proper sequence, and to perform the resistance training that stimulates muscle gain. Thus, as much as I hate to say it, the caloric recommendations for weight gain are not based on a lot of hard science. Typically, to keep things simple and allow for a fudge factor of some sort, most practitioners use a figure of 3,500 calories to represent the cost of gaining one pound of muscle tissue.

We do, however, know quite a bit about the potent stimuli for promoting muscle growth, often called *anabolism,* which includes feeding (as compared to fasting) and resistance training. Although feeding alone is not sufficient to induce muscle growth—otherwise most people in the Western world would look like professional bodybuilders—it supplies the amino acid building blocks and elevates many anabolic hormones including insulin. Insulin is important because it helps muscles take up and use amino acids for growth. Resistance exercise, as you know, provides the stimulus for muscle hypertrophy by promoting protein synthesis, which may be elevated for up to 48 hours following just a single bout of strenuous exercise. Eating in close association with resistance exercise is important because protein breakdown also increases after exercise, and food intake helps the body make more muscle than it degrades. Thus, the timing of nutrient delivery relative to the bout of exercise is also important. The general thinking is that feeding should occur about 20 to 30 minutes after exercise.

Should You Really Be Trying to Gain Weight?

The ultimate goal for many athletes engaged in heavy strength training is to increase muscle mass. For some athletes—such as wrestlers and baseball players—an increase in muscle with minimal increase in fat mass is desirable. For others—such as powerlifters or football linemen—the absolute mass is important. Vegetarian athletes are no different in this respect. Often included in the "trying to gain weight group" are athletes who "leaned up" after the transition to a vegetarian diet, most likely because they did not eat enough calories initially, and now want to put this weight back on. See box 13.2 to dispel the myth that vegetarian diets lower testosterone levels and are not compatible with gaining muscle mass.

Similar to athletes with weight-loss goals, many athletes have unrealistic expectations about weight gain. They or their coach have the idea that they can put on 20 to 30 pounds (9-13 kg) of muscle in the preseason. They also feel that bigger is almost always better, which follows the movement in certain sports like football and baseball for athletes to become increasingly bigger and more muscular. This movement has led to an increase in the number of athletes wanting to gain weight, sometimes at the expense of good health. An unfortunate example of this is a college football player I worked with for weight loss during my first year as a college team nutritionist. This athlete had deep red stretch marks over many areas of his body, including his chest and shoulders. Upon inquiry, he told me that last year he had been on "the weight-gain list." He had overdone it by eating a lot of pizza, burgers, fries, and sausage and now was on "the weight-loss list." Unfortunately, this athlete more than likely will now struggle with overweight issues for the rest of his life.

Although vegetarian athletes are not likely to overdo the sausage and burgers, athletes trying to gain weight should seriously consider whether their weight-gain goals are realistic based on their genetics, current training regimen, prior training regimen, age, sex, and sport. Expecting to look like Arnold Schwarzenegger when you come from a family of men who look like Fred Astaire is probably not a realistic goal. However, hoping to gain 20 pounds (9 kg) as a freshman—the first year you engage in heavy resistance training—certainly may be. One study of 18- to 25-year-old bodybuilders and football players showed that an increase of 20 percent in body mass was possible during one year of heavy resistance training (ref in [3]). And although most of the weight gain was in lean mass, individual responses were variable. Such initial gains, however, quickly taper off and may be as little as 1 to 3 percent after several years of training. This is most likely because people tend to reach their genetic potential early in a training program.

Adapting the Plan to Promote Weight Gain

As with weight reduction, the eating plan for weight gain should be similar to the meal plan you would follow if you were trying to maintain weight but contain extra calories to support lean-tissue gain. Exactly how much extra has not been

Box
13.2

The Low Testosterone Myth

The rumor is out in popular media that a vegetarian diet might not be appropriate for strength and power athletes because plant-based diets reduce testosterone levels. Although these reports might scare strength athletes, I can assure you that they mean little to your performance and muscle-gaining abilities, and, in fact, may not be true at all.

➤ **Testosterone may be lowered when switching to a drastically different diet.** A handful of small-scale studies have found that the concentration of total testosterone in blood tends be lowered when people switch to either a vegetarian diet[9, 18] or a low-fat omnivorous diet.[19] Unbound testosterone concentrations—the small fraction that is free to enter target cells—are not typically affected, however, unless the diet is extremely low in fat. Why this drop in total concentration occurs is not well understood but may be related to the reduced fat and cholesterol content of the diet[19] or to the sudden and substantial change in dietary habits.[11, 18] Interestingly, testosterone levels were also found to drop in black South African men who switched from their usual vegetarian diet to a Western diet.[8]

➤ **Vegan and vegetarian men do not have lower testosterone levels.** Larger-scale comparisons between long-term vegetarians and meat eaters have found that neither total-testosterone nor free-testosterone concentrations are different among vegans, vegetarians, or meat eaters.[1, 10] In fact, if anything, total testosterone has been noted by several investigators to be slightly elevated in long-term vegetarians compared to omnivores,[10] and in vegans compared to both vegetarians and omnivores.[1] Thus, it appears that if testosterone levels are lowered during the transition to a vegetarian or vegan diet, this drop is probably short lived.

➤ **What does it mean if testosterone levels drop?** In the aforementioned studies, total testosterone was lowered when people switched to a different type of diet, but this reduction was just a small dip and did not fall below the normal range of 300 to 1,200 nanograms per deciliter (ng/dl) for total testosterone. Free testosterone did not drop and remained within the normal range for free testosterone of 9 to 30 ng/dl. Because there is no relationship between muscle gain or strength and total testosterone that varies within the normal range, this small dip is meaningless for athletic performance but may be advantageous for cancer prevention. Certainly, if testosterone drops below the normal range, muscle and bone loss may ensue. On the other hand, elevating testosterone beyond the normal physiological range through anabolic steroid use promotes gains in muscle mass. Neither, however, is the issue here.

➤ **What if I am concerned?** If you are concerned about your testosterone level, have your personal or team physician measure total and free testosterone during your next physical. (You may have to pay out of pocket for this.) If it is on the lower range of normal, assess your intake of dietary fat and total energy and increase smart fat choices as needed. Most likely, however, the test will put you at ease.

established, but the general recommendation is to increase energy intake by about 500 calories per day above daily needs, and to meet your protein and carbohydrate needs. Protein, of course, supplies the amino acids needed for growth, and carbohydrate spares the amino acids so that they can be used to build muscle rather than be converted to blood sugar.

Increasing calories above those of an already high intake, however, is easier said than done. You need to be diligent in your efforts, refrain from skipping meals, and pay attention to meal timing. I was always amazed when I asked the college athletes I counseled for weight gain about their food intake immediately before our appointment, which was typically in the late morning or early afternoon following practice. "Nothing for breakfast," they would say. "Nothing after practice," they would follow. "Really?" I always responded. "You are trying to gain weight but you have not eaten anything yet today." These athletes were ignoring some of the basics of gaining weight, which include spreading food intake throughout the day and taking advantage of postexercise meal timing. Ingesting carbohydrate and protein following training promotes muscle protein synthesis, so you don't want to miss this window when your goal is to maximize weight gain.

You can take in an extra 500 or so calories each day by eating larger-than-normal portions of healthy foods as part of a well-balanced diet or by adding an extra snack or two (of approximately 250 calories each) to your current intake. Keep bulky low-calorie foods such as whole-grain cereal, salads, and soup to a minimum because they are too filling in relation to the calories they provide. In contrast, healthy shakes, smoothies, fruit juice, and other liquid supplements along with dried fruit and nuts provide an easy way to squeeze the calories in (see box 2.4 on page 22). Healthy sources of fat, including olive oil, avocado, flaxseed oil, low-trans-fat margarine, and nuts and seeds, can be added if you have already met your carbohydrate and protein needs (see box 13.3).

Beyond that, how much weight you gain depends on the many factors discussed earlier, including your genetics, body type, and training regimen and the number of years you have been training. These are factors I typically review with athletes during their initial visit. Athletes who are just starting a new training regimen, such as freshman football players, are more likely to note significant gains in muscle mass as a result of their resistance training than are more senior players. Along these same lines, athletes who come from families with more muscular (or mesomorphic) body types are more likely to show results than those who come from families with lean (ectomorphic) body types. To this day I still recall working with an African American football player who had been trying to gain weight for several years. At our first session, we discussed his family background and I learned that not only were his dad, brother, and uncle trying to gain weight, but so was his mother. Although I was able to help him gain about five pounds (2.25 kg) before the spring game, which protected him a bit more from the contact on the field—it was apparent he was fighting his genes.

A ton of weight-gain formulas are out there promising immediate benefits. These formulas may work simply by increasing an athlete's energy intake. Remember,

Box
13.3

Tips for Adopting a Plan to Promote Weight Gain

➢ Eat a well-balanced vegetarian diet that provides approximately 500 calories per day more than you need in combination with an intense strength or resistance-training program.

➢ Ensure adequate protein intake. Intake beyond this, however, will not promote muscle growth.

➢ Increase energy intake by selecting larger portion sizes of healthy foods or by adding one or two 250-calorie snacks to your current eating regimen.

➢ Spread food intake throughout the day and don't skip meals. Eating three meals a day plus two to four snacks is typically needed.

➢ Consume a high-carbohydrate, protein-containing snack or liquid meal 20 to 30 minutes after exercise.

➢ Sneak in additional calories by consuming liquids, including smoothies, shakes, and fruit juice. Grape and cranberry juice typically have more calories per cup than other juices.

➢ Add healthy fats to your diet by snacking on peanuts, nuts, and seeds. Dipping bread in olive oil; spreading peanut butter, other nut butters, or no-trans-fat margarine on crackers, toast or bagels; and adding avocado slices to salads and sandwiches or as a topping on crackers are all great options.

➢ Keep bulky low-calorie foods such as whole-grain cereal, salads, and soup to a minimum. They are too filling in relation to the calories they provide.

➢ Do not go overboard. Consuming more than 1,000 calories per day in excess of your normal required intake will lead to fat deposition.

➢ Strength train, strength train, strength train.

➢ Remember that muscle can only be gained through intense strength or resistance training several times a week, coupled with the consumption of additional calories.

they are liquid and a bit easier to consume than solids. Liquid supplements for weight gain, however, are also packed with various combinations of amino acids that not only taste "supplementy" but also may be produced using nonvegan or nonvegetarian sources. The best bet for a health-conscious vegetarian athlete is to make smoothies and shakes at home (a recipe is in chapter 14) so you can control the ingredients. If you want to try a dietary supplement, evaluate it with great scrutiny as discussed in chapter 10.

This chapter has focused on how you can alter your vegetarian meal or nutrition plan if necessary to promote weight loss or weight gain, and also provided tips for changing your habits to maintain a healthy body weight. You are now ready for the remaining step—learning how to whip up quick meals and snacks that fit into your customized meal plan.

14

Whipping Up Quick Vegetarian Meals and Snacks

She was an upperclassman on the women's soccer team and came to see me in hopes of improving her eating habits. "I don't feel good about myself," she said as she walked in the door to my office, "I need to eat better." Indeed, when we started through her typical day, it was easy to see that her eating habits were irregular and inconsistent. She typically skipped breakfast and admitted it was because she liked to leave the house quickly. She then found herself having to grab a vending-machine snack right before practice because she was ravenous. Lunch was equally haphazard. "I eat a good meal with my roommate at night," she told me. As we discussed things further, I realized that she had a good understanding of nutrition and knew what she needed to do, but that she just needed specific how-tos. Simple how-tos at that because she claimed she could not cook. We came up with a list of ideas for high-carbohydrate, nutrient-dense meals that were easy to prepare on a budget and scheduled a grocery store tour emphasizing how to select nutritious snacks and foods for use in quickly prepared meals. Our most immediate goal, however, was to come up with ideas for quick healthy breakfasts that she could eat while running out the door. This simple but important change would start her off on the right track nutritionally.

Many athletes get off track when faced with preparing their own meals. In fact, for many athletes it is easy to eat right when their only responsibility is to make good choices from the training table, mess hall, cafeteria, or sorority dining room—unless of course the quality of the food is not up to par. Entering the kitchen and having to prepare healthy meals on a schedule, a budget, or both, however, is a bit more challenging. Wouldn't it be great if we could just hire a personal vegetarian chef? Because this is unlikely, this last chapter provides tips and ideas to help you set a kitchen PR (preparation record) creating healthy vegetarian meals. If you are a novice or feel you just can't cook, this chapter will take some of the uncertainty out of meal preparation and start you on your way to performing your best—in the kitchen.

Different Tastes for Different Folks

Although nearly everyone reading this book is an active vegetarian, you all have different taste preferences, eating philosophies, and lifestyles. Therefore, you may find many of the following tips helpful and directed right at you and find others completely futile. This is, of course, to be expected given that some of you are in college or even high school, some are single, some are married, and some have 10 kids (or on some days it seems like there are 10). Some of you frequent your city supermarket and others shop exclusively at the local co-op or health food store. Some of you train in the early-morning hours, and others sneak in workouts before dinner or whenever the 10 kids allow. Some of you are trying to shed a few pounds and others need ideas to keep them eating healthfully. No matter your situation, pick and choose the tips most helpful to you now, remembering that things can and do change, and you will be well on your way to whipping up healthy vegetarian meals.

Getting Started

As with most exercise and sport training, it is a good idea to start with a plan rather than to dive right in unprepared. Although you won't be concerned with purchasing properly fitting sport equipment, you will need to evaluate the organization of your kitchen, pantry, and cupboards; learn the layout of your favorite food store; and get in the habit of making a weekly game plan.

Organize the Pantry   Louis Parrish, a general medicine practitioner who promotes cooking as therapy, says, "If you can organize your kitchen, you can organize your life." This is especially true for the vegetarian athlete. It may take an entire weekend, but it is definitely worth the effort. If your pantry is organized and well stocked you can easily find the ingredients needed for quick meal preparation. Start by taking everything out of the cupboards and putting things back so that they are easy to see and reach and fit logically into the flow of how you cook and eat in the kitchen. Oh, and while you're at it, toss out those spices and ingredients you have held onto for years.

Think Ergonomics   Athletes are well aware of ergonomics in their own sport but not necessarily in their kitchen. Cyclists are trained to cut corners closely during criterium races, and team athletes intuitively know the shortest path to take to the ball or the opponent. Apply this same type of thinking to your kitchen. Before putting things back into your cupboard, think about where in the kitchen you cook, where you clean up, and where you eat—the three principal work centers in the kitchen. Ideally, your cooking or food-preparation center should be close to the stove, have adequate counter space for chopping and mixing, and be close to the sink and refrigerator. The most-used items—pots and pans, mixing bowls, spices, and cooking utensils—should be stored in the cooking and prep area so that you do not have to do intervals across your kitchen during food preparation. Ideally, the storage pantry should be close to the work area, but because this is not always possible, you should stock it with the foods and ingredients you use least often during day-to-day food preparation. These might include items such as flour, cornmeal, dried beans, dried fruit, and snack foods.

If you are not sure how to come up with a plan, try thinking about the way your coach comes up with playing strategies. It may help to diagram things and trace the path you would walk during dinner preparation. Also, consider the clean-up and serving areas. Cleaning supplies and the dish drainer should be close to the sink; silverware, plates, and glasses should be close to the table. If you have to walk across the kitchen to get a spatula or spices while prepping foods, they're not stored in the most ergonomic spot. If your kitchen is not ideally laid out and you cannot devise "the perfect plan," your goal then should be to come up with the most logical plan. For example, if your sink, refrigerator, and pantry are not close to the prep area, then your plan could be to wash all the vegetables and place them in the prep area by the stove, then gather everything from the pantry and refrigerator and put them in the prep area. Right now we live in an old Victorian-style house and my storage pantry is down some stairs. Although I sometimes welcome the idea of an extra stair workout, I have to be organized if I want to prepare dinner in a timely manner. Luckily, my sink, stove, and chopping block form a nice triangle close to the refrigerator.

Invest in Storage Containers   There is a lot to be said for storing ingredients in clear, airtight containers that fit neatly into cupboards and pantries. To conserve space, they should be square or rectangular, not round. They should also be well labeled. Six or seven years ago, I purchased clear stackable containers that fit in my panty in a modular fashion. I filled them with dry goods and have never regretted the time investment. In my downstairs pantry I store rice, bulgur, barley, oatmeal, dried beans, egg substitute, gluten, agar (vegetarian gelatin), and bread crumbs, among other things, in these containers. I also store roasted walnuts, almonds, pecans, and flaxseed in the same type of containers in my upstairs cupboard because we consume these items almost daily. Pasta, which we use more than rice, is stored upstairs in cupboards in the prep area as are the spices, oils, vinegars, and other basic ingredients. My flour, sugar, cornmeal, and master mix, a homemade all-purpose baking mix, are stored in a roundabout in my prep area both because these ingredients fit there and because I use these items with surprising regularity.

Don't Bury the Herbs and Spices Another hint I learned when we lived in a new home in Louisiana that had lots of kitchen drawers was the concept of the spice drawer. Keeping spices and herbs in similarly sized containers in a drawer near the stove is a tremendous time saver because you can easily locate the spices you need without having to take everything out of the spice cupboard. My favorite containers are the small glass jars that are round on top with slightly squared bottoms that keep them from rolling. Organizing them in the drawer, however, should be done by personal preference. I typically go with the Simon and Garfunkel approach and put parsley next to sage, rosemary, and thyme and follow with basil and the other spices in a functional order that is probably only logical to me. Others simply alphabetize.

Take a Self-Guided Grocery Store Tour Somewhere in the process of organizing, it might be wise to visit your favorite supermarket or health food store both to stock up on ingredients and familiarize yourself with products for vegetarians. This is a great idea even for veteran vegetarians because new foods come onto the market regularly. Before making this trip, take stock of what you have in your pantry and what type of items you are looking for. For example, you might be curious about which food products are fortified with vitamin B_{12} or have added flax, or what healthy snacks, premixes, or bean varieties are available. You may be interested in everything, which is fine; just go prepared to be there a while (and don't take the kids). Table 14.1 lists basic items to keep stocked in your pantry or freezer. Box 14.1 provides ideas for your self-guided grocery store tour.

TABLE 14.1 Suggestions for Stocking a Healthful Pantry

Grains	Vegetables	Fruit	Protein	Nuts and oils
Pasta	Onions	Dried fruit (cranberries, raisins, cherries, apricots, prunes, dates, figs)	Textured vegetable protein (TVP)	Almonds
Couscous	Garlic		Black beans	Cashews
Brown rice	Potatoes		Chickpeas	Peanuts
White rice	Sweet potatoes	Selected canned fruit (in its own juice)	Kidney beans	Pecans
Wild rice	Canned tomato products (whole and chopped tomatoes, tomato puree, tomato sauce, and tomato paste)	Frozen strawberries, berries, and peaches	Pinto beans	Pine nuts
Polenta			White beans	Pumpkin seeds
Bulgur			Dry beans (lentils, split peas, black, pinto, white, black-eyed, navy, fava, and adzuki)	Sunflower seeds
Barley				Nut butters
Whole-grain and healthy crackers				Tahini
Millet	Canned corn			Olive oil
Whole-wheat flour	Dried mushrooms		Frozen meat analogues (vegetarian chicken and sausage)	Canola oil
Enriched, unbleached white flour	Sundried tomatoes			Flaxseed oil
Cornmeal	Frozen vegetables (including leafy greens)			Flax seeds
All-purpose baking mix (homemade or commercially available)	Frozen sweet peppers			Hemp oil
				Sesame seed oil
				Other flavorful oils

Note: Because many of these items have a limited shelf life, it is a good idea to date foods when purchased and stock only those that you use regularly.

Box
14.1

Taking a Self-Guided Grocery Store Tour

Spending a little time in your grocery store or health food store will help make you aware of the vegetarian products available and their nutritional value. Although the layout of each store differs, the following will help as you take your tour.

Fresh Produce

> ➤ Fresh produce is always a good choice.
> ➤ Look for a variety of fruits and vegetables and make the effort to try those you have not tasted before.
> ➤ Most stores now sell organic produce, which is slightly more expensive. You can also check with the produce manager to learn where produce is purchased and whether the store buys goods from local farmers.
> ➤ Look for time-savers such as presliced mushrooms and packages of mixed greens and baby spinach. Major grocery stores regularly sell these at reasonable prices, e.g., buy one, get one free.

Bread and Cereal Shelves

> ➤ Look for cereal with at least two grams of fiber, eight grams or less of sugar, and two grams or less of fat per serving. Compare portion sizes and carbohydrate content on the nutrition facts label; servings range from a 0.25 cup to 1.25 cups. Many cereals are now available with added flax or hemp.
> ➤ Look for bread that is made from whole grain or partially whole grain. If selecting white bread, choose enriched or unmilled versions.
> ➤ Check ingredient labels for animal products.

Canned-Food Aisle

> ➤ Canned beans, peas, and tomato products are a must for the vegetarian pantry. Choose brands with firm beans or peas of good quality. Use reduced-sodium products if desired, but remember to rinse all beans before use. Also look for vegetarian varieties of baked beans.
> ➤ Choose 100 percent pure fruit juices instead of fruit cocktails or punches. If you select a juice that needs sugar, for example cranberry juice, look for brands with less high-fructose corn syrup.
> ➤ Look for canned fruit in is own juice and unsweetened applesauce. These make good staples in the winter months.

Cracker and Cookie Aisle

> ➤ Check out the selection of cookies and crackers. Several brands are healthy, but most are loaded with high-fructose corn syrup, sugar, or hydrogenated oil.

(continued)

(continued)

> Good bets for crackers include water crackers and whole-grain crackers made with no hydrogenated oils.

> Best bets for cookies include fruit newtons, oatmeal cookies, cookies sweetened without sugar, and cookies that contain whole grains, nuts, or dried fruit. With cookies, you can usually justify making a healthy batch at home.

Bulk-Foods Section

> The bulk foods section is a great place to find muesli, granola, and other interesting and healthy cereals; hard-to-find grains; dried fruit; TVP; nutritional yeast; fair-trade teas; and organic candy.

> It is worth a stop every time you are in the store.

Dairy Case

> Milk, buttermilk, cottage cheese, and yogurt that are nonfat or have 1 percent milk fat are good low-saturated fat choices for vegetarians.

> Some brands of soy milk are now refrigerated and available in the dairy case.

> Look for strongly flavored cheeses, where a little cheese goes a long way, or cheeses that are made partly with nonfat milk.

Frozen Foods

> Check out the selection of frozen fruits and vegetables. Because these foods are frozen soon after picking, their nutritional value is often higher than that of fresh. Frozen vegetables are also convenient to keep on hand and lower in sodium than canned. In addition, some stores do not carry certain varieties of fresh products, for example turnip greens, but do offer frozen versions.

> Look for vegetarian meat analogues and vegetarian frozen entrees. Many health food store brands have gone mainstream and can be found in local grocery stores.

> The varieties of meat analogues continue to grow. Check out new and interesting products.

Other

> Learn the layout of your store and which foods are stocked where; this facilitates quick shopping.

> Meander the aisles and read nutrition labels on new or interesting-looking foods. Some seemingly nonvegetarian items, such as premixes, might be vegetarian and might even have vegetarian cooking suggestions on the back.

> In your wanderings, also check out salad dressing and vegetarian broth offerings. Finding a flavorful salad dressing made with healthy oils and no high-fructose corn syrup and flavorful not-so-salty broth will drastically improve how your meals and foods taste.

Keep the Cookbooks in Check   The last things you need to organize—and this will take some time—are your recipes and cookbooks. Although I would bet many of you have quite a cookbook collection and are maybe even considering purchasing a few more, having cookbooks does not mean you will be efficient cooks with many healthy meal ideas. If only it were that simple. Instead, just the opposite often occurs because people either become overwhelmed with their collection or spend valuable time looking through cookbooks but are somehow unable to make the connection between the cookbook and the dinner table. What my husband and I started doing years ago, because he wanted a list of tried-and-true recipes he could pass on to colleagues or patients, was to keep files of practical recipes we wanted to try that I organized by categories, such as main dish beans, main dish pasta, main dish other, vegetables, salads, breads, and holiday. When we wanted to try a new recipe, one of us would pull it from the file or look one up in a cookbook and prepare it. If we loved it and it was easy to prepare, I would type it into a word-processing program, noting modifications, meal serving suggestions, and the original source. If we thought it was *just OK* or did not really enjoy it, we tossed it into the recycling bin. If we loved it but found it too tedious, it went back into the file drawer in a folder labeled special occasion.

Over the years we have developed our collection of easy-to-prepare preferred recipes. Although we keep adding to the file, I print it out periodically and stick the pages in plastic protectors that we keep in a stainless steel file holder right in the work area. And the word-processed files are easy to e-mail to my mother-in-law and interested friends (in a way silently recruiting them into the vegetarian world). Although I occasionally consult my favorite cookbooks, it is typically only to look up a standard recipe like cornbread or bran muffins, or to seek out a new recipe idea. I have also narrowed my collection tremendously and only keep the cookbooks that have recipes we *love.* After a while you begin to notice that there are some cookbooks you always reach for and others that collect dust.

Keeping the Basics

Although you certainly don't want to wait until you are fully organized to start whipping up healthy meals, it certainly helps to start out somewhat on the right foot. Once you are organized or are in the process of organizing, you can begin thinking about daily meal preparation.

Work Out the Plan   The number one reason athletes eat haphazardly is that they fail to plan. Although we discussed custom meal plans—which help you learn to eat right—you also need a weekly or bimonthly menu plan to assist with dinner, portable lunches, and quick-and-go breakfasts. Unlike the eating plan, however, the meal plan is something you, along with the rest of the members of your household, should create regularly. Although there are many different ways to go about this, it is less daunting if you dedicate time once a week for menu planning and follow a basic structure. The basic structure might look something like the sample shown in table 14.2 where you would tentatively plan to serve certain types of dishes once a week and even on specific nights if it helps. Alternately, you might decide to have a soup and salad night, healthy pizza night, stir-fry night, Mexican night, pasta night, and quick-skillet night. It depends on your preferences. Once you have a workable form, select main dish recipes that fits the theme and add in—just like you did with your eating plan—bread, side vegetables and salads, fruits, and healthy desserts as appropriate. Often with vegetarian cuisine, the vegetables are part of the main dish so you may simply need to add an additional bread or a fruit or leafy green salad and you are done. For example, a bowl of vegetarian chili goes great with soda crackers or homemade corn bread and sliced fresh fruit drizzled with fresh lime juice, whereas most bean and vegetable soups and pasta dishes need just a leafy green salad and some bread. A tofu and vegetable stir-fry with fresh ginger is complete. Just serve it over rice or Asian noodles with a glass of water and white wine if desired. Add a fresh or baked pear for dessert if you are still hungry.

Think About Planned-Overs   Give yourself a break at least once a week by eating planned-overs. You can do this simply by eating vegetarian chili on both Monday and Wednesday or creatively by serving Monday's chili over a baked or microwaved potato on Wednesday or even freezing Monday's chili and eating it on Wednesday a few weeks later. I do this a lot with vegetable soups, such as pumpkin or butternut squash. I cook up a few small pumpkins or squash with sauteed onions, sage, and olive oil in some vegetable broth and, after pureeing, I freeze quite a bit in pint or quart bags. I then stir in the milk, soy milk, or silken tofu for the current night's dinner and do the same with the defrosted mixture for a quick meal a few weeks later. Another way to use planned-overs is to cook up a huge pot of dried beans and use them in several meals throughout the week, giving you black bean week, pinto bean week, and aduki bean week.

Keep the Plans Quick and Simple   During the week and on busy race or game weekends, don't be afraid to keep the plan simple. Although I cook from our recipe list many nights, I also make many throw-together meals such as vegetarian burgers and sweet potato fries or simple skillet meals or casseroles (see table 14.3). Lately, I have also been making quick meals by adding frozen vegetables and either tofu or canned and rinsed beans to commercially available premixes. For several of my current favorites, I toss tofu into Thai peanut or other Thai-style mixes and steam some Chinese greens. Or I whip up one of the "impossible pies" or pizza bakes listed on the Bisquick box (using the new Bisquick Heart Smart made with canola oil, or master mix—see box 14.2). My kids love salsa chicken fiesta, which I prepare with one can of pinto beans and one can of light-red kidney beans instead of chicken. Other ideas include making fajitas with a commercial fajita mix and tofu, onion, bell pepper, and summer squash; tossing black-eyed peas into a dirty-rice mix or pinto beans into a smoked-chipotle rice mix; or using textured vegetable protein (TVP) instead of hamburger in noodle or rice dishes.

TABLE 14.2 Sample Menu Rotation

Sunday	Monday	Tuesday	Wednesday	Thursday	Friday	Saturday
Hearty bean dish	Tofu or tempeh	Pasta	Planned-overs	Vegetable dish	Meat analogue	Rice or grain

YEAR-ROUND AND WINTER SUGGESTIONS

Hearty bean dishes

Lentil tacos

Three-bean chili

Red beans and rice

Hoppin' John

White-bean soup

Dahl over Indian rice

Spicy chickpeas over rice

Jamaican black beans with broiled plantain

Tofu or tempeh dishes

Tofu vegetable stir-fry with cashews

Tofu with peanut sauce and Asian noodles

Tofu, onion, and vegetable fajitas

Tofu and vegetable pot pie

Baked tempeh with mashed potatoes and mushroom gravy

Asian noodles with marinated tempeh and snow peas

Pasta dishes

Spaghetti with marinara sauce or lentil–tomato sauce

Pasta primavera

Penne with roasted vegetables

Spinach lasagna

Pasta with leeks, goat cheese, and walnuts

Capas tasta (pasta with cabbage slaw)

Vegetable dishes

"Cream" of carrot soup

Minestrone

Potato dill soup

Parsnip and carrot soup with leeks

Beet greens and vegetarian sausage soup

Winter squash stuffed with pine nuts and feta cheese (served over brown rice)

Stuffed peppers (served with rice)

Spaghetti squash with red or white pasta sauce and toasted pine nuts

Meat-analogue dishes

Vegetarian burger on whole-grain bun with sweet potato fries

Vegetarian chicken nuggets with broccoli slaw and pumpernickel rolls

Mushroom and "burger" crumbles stroganoff

Vegetarian sausage with potato pancakes and homemade applesauce

Tofu pigs in a blanket

Rice or grain dishes

Couscous with winter vegetable stew

Mushroom and barley soup

Spinach risotto (made in pressure cooker)

Smoked chipotle rice with pinto beans

SUMMER SUGGESTIONS

Hearty bean dishes

Three-bean salad

Black-bean and corn salad

White bean and goat cheese tostadas with tomato mango salsa

Tofu or tempeh dishes

Greek tofu salad

Chinese noodle salad with tofu

Sesame tofu over cold rice noodles

Tofu and vegetable kabobs

Tofu, grapes, and red-leaf lettuce salad (served with toasted flat bread)

Pasta dishes

Penne and roasted pepper and tomato salad

Italian pasta salad (with chickpeas)

Pasta with homemade pesto

Vegetable dishes

Main dish chef's salad (with greens, beans, cottage cheese, and vegetables)

Tomato gazpacho with avocado

Grilled portobello mushroom burger

Baked (or microwaved) potato with fresh vegetables and soy sour cream

Meat-analogue dishes

Grilled vegetarian burgers with grilled summer vegetables

Coney Island vegetarian dogs and slaw

Rice or grain dishes

Couscous salad with cucumber, peppers, and tomatoes

Tabouli

Wheat-berry and orange salad

Polenta triangles with fresh saffron tomatoes

TABLE 14.3 Quick Skillet Meals

Grains (1 cup uncooked)	Sauce (1 can soup plus 1 1/2 cans water or milk)	Beans, textured vegetable protein (TVP), or "burger" recipe crumbles (1 can beans, 3/4 cup dry TVP, 1 1/2 cups burger recipe crumbles; 1 package tofu)	Vegetables (1 1/2-2 cups frozen or raw)	1. Choose one food from each of the four groups in the table. If desired, saute vegetables first. Stir in remaining ingredients.
Whole-wheat macaroni Shells, fiore, rotini, or other small pasta Brown rice Bulgur	Cream of celery soup Cream of mushroom soup Tomato soup Onion soup Vegetable soup or broth	Kidney beans Pinto beans Black beans White beans Chickpeas Black-eyed peas TVP "Burger" recipe crumbles Extra-firm tofu	Onions, celery, green peppers Mushrooms Carrots Peas Corn Green beans Broccoli Spinach Mixed vegetables	2. Season to taste with salt, pepper, soy sauce, fresh or dehydrated minced onion, and fresh garlic. 3. Bring to boil. 4. Reduce heat to lowest setting; cover and simmer 30-40 min until pasta or rice is tender. Stir occasionally to prevent sticking. 5. Stir in up to 1/2 cup cheese at the very end (optional). Example 1: Macaroni mixed with tomato soup, kidney beans, and a combination of onion, celery, and green pepper. Example 2: Shells mixed with mushroom soup, TVP, and mixed vegetables (no cheese) *Note:* These ingredients also work well in a casserole. Mix all ingredients and bake in a covered casserole dish at 350 °F for 35-45 min.

Adapted from Wyoming Cent$ible Nutrition News, a publication of the Wyoming Food Stamp Nutrition Education Program, University of Wyoming.

Although a clear disadvantage to some of these mixes is their sodium or trans fat content or both, you can look for brands that have no monosodium glutamate or added hydrogenated oils and use just half to three-quarters of the salt-containing flavor packet. For the Bisquick meals, you can also make your own baking premix (see box 14.2) using a combination of whole and white flours and healthy oils. This works perfectly for making quick meals and breads for dinner as well as breakfast.

Add a Salad to the Menu   Add a mixed green salad to dinner or lunch at least a few times a week. Salads are easy to make—particularly if you use the prepared green mixes—and pack in the nutrients, including calcium, vitamin C, vitamin E, vitamin K, vitamin A and the carotenoids, iron, zinc, magnesium, and healthy fats. Tossing in fresh and dried fruit adds more carbohydrate. If you are tired of the traditional lettuce and tomato salad, try some of the following salads made with greens, fruits, vegetables, nuts, healthy oils, and optional cheese.

- Mixed greens with tangerines, dried cranberries, and slivered almonds. Serve with honey and dijon mustard dressing.
- Spinach and arugula with chopped apple, dried cranberries, and toasted walnuts. Serve with red wine and olive oil vinaigrette.
- Spinach and red leaf lettuce with strawberries, red onions, and toasted walnuts. Serve with champagne and olive oil vinaigrette.

Box
14.2

Master Mix and Recipes

Master Mix (MIX)

4 cups enriched flour

3 3/4 cups whole-wheat flour

1/4 cup double-acting baking powder

3 Tbsp sugar

1 Tbsp iodized salt

1 1/3 cups nonfat dry milk powder*

1 cup canola oil

Sift enriched flour with baking powder, sugar, and salt. Stir in dry milk. Cut in oil with pastry blender or fingers until it looks like coarse cornmeal. Stir in whole-wheat flour; stir well. Makes about 10 cups.

Note: Keeps about three months in refrigerator.

To measure MIX: Stir lightly and pile into cup (do not shake or level off).

Corn Bread

1 cup MIX

1 cup cornmeal

2 Tbsp sugar

1/2 tsp baking soda

1 egg beaten**

1 cup buttermilk, sour milk, or soymilk

Blend dry ingredients thoroughly. Combine beaten egg and buttermilk; stir into dry ingredients. Pour into greased 8-inch (20 cm) square pan. Bake at 425 °F (218 °C) for 25 to 30 minutes.

Muffins

3 cups + 2 Tbsp MIX

3 Tbsp sugar or brown sugar

1 egg, beaten**

1 cup water

1 cup fruit (mashed banana, blueberries, applesauce, and so on)

1 tsp cinnamon or vanilla (optional)

Combine MIX and sugar. Blend egg and water; add to MIX. Stir gently just until dry ingredients are moistened. Mixture should be lumpy. Bake in well-greased muffin pans at 425 °F (218 °C) for about 20 minutes. Makes 12 muffins.

Biscuits

2 cups MIX

1/3 to 1/2 cup water

Stir MIX and water together in bowl. Knead gently about 12 times on floured surface. Roll or pat to 1/2-inch (12 mm) thickness. Cut into circles using a floured biscuit cutter or glass. Bake at 450 °F (232 °C) for 12 to 15 minutes. Makes 10 to 12 biscuits.

Banana Bread

2 eggs**

1/4 cup sugar

1/2 tsp baking soda

1 1/4 cups mashed banana

2 1/2 cups MIX

Beat eggs and sugar together in a bowl until well blended. Mix in soda and mashed banana. Stir in MIX just until all dry ingredients are coated. Pour into a greased loaf pan that is 9 × 5 × 3 inches (23 × 13 × 8 cm). Bake at 350 °F (121 °C) for 45 to 55 minutes or until brown.

Variation: For pumpkin bread, use 1/2 cup sugar plus 1/2 tsp cinnamon, 1/4 tsp nutmeg, 1/4 tsp ginger, 1/4 cup water, and 1 cup canned or cooked mashed pumpkin or squash. For zucchini bread use 1 1/2 cups shredded zucchini and 2/3 cup sugar.

Refer to appendix E for guidance on converting English units to metric.

*May use nondairy dry milk substitutes such as Vance's DairFree or Ener-G SoyQuick or NutQuick powder. **May use vegan egg replacer.

Additional recipes for using homemade master mix or Bisquick Heart Smart (made with canola oil) can be found at www.bettycrocker.com/products/prod_bisquick.aspx.

Adapted from Wyoming Cent$ible Nutrition News, a publication of the Wyoming Food Stamp Nutrition Education Program, University of Wyoming.

- Arugula with grilled apple, bread, blue cheese, and grapes. Serve with basic or raspberry vinaigrette.
- Watercress with fennel, oranges, and walnuts. Serve with sweet orange dressing (made with orange juice and olive or hemp oil).
- Arugula with Bartlett pears and grated fresh Parmesan or Gorgonzola cheese. Serve with lemon juice and hazelnut oil or walnut oil vinaigrette.
- Watercress with red pears and walnuts. Serve with honey and dijon mustard dressing.
- Mixed greens with caramelized onions, baked goat cheese, toasted walnuts, and fresh or dried figs. Serve with rosemary honey vinaigrette.
- Boston or Bibb lettuce and dandelion greens with chopped apricots, toasted pecans, and smoked Gouda. Serve with raspberry vinaigrette.
- Mixed greens with blueberries, toasted pecans, and Gorgonzola or blue cheese. Serve with white wine and olive oil vinaigrette.
- Mixed greens with avocado, grated carrot, and sunflower seeds. Serve with tomato and herb dressing.

Keep in mind, however, that because the dressing can make or break the salad, you should use fresh homemade vinaigrettes or your favorite commercial dressing prepared with healthy oils and without high-fructose corn syrup. The basic dressing has one part vinegar plus juice, if desired, and one to two parts oil plus added favorites such as black pepper, herbs, chopped scallions, dijon mustard, maple syrup, honey, or other flavorings.

Prepare Grab-and-Go Breakfasts   Because many athletes struggle with the need for grab-and-go breakfasts, coming up with a list of options and keeping these on hand is a big help. See box 14.3 for a list of ideas to get you started. Believe it or not, this is much easier than planning lunch or dinner. Before you go to the store each week, simply take stock of what you have and make your list accordingly. For example, if you are happy having English muffins all week, you just need to add fresh fruit and English muffins to your list and make sure you are not out of jam or low-trans-fat margarine. If you like the idea of homemade muffins, set aside time on the weekend and make up a batch or two and freeze them. You can then pop one or two in the microwave before leaving the house or when you get to work. Just remember to add juice or fresh fruit. Also remember that when there is more time—like on Sunday morning after your long run—you might enjoy experimenting with cooked hearty grains or tofu or egg and vegetable skillet dishes. Ideas include fruit crepes, waffles with apricot and ginger compote, scrambled tofu with vegetables, tofu breakfast burrito, and hot porridge with fruit puree and roasted nuts.

Plan Portable Lunches   Lunches are also a challenge for many vegetarian athletes, myself included. I remember living in Birmingham, Alabama, where there were many restaurants that served delicious and reasonably priced vegetarian fare just a short walk from my lab. Currently, however, I have no such luxury. If I

Box
14.3

Ideas for Grab-and-Go Breakfasts

Keep fresh or dried fruit and juice in small reusable containers on hand, ready to grab along with one of the following:

> Homemade muffins, made with canola oil and whole or unmilled grains

> Trail mix or granola in portion-sized baggies

> Whole English muffin with low-trans-fat margarine and jam (making a sandwich using both halves reduces the mess)

> Fresh or toasted bagels either plain or with nut butter or Neufchatel cheese

> Fruit bread such as pumpkin, zucchini, or banana, made with canola oil

> Toaster sticks or waffles (hold the syrup); some versions now add flax

> Fruit smoothie with added flax or flaxseed oil (see table 14.4)

> Dairy or soy yogurt, fruit, and granola parfait (made the night before in a to-go container)

> Breakfast cookies (make your favorite oatmeal cookies with orange juice as the liquid and added dried fruit, ground flaxseed and half the sugar—who said you can't have cookies for breakfast?)

> Healthier granola or breakfast bars made with whole grains and healthy oils and without high-fructose corn syrup (usually available at health food stores)

> Cereal and soy milk in a large plastic cup (Believe it or not, I used to run down a huge hill in Brookline, Massachusetts, with cereal and sliced banana in a cup to catch the mass-transit train. I then devoured it seated or standing. Don't try this while driving, however.)

am not prepared, I end up eating sport bars and dried fruit and coming home starved. Although I can get away with this on rest days, it is worse than awful on days I run at noon or stop at the dance studio after work for Irish dance practice. The solution of course is to stock your pantry with lunch options and spend five minutes after dinner preparing tomorrow's lunch (see box 14.4 for ideas). If you need to, it may help to set up a rotating lunch schedule. Remember that leftovers are also a great lunch option.

Think Healthy Snacks   Thinking about healthy snacks is similar to planning a grab-and-go breakfast and a portable lunch. Make a list of healthy snacks and keep several varieties in stock at home, at your office, and in your gym bag. Because your energy needs vary considerably from day to day, it helps to have healthy snacks available when you are hungry. If you are a fan of less-healthy snacks, it is best to buy them in individual-sized portions.

TABLE 14.4 Whipping Up Healthy Smoothies

Fruit (~1 cup fresh or frozen)	Fruit juice (~1/2 cup)	Tofu or dairy	Extras (small amounts for flavor)	
Banana Pineapples Mangos Berries Kiwi fruits Nectarines Cherries Papayas Peaches Apricots Melon Fruit cocktail	Apple Orange Pineapple Grape Cranberry	Milk—1 cup Buttermilk Yogurt—1 cup Silken tofu—1 cup Soy milk—1 cup Powdered milk—2 Tbsp Isolated soy protein—1-3 Tbsp	Honey Maple syrup Vanilla Flaxseed or Peanut butter (1 Tbsp) Flaxseed oil (1-3 tsp) Grape nuts or wheat germ (1-2 tbsp) Fresh mint Fresh lime Fresh lemon	1. Select ingredients. 2. If using flaxseeds, blend on high until ground, add additional ingredients, and blend until smooth. 3. If using flax or hemp oils, blend all ingredients except oil until smooth. Turn blender to low and slowly drizzle in oil. 4. For all other combinations, place all ingredients in blender and mix until smooth. 5. Enjoy. Example 1: bananas with orange juice, yogurt, and flaxseed Example 2: peaches with cranberry juice, tofu, and fresh mint *Note:* Ice cubes or crushed ice may be added to make a slushier frozen smoothie.

Refer to appendix E for guidance on converting English units to metric.

Adapted from WIN the Rockies (Wellness IN the Rockies). Available: http://www.uwyo.edu/wintherockies.

Box
14.4

Ideas for Quick Portable Lunches

Pack one of the following lunches with fresh fruit, whole-grain crackers, whole-wheat pretzels, or chips baked or made with healthy oils, and/or healthy cookies. Add water, soy milk, fruit juice, or Gatorade to drink.

Tomato, avocado, and spicy sprouts on a bagel

Black beans, lettuce, Neufchatel cheese, and salsa in a spinach or whole-wheat roll-up

Home-grown tomato, fresh large-leaf basil, and mozzarella on sour dough (my favorite in the summer)

Hummus and sliced vegetables in a pita

Chickpeas, vegetables, cottage cheese (optional), and Italian dressing in a whole-wheat pita

Black-eyed-peas spread (1 can beans, 1/2 cup parsley, 2 Tbsp olive oil, 2 Tbsp lemon juice, 1/2 tsp tarragon, and garlic and pepper to taste) on flat bread or leftover corn bread

(continued)

(continued)

Chili bean spread (1 cup pinto beans, 1 tsp chili powder, 1 tsp onion powder, 1 tsp chopped green chili peppers, and 1/4 tsp red-pepper flakes) on flat bread or in a whole-wheat roll-up

Red-pepper bean spread (1 cup white beans, 3 tsp finely chopped roasted sweet peppers, 1 tsp finely chopped scallions) on focaccia or flat bread

Kidney beans, chopped sweet peppers, and celery with Italian dressing in a pita

Fresh spinach, cashews, cranberry sauce, and chickpeas in a roll-up

Grilled or roasted peppers, eggplant, and squash with olive oil and feta on sour dough or Italian bread

Tofu "egg" salad (firm tofu mixed with celery, sweet peppers, mustard, mayonnaise, and dill) in a whole-wheat pita with lettuce and tomato

Marinated tofu, lettuce, and vegetables in a whole-grain pita

Dilly cottage cheese filling (1/2 cup cottage cheese, 1 tsp lemon juice, 1 Tbsp minced green onion, 1 tsp dill) in whole-wheat pita with shredded vegetables

Tempeh-salad sandwich (tempeh mixed with mayonnaise, yogurt, celery, and mustard) on whole-grain bread or in whole-wheat pita with lettuce and tomato

Grilled or roasted eggplant spread (1 large roasted eggplant blended with 1/4 cup chopped parsley, 1 Tbsp green onion, 2 tsp lemon juice, 1 Tbsp olive oil, and salt and pepper to taste) on sourdough or Italian bread.

Dark leafy greens in pita with chickpeas, kidney beans, or white beans and honey-mustard dressing.

Peanut butter, sliced banana, raisins, and walnuts on whole-wheat bread

Nut butter and jam on whole-wheat bread

Peanut butter and pickles on mixed-grain bread (delicious after long endurance races or when pregnant)

Refer to appendix E for guidance on converting English units to metric.

For other ideas, take note of the menu next time you eat at your favorite restaurant, deli, coffee shop, or natural food store.

Compose a Store List The final piece of weekly meal planning is to make a grocery store list, but you probably saw this coming. To do this properly, quickly check your organized pantry for what is in stock and make a quick list of what you will need to make quick breakfasts and lunches and prepare dinner meals. If you always shop at the same grocery store, you may find that it is easiest to make up your list based on the store layout. For example, when I make my list, I try to list the foods in the order I find them as I walk through the store: bakery section, breakfast cereal, canned vegetables, dairy, produce, and the vegetarian section. Believe me, it takes me almost twice as long to shop at the store across town where I am not familiar with the layout.

Keeping It Exciting

Creating healthy meals is a lifelong process and one you need to fit into your regular routine—just like your training. Once you have the basics down, however, you will find that it does not take much work, and the work is, for the most part, enjoyable. Although I must admit, my favorite meals are those I prepare with my husband on relaxed nights, perhaps while enjoying a glass of wine, after we have both had good workouts earlier in the day, I also heartily enjoy making quick meals my little vegetarians can help with. The following information provides a few more suggestions for effective meal planning for vegetarian athletes.

Periodize Your Meal Plan   Eating the same thing every week can get pretty boring. This and the fact that different foods are available during different seasons— particularly locally grown foods—are reasons to periodize your menus, much like you periodize your training. In our family, we tend to eat a lot of soups in the winter, which we serve with salad and bread. In the summer, we make a lot of hearty salads and meals that can be prepared without heating the house (see table 14.2). We also take advantage of seasonal produce, whether it comes from our garden, the farmers' market, or the store. As an athlete, however, you may also find your menu choices vary a bit depending on your training season. If you are training at a high volume, you may find that you prefer eating main dishes with pasta or rice most of the time and then enjoy soup and salad when your training volume is lower. This is also something to consider when planning your weekly menus. Think about what you prefer to eat after a weight workout compared to an aerobic workout. Hopefully, if you live with a roommate, spouse, or partner, your training schedules and menu preferences will coincide.

Try a Class or a New Cooking Technique   There is much more to cooking than an oven, a skillet, and a microwave. If you are not using them already, try experimenting with a slow cooker, pressure cooker, grill, or wok or enroll in a cooking class. Slow cookers are great if you have time in the morning; you can throw in a vegetarian stew, soup, or pasta sauce and come home to find dinner ready to go. On the other hand, pressure cookers can cook a meal, including risotto, quinoa, or bean soup in less than 20 minutes. Unlike your grandma's pressure cooker, new technology makes current models safer to use. Grills—both outdoor or the indoor George Foreman type—are perfect for grilling tasty fresh veggies, marinated tofu, and even fruit—yum! Woks and rice cookers are convenient if you make a lot of stir-fries and cook a lot of rice. I still make my rice in the pan and stir-fries in the skillet; however, learning to use a wok is on my list, after I take a Chinese cooking class, that is. To enroll in a class, check out those offered by hospitals, cooking stores, or college or university outreach programs. And, don't be afraid to take a class if it is not specifically vegetarian. Many times the instructor will provide vegetarian suggestions if he or she knows up front that you are vegetarian. And usually you can modify the recipes so that they are vegan or vegetarian. Cooking classes not only give you ideas but often also improve your chopping and cooking skills. When was the last time you sharpened your vegetable-chopping knives?

Don't Be Afraid to Modify Delicious-Sounding Omnivorous Recipes   Several of our favorite recipes in our recipe packet are ones I modified from meat-based recipes or dishes I saw on restaurant menus. Although you will get better at this the more you cook and eat vegetarian meals, here are a few tricks of the trade. Marinated tofu works well in place of chopped chicken or turkey. Marinate the tofu in the sauce or spices used in the recipe and if desired use frozen tofu. Freezing the tofu removes some of the water and makes the texture a bit chewier. TVP, tempeh, or "burger" recipe crumbles, a ground-beef analogue, typically work well in place of ground beef in many dishes. The burger crumbles have more flavor but also add salt. Thus, TVP works better in dishes with stronger flavors and burger crumbles work better when the flavor of the dish depends on the quality of the meat analogue. Fresh or dried mushrooms, particularly porcini, portabello, or crimini, also work well as beef substitutes. In many recipes, different beans work well either alone or in combination with TVP. Just experiment, and it should become second nature. Finally, many spicy versions of vegetarian sausages can be sliced and added in place of meat sausage. However, these dishes will taste fine without sausage as long as you add a flavorful lower-salt vegetarian broth.

Grow Herbs and Leafy Greens   Although many vegetarian athletes may also be master gardeners, some do not have the space or the time. My suggestion for all athletes, however, is to figure out how to grow the minimal amount during the growing season in your area. This includes herbs such as basil, cilantro, mint, and darker leafy greens such as California mix, arugula, spinach, and dandelion greens. In just a small space you can have access to fresh herbs and greens. And you can grow herbs year-round in pots in your house.

Congratulations on making healthy choices and going for the vegetarian advantage. Good planning and attention to food and diet details are hard work but worth it! Good luck. You should be well on your way to better health and performance.

Selected Cookbooks and References

Favorite Cookbooks

A variety of great vegan and vegetarian cookbooks are available. These are my favorite and most used.

Bishop, J. *Vegetables Every Day: The Definitive Guide to Buying and Cooking Today's Produce, With More than 350 Recipes.* New York, NY: HarperCollins, 2001.

Bronfman, D. and R. Bronfman. *CalciYum! Delicious Calcium-Rich Dairy-Free Vegetarian Recipes.* Toronto, Ontario: Bromedia, 1998.

Graimes, N. *The Greatest Ever Vegetarian Cookbook.* New York: Hermes House, 1999.

McIntosh, S.M. (editor). *Low-Fat Ways to Cook Vegetarian.* Birmingham, AL: Oxmore House, 1996.

Ray, R. *Rachael Ray's 30-Minute Veggie Meals.* New York: Lake Isle Press, 2001.

Rivera, M. *The Simple Little Vegan Slow Cooker.* Summertown, TN: Book Publishing Co., 2005.

Sass, L.J. *Great Vegetarian Cooking Under Pressure: Over 150 Exceptional Recipes to Make Today's Safe Pressure Cooker the Essential Tool in Your Kitchen.* New York: William Morrow, 1994.

Shaw, D. *The Essential Vegetarian Cook Book: Your Guide to the Best Foods on Earth. What to Eat. Where to Get It. How to Prepare It.* New York: Clarkson Potter, 1997.

Williams, C. (editor). *Williams-Sonoma Kitchen Library: Vegetarian.* San Francisco: Time-Life Custom Publishing, 1996.

Resources and Organizations

Vegetarian Resource Group, Baltimore, MD, www.vrg.org

Vegetarian Resource Group. *Vegetarian Journal's Guide to Natural Food Restaurants in the U.S. and Canada*, Vegetarian Resource Group: Baltimore, 2005.

Vegetarian Resource Group. *Guide to Food Ingredients.* Vegetarian Resource Group: Baltimore, 2003.

Appendix A

Energy Costs
of Physical Activity

Approximate Caloric Expenditure (above rest) per Minute for Rest and Various Exercise and Sport Activities

Weight in kg	45	52	59	66	73	80	86	93	100
Weight in lb	100	115	130	145	160	175	190	205	220
Baseball, player	2.1	2.5	2.8	3.0	3.4	3.8	4.0	4.4	5.7
Baseball, pitcher	2.9	3.4	3.8	4.2	4.7	5.2	5.5	6.0	6.4
Basketball, vigorous or competition	5.5	6.4	7.2	8.0	8.9	9.8	10.6	11.5	12.3
Bicycling, 15 mph	6.3	7.3	8.2	9.0	10.0	11.0	11.9	12.9	13.8
Bicycling, 20 mph	9.7	11.2	12.6	14.0	15.5	17.0	18.4	19.9	21.3
Calisthenics, light	2.4	2.9	3.2	3.5	3.9	4.4	4.7	5.1	5.5
Calisthenics, timed, vigorous	8.7	10.0	11.3	12.6	14.0	15.4	16.7	18.0	19.3
Dancing, active (square/disco)	3.5	4.1	4.6	5.1	5.7	6.2	6.7	7.3	7.8
Dancing, aerobic (vigorously)	5.0	5.9	6.6	7.3	8.1	8.9	9.6	10.4	11.1
Football, touch, vigorous	4.5	5.3	5.9	6.5	7.3	8.0	8.7	9.4	10.0
Hiking, 3 mph with pack	3.5	4.1	4.6	5.1	5.7	6.2	6.7	7.3	7.8
Hockey, field	4.0	5.9	6.6	7.3	8.1	8.9	9.6	10.4	11.1
Hockey, ice	5.6	6.5	7.4	8.2	9.1	10.0	10.8	11.8	12.6
Martial arts (judo/karate)	7.5	8.7	9.7	10.8	12.0	13.2	14.3	15.5	16.6
Mountain climbing	5.5	6.4	7.2	8.0	8.9	9.8	10.6	11.5	12.3
Racquetball	5.5	6.4	7.1	7.9	8.8	9.7	10.5	11.4	12.2
Running, steady state									
6 mph (10:00 min/mile)	6.2	7.3	8.2	9.1	10.1	11.1	11.9	13.0	14.0
7 mph (8:35 min/mile)	7.5	8.7	9.7	10.8	12.0	13.2	14.3	15.5	16.6
8 mph (7:30 min/mile)	8.7	10.1	11.3	12.6	14.0	15.4	16.6	18.0	19.3
9 mph (6:40 min/mile)	9.8	11.3	12.7	14.2	15.7	17.3	18.7	20.2	21.7
10 mph (6:00 min/mile)	11.1	12.8	14.4	16.1	17.8	19.6	21.2	22.8	24.5
11 mph (5:28 min/mile)	12.3	14.2	16.0	17.9	19.8	21.7	23.5	25.5	27.3
12 mph (5:00 min/mile)	13.5	15.6	17.6	19.6	21.7	23.9	25.9	28.0	30.0
Skating, ice, 9 mph	3.2	3.7	4.2	4.6	5.2	5.7	6.2	6.7	7.2
Skating, inline, 13 mph	8.5	9.8	11.1	12.4	13.7	15.1	16.2	17.5	18.8
Skiing, cross country, 5 mph	6.7	7.7	8.7	9.6	10.7	11.6	12.8	13.8	14.8
Skiing, downhill	5.5	6.4	7.2	8.0	8.9	9.8	10.6	11.5	12.3
Soccer	4.9	5.8	6.5	7.2	8.0	8.8	9.5	10.3	11.0
Weight in kg	45	52	59	66	73	80	86	93	100

Weight in lb	100	115	130	145	160	175	190	205	220
Swimming, yards/min									
Backstroke, 30	2.5	3.0	3.3	3.6	4.0	4.5	4.8	5.2	5.4
Backstroke, 35	3.5	4.1	4.6	5.1	5.7	6.2	6.7	7.3	7.6
Backstroke, 40	4.5	5.3	5.9	6.5	7.3	8.0	8.7	9.4	9.8
Breaststroke, 30	3.7	4.3	4.9	5.4	6.0	6.6	7.2	7.8	10.3
Breaststroke, 40	5.3	6.2	7.0	7.8	8.6	9.5	10.3	11.1	11.9
Front crawl, 25	3.0	3.5	3.9	4.3	4.8	5.3	5.7	6.2	6.4
Front crawl, 35	3.8	4.5	5.1	5.5	6.2	6.8	7.3	7.9	8.2
Front crawl, 45	4.7	5.5	6.2	6.9	7.7	8.4	9.1	9.9	10.3
Front crawl, 50	6.0	7.0	7.9	8.8	9.7	10.7	11.6	12.5	13.0
Tennis, competition	5.4	6.3	7.1	7.9	8.8	9.7	10.5	11.4	12.2
Volleyball, vigorous or competition	5.5	6.4	7.1	7.9	8.8	9.7	10.5	11.4	12.2
Walking, brisk or race									
4 mph (15:00 min/mile)	3.2	3.7	4.2	4.6	5.2	5.7	6.2	6.7	7.2
5 mph (12:00 min/mile)	4.4	5.2	5.8	6.4	7.1	7.8	8.5	9.2	9.8
5.8 mph (10:20 min/mile)	6.7	7.7	8.7	9.6	10.7	11.8	12.8	13.8	14.8
Weight training	4.2	4.9	5.5	6.1	6.7	7.4	8.0	8.7	9.3
Wrestling	8.5	8.7	9.7	10.8	12.0	13.2	14.3	15.5	16.6
Lying quietly	1.0*	1.1*	1.3*	1.5*	1.6*	1.7*	1.9*	2.0*	2.2*
Standing with light work	1.7	2.0	2.2	2.4	2.8	3.1	3.3	3.6	3.8

Keep the following in mind when using this table:

1. The figures are approximate values above rest or resting energy expenditure (REE) and thus can be calculated and added to your daily REE value as discussed in chapter 2. To obtain these values REE* was subtracted from the total cost of the activity to get net activity cost or calorie expenditure above rest.

2. The values in the table are only for the time you are performing the activity. For example, during an hour of a basketball game you may play strenuously for only 35 or 40 minutes, as you may take time-outs and rest during foul shots. In general, record only the amount of time that you are actually exercising during the activity. If desired, you can also include time spent standing but do not need to estimate time spent sitting.

3. The energy cost, expressed in calories per minute, will vary for different activities in a given individual depending on several factors. For example, the caloric cost of bicycling will vary depending on the type of bicycle, going uphill and downhill, and wind resistance. Energy cost for swimming at a certain pace will depend on swimming efficiency, so the less efficient swimmer will expend more calories. Thus, the values expressed here are approximations and may be increased or decreased depending on various factors that influence energy cost for a specific physical activity.

4. Not all body weights could be listed, but you may approximate by using the closest weight listed or using a value between the two closest values.

5. There may be small differences between males and females, but not enough to make a significant difference in the total caloric value for most exercises.

6. Not all physical activities and sports could be listed. For a more extensive list see the original source.

Adapted from M. Williams, 2005, *Nutrition for health, fitness & sport*, 7th ed. (New York, NY: McGraw-Hill), by permission of The McGraw-Hill Companies.

Appendix B

Food Guidance Systems

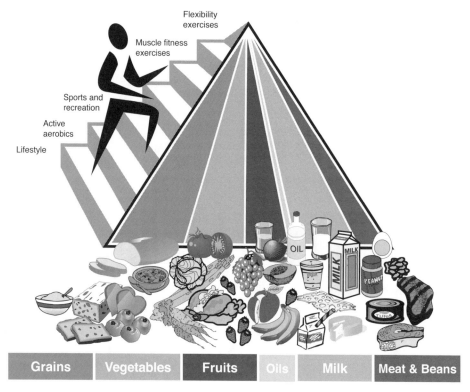

MyPyramid.
From the United States Department of Agriculture (USDA). Available: www.MyPyramid.gov.

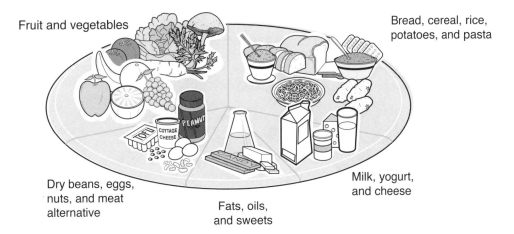

Fruit and vegetables

Bread, cereal, rice, potatoes, and pasta

Dry beans, eggs, nuts, and meat alternative

Fats, oils, and sweets

Milk, yogurt, and cheese

Food plate model.

Appendix C

Glycemic Index of Common Foods

HIGH GLYCEMIC–INDEX FOODS (GI >85)
Angel food cake
Croissant
Muffins
Melba toast
Cake doughnut
Soft drinks
Waffles
Cheese pizza
Bagel, white
Barley flour bread
White bread
Rye flour bread
Whole wheat bread
Cheerios
Corn bran cereal
Corn Chex cereal
Cornflakes
Cream of wheat
Crispix cereal
Grape-Nuts
Raisins
Mueslix
Rice Krispies
Shredded wheat
Cornmeal
Millet
Ice cream
Brown rice
Rice cakes
Soda crackers
Oatmeal
Total cereal
Couscous

Watermelon
Potatoes
Hard candy
Sucrose
Carrots
Glucose
Maltose
Corn chips
Honey and syrups
Sport drinks
Molasses
MODERATE GLYCEMIC– INDEX FOODS (GI = 60-85)
Sponge cake
Pastry
Popcorn
Oat bran bread
Rye kernel bread
Pita bread, white
Bulgur bread
Mixed grain bread
All-Bran cereal
Bran Chex cereal
Oat bran cereal
Special K cereal
Cracked barley
Buckwheat
Bulgur
Sweet corn
White rice (long-grain)
Basmati rice
Parboiled rice
Wild rice
Sweet potato/yams
Wheat, cooked

Ice cream, low-fat
Banana
Fruit cocktail
Grapefruit juice
Grapes
Kiwi fruit
Mango and papaya
Orange (whole or juice)
Durum spaghetti
Linguine
LOW GLYCEMIC–INDEX FOODS (GI <60)
Barley kernel bread
Barley
Rice bran
Wheat kernels
Milk (whole or skim)
Yogurt (all types)
Apples
Apricots (dried)
Cherries
Grapefruit
Peaches (fresh)
Pears (fresh)
Plums
Beans (all types)
Lentils
Dried peas
Spaghetti
Peanuts
Tomato soup
Fructose

White bread (50 g) was used as the reference food and has a GI of 100.

From K. Foster-Powell and J.B. Miller, 1995, "International table of glycemic indices," *The American Journal of Clinical Nutrition* 62(suppl): 871S-893S. Adapted from *The American Journal of Clinical Nutrition*.

Dietary Reference Intakes for Vitamins and Minerals

Dietary Reference Intakes:
Recommended Intakes for Individuals for Vitamins

Age	Males			Females			Pregnancy (19-50)	Lactation (19-50)
	19-50	51-70	Over 70	19-50	51-70	Over 70		
Vitamin A (mcg/day)[a]	900	900	900	700	700	700	770	1,300
Vitamin C (mg/day)	90	90	90	75	75	75	85	120
Vitamin D (mcg/day)[b,c]	5*	10*	15*	5*	10*	15*	5*	5*
Vitamin E (mg/day)[d]	15	15	15	15	15	15	15	19
Vitamin K (mcg/day)	120*	120*	120*	90*	90*	90*	90*	90*
Thiamin (mg/day)	1.2	1.2	1.2	1.1	1.1	1.1	1.4	1.4
Riboflavin (mg/day)	1.3	1.3	1.3	1.1	1.1	1.1	1.4	1.6
Niacin (mg/day)[e]	16	16	16	14	14	14	18	17
Vitamin B$_6$ (mg/day)	1.3	1.7	1.7	1.3	1.5	1.5	1.9	2.0
Folate (mcg/day)[f]	400	400	400	400[i]	400	400	600[j]	500
Vitamin B$_{12}$ (mcg/day)	2.4	2.4[i]	2.4[i]	2.4	2.4[h]	2.4[h]	2.6	2.8
Pantothenic acid (mg/day)	5*	5*	5*	5*	5*	5*	6*	7*
Biotin (mcg/day)	30*	30*	30*	30*	30*	30*	30*	35*
Choline (mg/day)[g]	550*	550*	550*	425*	425*	425*	450*	550*

Note: This table (taken from the DRI reports; see www.nap.edu) presents Recommended Dietary Allowances (RDAs) in **bold type** and Adequate Intakes (AIs) in ordinary type followed by an asterisk (*). RDAs and AIs may both be used as goals for individual intake. RDAs are set to meet the needs of almost all (97 to 98 percent) individuals in a group. For the ages presented here, the AI is believed to cover needs of all individuals in the group, but lack of data or uncertainty in the data prevent being able to specify with confidence the percentage of individuals covered by this intake.

[a]As retinol activity equivalents (RAEs). 1 RAE = 1 mcg retinol, 12 mcg beta-carotene, 24 mcg alpha-carotene, or 24 mcg beta-cryptoxanthin. The RAE for dietary provitamin A carotenoids is twofold greater than retinol equivalents (RE), whereas the RAE for preformed vitamin A is the same as RE.

[b]As cholecalciferol. 1 mcg cholecalciferol = 40 IU vitamin D.

[c]In the absence of adequate exposure to sunlight.

[d]As α-tocopherol. α-tocopherol includes *RRR*-α-tocopherol, the only form of α-tocopherol that occurs naturally in foods, and the *2R*-stereoisomeric forms of α-tocopherol (*RRR*-, *RSR*-, *RRS*-, and *RSS*-α-tocopherol) that occur in fortified foods and supplements. It does not include the *2S*-stereoisomeric forms of α-tocopherol (*SRR*-, *SSR*-, *SRS*-, and *SSS*-α-tocopherol), also found in fortified foods and supplements.

[e]As niacin equivalents (NE). 1 mg of niacin = 60 mg of tryptophan.

[f]As dietary folate equivalents (DFE). 1 DFE = 1 mcg food folate = 0.6 mcg of folic acid from fortified food or as a supplement consumed with food = 0.5 mcg of a supplement taken on an empty stomach.

[g]Although AIs have been set for choline, there are few data to assess whether a dietary supply of choline is needed at all stages of the life cycle, and it may be that the choline requirement can be met by endogenous synthesis at some of these stages.

[h]Because 10 to 30 percent of older people may malabsorb food-bound B$_{12}$, it is advisable for those older than 50 years to meet their RDA mainly by consuming foods fortified with B$_{12}$ or a supplement containing B$_{12}$.

[i]In view of evidence linking folate intake with neural tube defects in the fetus, it is recommended that all women capable of becoming pregnant consume 400 mcg from supplements or fortified foods in addition to intake of food folate from a varied diet.

[j]It is assumed that women will continue consuming 400 mcg from supplements or fortified food until their pregnancy is confirmed and they enter prenatal care, which ordinarily occurs after the end of the periconceptional period—the critical time for formation of the neural tube.

Adapted with permission from *Dietary Reference Intakes for Vitamin A, Vitamin K, Arsenic, Boron, Chromium, Copper, Iodine, Iron, Manganese, Molybdenum, Nickel, Silicon, Vanadium and Zinc,* © 2000 by the National Academy of Sciences, courtesy of the National Academies Press, Washington, D.C.

Dietary Reference Intakes:
Recommended Intakes for Individuals for Elements

Age	Males			Females			Pregnancy (19-50)	Lactation (19-50)
	19-50	51-70	Over 70	19-50	51-70	Over 70		
Calcium (mg/day)	1,000*	1,200*	1,200*	1,000*	1,200*	1,200*	1,000*	1,000*
Chromium (mcg/day)	35*	30*	30*	25*	20*	20*	30*	45*
Copper (mcg/day)	900	900	900	900	900	900	1,000	1,300
Fluoride (mg/day)	4*	4*	4*	3*	3*	3*	3*	3*
Iodine (mcg/day)	150	150	150	150	150	150	220	290
Iron (mg/day)	8	8	8	18	8	8	27	9
Magnesium (mg/day)	400 (19-30) 420 (31-50)	420	420	310 (19-30) 320 (31-50)	320	320	350 (19-30) 360 (31-50)	310 (19-30) 320 (31-50)
Manganese (mg/day)	2.3*	2.3*	2.3*	1.8*	1.8*	1.8*	2.0*	2.6*
Molybdenum (mcg/day)	45	45	45	45	45	45	50	50
Phosphorus (mg/day)	700	700	700	700	700	700	700	700
Selenium (mcg/day)	55	55	55	55	55	55	60	70
Zinc (mg/day)	11	11	11	8	8	8	11	12
Potassium (g/day)	4.7*	4.7*	4.7*	4.7*	4.7*	4.7*	4.7*	5.1*
Sodium (g/day)	1.5*	1.3*	1.2*	1.5*	1.3*	1.2*	1.5*	1.5*
Chloride (g/day)	2.3*	2.0*	1.8*	2.3*	2.0*	1.8*	2.3*	2.3*

Note: This table presents Recommended Dietary Allowances (RDAs) in **bold type** and Adequate Intakes (AIs) in ordinary type followed by an asterisk (*). RDAs and AIs may both be used as goals for individual intake. RDAs are set to meet the needs of almost all (97 to 98 percent) individuals in a group. For the ages presented here, the AI is believed to cover needs of all individuals in the group, but lack of data or uncertainty in the data prevent being able to specify with confidence the percentage of individuals covered by this intake.

Sources: Dietary Reference Intakes for Calcium, Phosphorous, Magnesium, Vitamin D, and Fluoride (1997); Dietary Reference Intakes for Thiamin, Riboflavin, Niacin, Vitamin B_6, Folate, Vitamin B_{12}, Pantothenic Acid, Biotin, and Choline (1998); Dietary Reference Intakes for Vitamin C, Vitamin E, Selenium, and Carotenoids (2000); Dietary Reference Intakes for Vitamin A, Vitamin K, Arsenic, Boron, Chromium, Copper, Iodine, Iron, Manganese, Molybdenum, Nickel, Silicon, Vanadium, and Zinc (2001); and Dietary Reference Intakes for Water, Potassium, Sodium, Chloride, and Sulfate (2004). These reports may be accessed via www.nap.edu.

Adapted with permission from *Dietary Reference Intakes for Vitamin A, Vitamin K, Arsenic, Boron, Chromium, Copper, Iodine, Iron, Manganese, Molybdenum, Nickel, Silicon, Vanadium and Zinc*, © 2000 by the National Academy of Sciences, courtesy of the National Academies Press, Washington, D.C.

Appendix E

Metric Conversions for Common Measures

Measurement		Conversion formula	Metric equivalent
Teaspoon	Liquid	× 5 =	5 ml
	Solid	× 4.7 =	4.7 grams
Tablespoon	Liquid	× 15 =	15 ml
	Solid	× 14.2* =	14.2 grams
Cup	Liquid	× 236 =	236 ml
	Solid	× 230* =	230 grams
Ounce	Liquid	× 29 =	29 ml
	Solid	× 28* =	28 grams
Inch		× 2.5 =	2.5 cm

*These are general conversion factors. To accurately convert cups to grams, a different factor is necessary depending on the type of food. For example, one cup of flour is 120 grams, and one cup of peanut butter is 258 grams. To accurately convert measurements for specific foods, use an online conversion tool such as the one at GourmetSleuth.com (www.gourmetsleuth.com/cookingconversions. asp?Action=find).

Bibliography

Chapter 1

1. American Dietetic Association and Dietitians of Canada. Position of the American Dietetic Association and Dietitians of Canada: Vegetarian diets. *Journal of the American Dietetic Association.* 103:748-765, 2003.

2. *Tracking nutrition trends 1989-1994-1997.* Toronto: Canadian Facts and National Institute of Nutrition, 1997.

3. Appleby, P.N., T.J. Key, M. Thorogood, M.L. Burr, and J. Mann. Mortality in British vegetarians. *Public Health Nutrition.* 5:29-36, 2002.

4. Barr, S.I. and G.E. Chapman. Perceptions and practices of self-defined current vegetarian, former vegetarian, and nonvegetarian women. *Journal of the American Dietetic Association.* 102:354-360, 2002.

5. Berkow, S.E. and N. Barnard. Vegetarian diets and weight status. *Nutrition Reviews.* 64, 2006.

6. Berry, E. The effects of a high and low protein diet on physical efficiency. *American Physical Education Review.* 14:288-297, 1909.

7. Block, G., B. Patterson, and A. Subar. Fruit, vegetables, and cancer prevention: A review of the epidemiological evidence. *Nutrition and Cancer.* 18:1-29, 1992.

8. Boyle, M.A. and D.H. Holben. *Community Nutrition in Action: An Entrepreneurial Approach.* 4th ed. Belmont, CA: Thomson Wadsworth, 2006, 8.

9. Campbell, W.W., M.L. Barton, Jr., D. Cyr-Campbell, S.L. Davey, J.L. Beard, G. Parise, and W.J. Evans. Effects of an omnivorous diet compared with a lactoovovegetarian diet on resistance-training-induced changes in body composition and skeletal muscle in older men. *American Journal of Clinical Nutrition.* 70:1032-1039, 1999.

10. Clarkson, P. Antioxidants and physical performance. *Critical Reviews in Food Science and Nutrition.* 35:131-141, 1995.

11. Eisinger, M., M. Plath, L. Jung, and C. Leitzmann. Nutrient intake of endurance runners with ovo-lacto-vegetarian diet and regular western diet. *Zeitschrift für Ernahrungswissenschaft.* 33:217-229, 1994.

12. Fisher, I. The influence of flesh eating on endurance. *Yale Medical Journal.* XIII:204-221, 1907.

13. Fraser, G.E. Associations between diet and cancer, ischemic heart disease, and all-cause mortality in non-Hispanic white California Seventh-day Adventists. *American Journal of Clinical Nutrition.* 70:532S-538S, 1999.

14. Fraser, G.E., J. Sabate, W.L. Beeson, and T.M. Strahan. A possible protective effect of nut consumption on risk of coronary heart disease. The Adventist Health Study. *Archives of Internal Medicine.* 152:1416-1424, 1992.

15. Giem, P., W.L. Beeson, and G.E. Fraser. The incidence of dementia and intake of animal products: Preliminary findings from the Adventist Health Study. *Neuroepidemiology.* 12:28-36, 1993.

16. Giovannucci, E., E.B. Rimm, M.J. Stampfer, G.A. Colditz, A. Ascherio, and W.C. Willett. Intake of fat, meat, and fiber in relation to risk of colon cancer in men. *Cancer Research.* 54:2390-2397, 1994.

17. Grandjean, A.C. Diets of elite athletes: Has the discipline of sports nutrition made an impact? *Journal of Nutrition.* 127:874S-877S, 1997.

18. Vegetarian Resource Group. *How many vegetarians are there?* Retrieved January 3, 2003, from: www.vrg.org/journal/vj2003issue3/vj2003issue3poll.htm.

19. Hanne, N., R. Dlin, and A. Rotstein. Physical fitness, anthropometric and metabolic parameters in vegetarian athletes. *Journal of Sports Medicine and Physical Fitness.* 26:180-185, 1986.

20. Harris, H.A. Nutrition and physical performance. The diet of Greek athletes. *Proceedings of the Nutrition Society.* 25:87-90, 1966.

21. Haub, M.D., A.M. Wells, M.A. Tarnopolsky, and W.W. Campbell. Effect of protein source on resistive-training-induced changes in body composition and muscle size in older men. *American Journal of Clinical Nutrition.* 76:511-517, 2002.

22. Hu, F.B., M.J. Stampfer, J.E. Manson, E.B. Rimm, G.A. Colditz, B.A. Rosner, F.E. Speizer, C.H. Hennekens, and W.C. Willett. Frequent nut consumption and risk of coronary heart disease in women: Prospective cohort study. *British Medical Journal.* 317:1341-1345, 1998.

23. Jacobs, D.R., Jr., L. Marquart, J. Slavin, and L.H. Kushi. Whole-grain intake and cancer: An expanded review and meta-analysis. *Nutrition and Cancer.* 30:85-96, 1998.

24. Jacobs, D.R., Jr., K.A. Meyer, L.H. Kushi, and A.R. Folsom. Whole-grain intake may reduce the risk of ischemic heart disease death in postmenopausal women: The Iowa Women's Health Study. *American Journal of Clinical Nutrition.* 68:248-257, 1998.

25. Kanter, M. Free radicals and exercise: Effects of nutritional antioxidant supplementation. *Exercise and Sport Sciences Review.* 12:375-397, 1995.

26. Key, T.J., G.E. Fraser, M. Thorogood, P.N. Appleby, V. Beral, G. Reeves, M.L. Burr, J. Chang-Claude, R. Frentzel-Beyme, J.W. Kuzma, J. Mann, and K. McPherson. Mortality in vegetarians and nonvegetarians: Detailed findings from a collaborative analysis of 5 prospective studies. *American Journal of Clinical Nutrition.* 70:516S-524S, 1999.

27. Krajcovicova-Kudlackova, M. and M. Dusinska. Oxidative DNA damage in relation to nutrition. *Neoplasma.* 51:30-33, 2004.

28. Krajcovicova-Kudlackova, M., V. Spustova, and V. Paukova. Lipid peroxidation and nutrition. *Physiological Research/Academia Scientiarum Bohemoslovaca.* 53:219-224, 2004.

29. Krajcovicova-Kudlackova, M., M. Ursinyova, P. Blazicek, V. Spustova, E. Ginter, V. Hladikova, and J. Klvanova. Free radical disease prevention and nutrition. *Bratislavské Lekárske Listy.* 104:64-68, 2003.

30. Kushi, L.H., L.A. Meyer, and D.R. Jacobs. Cereals, legumes, and chronic disease risk reduction: Evidence from epidemiologic studies. *American Journal of Clinical Nutrition.* 70:451S-458S, 1999.

31. Morillas-Ruiz, J.M., J.A. Villegas Garcia, F.J. Lopez, M.L. Vidal-Guevara, and P. Zafrilla. Effects of poly-phenolic antioxidants on exercise-induced oxidative stress. *Clinical Nutrition.* 25(3):444-453, 2006.

32. Newcomer, B.R., B. Sirikul, G.R. Hunter, E. Larson-Meyer, and M. Bamman. Exercise over-stress and maximal muscle oxidative metabolism: A 31P magnetic resonance spectroscopy case report. *British Journal of Sports Medicine.* 39:302-306, 2005.

33. Nieman, D. Vegetarian dietary practices and endurance performance. *American Journal of Clinical Nutrition.* 48:754-761, 1988.

34. Nieman, D.C. Physical fitness and vegetarian diets: is there a relation? *American Journal of Clinical Nutrition.* 70:570S-575S, 1999.

35. Powers, S.K., K.C. DeRuisseau, J. Quindry, and K.L. Hamilton. Dietary antioxidants and exercise. *Journal of Sports Sciences.* 22:81-94, 2004.

36. Raben, A., B. Kiens, E.A. Richter, L.B. Rasmussen, B. Svenstrup, S. Micic, and P. Bennett. Serum sex hormones and endurance performance after a lacto-ovo vegetarian and a mixed diet. *Medicine and Science in Sports and Exercise.* 24:1290-1297, 1992.

37. Rauma, A.L. and H. Mykkanen. Antioxidant status in vegetarians versus omnivores. *Nutrition.* 16:111-119, 2000.

38. Richter, E.A., B. Kiens, A. Raben, N. Tvede, and B.K. Pedersen. Immune parameters in male athletes after a lacto-ovo vegetarian diet and a mixed Western diet. *Medicine and Science in Sports and Exercise.* 23:517-521, 1991.

39. Rimm, E.B., A. Ascherio, E. Giovannucci, D. Spiegelman, M.J. Stampfer, and W.C. Willett. Vegetable, fruit, and cereal fiber intake and risk of coronary heart disease among men. *Journal of the American Medical Association.* 275:447-451, 1996.

40. Sabate, J. Nut consumption, vegetarian diets, ischemic heart disease risk, and all-cause mortality: Evidence from epidemiologic studies. *American Journal of Clinical Nutrition.* 70:500S-503S, 1999.

41. Simopoulos, A.P. Opening address. Nutrition and fitness from the first Olympiad in 776 BC to 393 AD and the concept of positive health. *American Journal of Clinical Nutrition*. 49:921-926, 1989.

42. Snowdon, D.A. and R.L. Phillips. Does a vegetarian diet reduce the occurrence of diabetes? *American Journal of Public Health*. 75:507-512, 1985.

43. Steinmetz, K.A. and J.D. Potter. Vegetables, fruit, and cancer prevention: A review. *Journal of the American Dietetic Association*. 96:1027-1039, 1996.

44. Steinmetz, K.A. and J.D. Potter. Vegetables, fruit, and cancer. I. Epidemiology. *Cancer Causes and Control*. 2:325-357, 1991.

45. Urso, M.L. and P.M. Clarkson. Oxidative stress, exercise, and antioxidant supplementation. *Toxicology*. 189:41-54, 2003.

46. Willett, W.C. Convergence of philosophy and science: the third international congress on vegetarian nutrition. *American Journal of Clinical Nutrition*. 70:434S-438S, 1999.

Chapter 2

1. Bahr, R. and O. Sejersted. Effect of intensity of exercise on excess postexercise O_2 consumption. *Metabolism*. 40:836-841, 1991.

2. Barr, S.I. Vegetarianism and menstrual cycle disturbances: Is there an association? *American Journal of Clinical Nutrition*. 70:549S-554S, 1999.

3. Brooks, S., C. Sanborn, B. Albrecht, and W. Wagner. Diet in athletic amenorrhoea [letter]. *Lancet*. 2:559-560, 1984.

4. Brouns, F. and W.H. Saris. Diet manipulation and related metabolic changes in competitive cyclists. In *American College of Sports Medicine Annual Meeting*, 1990.

5. Cunningham, J. A reanalysis of the factors influencing basal metabolic rate in normal adults. *American Journal of Clinical Nutrition*. 33:2372-2374, 1980.

6. Deuster, P.A., S.B. Kyle, P.B. Moser, R.A. Vigersky, A. Singh, and E.B. Schoomaker. Nutritional intakes and status of highly trained amenorrheic and eumenorrheic women runners. *Fertility and Sterility*. 46:636-643, 1986.

7. Goran, M. Variation in total energy expenditure in humans. *Obesity Research*. 3:59-66, 1995.

8. Goran, M., E. Poehlman, and R. Johnson. Energy requirements across the life span: New findings based on measurement of total energy expenditure with doubly labeled water. *Nutrition Research*. 15:115-150, 1994.

9. Hill, R.J. and P.S. Davies. Energy expenditure during 2 wk of an ultra-endurance run around Australia. *Medicine and Science in Sports and Exercise*. 33:148-151, 2001.

10. Hill, R.J. and P.S. Davies. Energy intake and energy expenditure in elite lightweight female rowers. *Medicine and Science in Sports and Exercise*. 34:1823-1829, 2002.

11. Huse, D.M. and A.R. Lucas. Dietary patterns in anorexia nervosa. *American Journal of Clinical Nutrition*. 40:251-254, 1984.

12. Kaiserauer, S., A. Snyder, M. Sleeper, and J. Zierath. Nutritional, physiological, and menstrual status of distance runners. *Medicine and Science in Sports and Exercise*. 21:120-125, 1989.

13. Lloyd, T., J. Buchanen, S. Bitzer, C. Waldman, C. Myers, and B. Ford. Interrelationship of diet, athletic activity, menstrual status, and bone density in collegiate women. *American Journal of Clinical Nutrition*. 46:681-684, 1987.

14. Loucks, A.B. Physical health of the female athlete: Observations, effects, and causes of reproductive disorders. *Canadian Journal of Applied Physiology*. 26 Suppl:S176-185, 2001.

15. Manore, M. and J. Thompson. *Sport Nutrition for Health and Performance*. Champaign, IL: Human Kinetics, 2000.

16. Messina, V., V. Melina, and A.R. Mangels. A new food guide for North American vegetarians. *Journal of the American Dietetic Association*. 103:771-775, 2003.

17. Messina, V., V. Melina, and A.R. Mangels. A new food guide for North American vegetarians. *Journal of the American Dietetic Association*. 103:771-775, 2003.

18. Nelson, M., E. Fisher, P. Catsos, C. Meredith, R. Turksoy, and W. Evans. Diet and bone status in amenor-rheic runners. *American Journal of Clinical Nutrition.* 43:910-916, 1986.

19. Neumark-Sztainer, D., M. Story, M.D. Resnick, and R.W. Blum. Adolescent vegetarians: A behavioral profile of a school-based population in Minnesota. *Archives of Pediatrics and Adolescent Medicine.* 151:833-838, 1997.

20. O'Connor, M.A., S.W. Touyz, S.M. Dunn, and J.V. Beumont. Vegetarianism in anorexia nervosa? A review of 116 consecutive cases. *Medical Journal of Australia.* 147:540-542, 1987.

21. Slavin, J., J. Lutter, and S. Cushman. Amenorrhea in vegetarian athletes [letter]. *Lancet.* 1984:1474-1475, 1984.

22. Thompson, J. and M. Manore. Predicted and measured resting metabolic rate of male and female endurance athletes. *Journal of the American Dietetic Association.* 96:30-34, 1996.

23. Toth, M. and E. Poehlman. Sympathetic nervous system activity and resting metabolic rate in vegetarians. *Metabolism.* 43:621-625, 1994.

Chapter 3

1. Achten, J., S.L. Halson, L. Moseley, M.P. Rayson, A. Casey, and A.E. Jeukendrup. Higher dietary carbohydrate content during intensified running training results in better maintenance of performance and mood state. *Journal of Applied Physiology.* 96:1331-1340, 2004.

2. Balsom, P.D., K. Wood, P. Olsson, and B. Ekblom. Carbohydrate intake and multiple sprint sports: With special reference to football (soccer). *International Journal of Sports Medicine.* 20:48-52, 1999.

3. Brewer, J., C. Williams, and A. Patton. The influence of high carbohydrate diets on endurance running performance. *European Journal of Applied Physiology.* 57:698-706, 1988.

4. Costill, D.L., W.M. Sherman, W.J. Fink, C. Maresh, M. Witten, and J.M. Miller. The role of dietary carbohydrates in muscle glycogen resynthesis after strenuous running. *American Journal of Clinical Nutrition.* 34:1831-1836, 1981.

5. Jenkins, D.J., C.W. Kendall, L.S. Augustin, S. Franceschi, M. Hamidi, A. Marchie, A.L. Jenkins, and M. Axelsen. Glycemic index: Overview of implications in health and disease. *American Journal of Clinical Nutrition.* 76:266S-273S, 2002.

6. Larson, D.E., R.L. Hesslink, M.I. Hrovat, R.S. Fishman, and D.M. Systrom. Dietary effects on exercising muscle metabolism and performance by ^{31}P-MRS. *Journal of Applied Physiology.* 77:1108-1115, 1994.

7. Livesey, G. Low-glycaemic diets and health: Implications for obesity. *Proceedings of the Nutrition Society.* 64:105-113, 2005.

8. American College of Sports Medicine, American Dietetic Association, and Dietitians of Canada. Nutrition and Athletic Performance. Joint Position Statement. *Medicine and Science in Sports and Exercise.* 32:2130-2145, 2000.

Chapter 4

1. American Diabetes Association. Evidence-based nutrition principles and recommendations for the treatment and prevention of diabetes and related complications. *Diabetes Care.* 25:202-212, 2002.

2. Executive summary of the third report of the National Cholesterol Education Program (NCEP) expert panel on detection, evaluation, and treatment of high blood cholesterol in adults (Adult Treatment Panel III). *Journal of the American Medical Association.* 285:2486-2497, 2001.

3. Ascherio, A. and W.C. Willett. Health effects of trans fatty acids. *American Journal of Clinical Nutrition.* 66:1006S-1010S, 1997.

4. Brown, R.C. and C.M. Cox. Effects of high fat versus high carbohydrate diets on plasma lipids and lipoproteins in endurance athletes. *Medicine and Science in Sports and Exercise.* 30:1677-1683, 1998.

5. Crist, D. M. and J.M. Hill. Diet and insulinlike growth factor I in relation to body composition in women with exercise-induced hypothalamic amenorrhea. *Journal of the American College of Nutrition.* 9, 1990.

6. Decombaz, J., M. Fleith, H. Hoppeler, R. Kreis, and C. Boesch. Effect of diet on the replenishment of intramyocellular lipids after exercise. *European Journal of Nutrition.* 39:244-247, 2000.

7. Decombaz, J., B. Schmitt, M. Ith, B. Decarli, P. Diem, R. Kreis, H. Hoppeler, and C. Boesch. Postexercise fat intake repletes intramyocellular lipids but no faster in trained than in sedentary subjects. *American Journal of Physiology. Regulatory, Integrative and Comparative Physiology.* 281:R760-769, 2001.

8. Deuster, P.A., S.B. Kyle, P.B. Moser, R.A. Vigersky, A. Singh, and E.B. Schoomaker. Nutritional intakes and status of highly trained amenorrheic and eumenorrheic women runners. *Fertility and Sterility.* 46:636-643, 1986.

9. Dyck, D.J., C.T. Putman, G.J. Heigenhauser, E. Hultman, and L.L. Spriet. Regulation of fat-carbohydrate interaction in skeletal muscle during intense aerobic cycling. *American Journal of Physiology.* 265:E852-859, 1993.

10. Food and Nutrition Board, Institute of Medicine. *Dietary Reference Intakes for Energy, Carbohydrate, Fiber, Fat, Fatty Acids, Cholesterol, Protein, and Amino Acids.* Washington D.C.: National Academy of Sciences, 2002.

11. Geppert, J., V. Kraft, H. Demmelmair, and B. Koletzko. Docosahexaenoic acid supplementation in vegetarians effectively increases omega-3 index: A randomized trial. *Lipids.* 40:807-814, 2005.

12. Hu, F.B., M.J. Stampfer, J.E. Manson, E. Rimm, G.A. Colditz, B.A. Rosner, C.H. Hennekens, and W.C. Willett. Dietary fat intake and the risk of coronary heart disease in women. *New England Journal of Medicine.* 337:1491-1499, 1997.

13. Hu, F.B. and W.C. Willett. Optimal diets for prevention of coronary heart disease. *Journal of the American Medical Association.* 288:2569-2578, 2002.

14. Krauss, R.M., R.H. Eckel, B. Howard, L.J. Appel, S.R. Daniels, R.J. Deckelbaum, J.W. Erdman, Jr., P. Kris-Etherton, I.J. Goldberg, T.A. Kotchen, A.H. Lichtenstein, W.E. Mitch, R. Mullis, K. Robinson, J. Wylie-Rosett, S. St Jeor, J. Suttie, D.L. Tribble, and T.L. Bazzarre. AHA Dietary Guidelines: Revision 2000: A statement for healthcare professionals from the Nutrition Committee of the American Heart Association. *Circulation.* 102:2284-2299, 2000.

15. Larson-Meyer, D.E., G.R. Hunter, and B.R. Newcomer. Influence of endurance running and recovery diet on intramyocellular lipid content in women: A ^{1}H-NMR study. *American Journal of Physiology.* 282:E95-E106, 2002.

16. Larson, D.E., G.R. Hunter, M.J. Williams, T. Kekes-Szabo, I. Nyikos, and M.I. Goran. Dietary fat in relation to body fat and intraabdominal adipose tissue: A cross-sectional analysis. *American Journal of Clinical Nutrition.* 64:677-684, 1996.

17. Larson, D.E., P.A. Tataranni, R.T. Ferraro, and E. Ravussin. Ad libitum food intake on a "cafeteria diet" in Native American women: Relations with body composition and 24-hour energy expenditure. *American Journal of Clinical Nutrition.* 62:911-917, 1995.

18. Laughlin, G.A. and S.S. Yen. Nutritional and endocrine-metabolic aberrations in amenorrheic athletes. *Journal of Clinical Endocrinology and Metabolism.* 81:4301-4309, 1996.

19. Leibel, R., J. Hirsch, B. Appel, and G. Checani. Energy intake required to maintain body weight is not affected by wide variation in diet composition. *American Journal of Clinical Nutrition.* 55:350-355, 1992.

20. Lissner, L. and B.L. Heitmann. Dietary fat and obesity: Evidence from epidemiology. *European Journal of Clinical Nutrition.* 49:79-90, 1995.

21. Mangels, R. Nutrition Hotline. Omega-3 Fatty Acids. *Vegetarian Journal.* Issue 3. Retrieved January 10, 2005, from: www.vrg.org/journal/vj2005issue3/vj2005issue3hotline.htm.

22. Muoio, D.M., J.J. Leddy, P.J. Horvath, A.B. Awad, and D.R. Pendergast. Effect of dietary fat on metabolic adjustments to maximal VO_2 and endurance in runners. *Medicine and Science in Sports and Exercise.* 26:81-88, 1994.

23. Pendergast, D.R., J.J. Leddy, and J.T. Venkatraman. A perspective on fat intake in athletes. *Journal of the American College of Nutrition.* 19:345-350, 2000.

24. Prentice, A.M. Manipulation of dietary fat and energy density and subsequent effects on substrate flux and food intake. *American Journal of Clinical Nutrition.* 67:535S-541S, 1998.

25. Romijn, J., E.F. Coyle, L.S. Sidossis, A. Gastaldelli, J.F. Horowitz, E. Endert, and R.R. Wolfe. Regulation of endogenous fat and carbohydrate metabolism in relation to exercise intensity and duration. *American Journal of Physiology--Endocrinology and Metabolism.* 265:E380-E391, 1993.

26. Romijn, J.A., E.F. Coyle, L.S. Sidossis, J. Rosenblatt, and R.R. Wolfe. Substrate metabolism during different exercise intensities in endurance-trained women. *Journal of Applied Physiology.* 88:1707-1714, 2000.

27. Rosell, M.S., Z. Lloyd-Wright, P.N. Appleby, T.A. Sanders, N.E. Allen, and T.J. Key. Long-chain n-3 polyunsaturated fatty acids in plasma in British meat-eating, vegetarian, and vegan men. *American Journal of Clinical Nutrition.* 82:327-334, 2005.

28. Simopoulos, A.P., A. Leaf, and N. Salem, Jr. Workshop on the essentiality of and recommended dietary intakes for omega-6 and omega-3 fatty acids. *Journal of the American College of Nutrition.* 18:487-489, 1999.

29. Spencer, E.A., P.N. Appleby, G.K. Davey, and T.J. Key. Diet and body mass index in 38000 EPIC-Oxford meat-eaters, fish-eaters, vegetarians and vegans. *International Journal of Obesity and Related Metabolic Disorders.* 27:728-734, 2003.

30. Venkatraman, J.T., J. Leddy, and D.R. Pendergast. Dietary fats and immune status in athletes: Clinical implications. *Medicine and Science in Sports and Exercise.* 32:S389-395, 2000.

31. Vukovich, M., D. Costill, M. Hickey, S. Trappe, K. Cole, and W. Fink. Effect of fat emulsion infusion and fat feeding on muscle glycogen utilization during cycle exercise. *Journal of Applied Physiology.* 75:1513-1518, 1993.

32. Willett, W.C. Is dietary fat a major determinant of body fat? [see comments]. *American Journal of Clinical Nutrition.* 67:556S-562S, 1998.

Chapter 5

1. American Dietetic Association and Dietitians of Canada. Position of the American Dietetic Association and Dietitians of Canada: Vegetarian diets. *Journal of the American Dietetic Association.* 103:748-765, 2003.

2. Boirie, Y., M. Dangin, P. Gachon, M.P. Vasson, J.L. Maubois, and B. Beaufrere. Slow and fast dietary proteins differently modulate postprandial protein accretion. *Proceedings of the National Academy of Sciences of the United States of America.* 94:14930-14935, 1997.

3. Butterfield, G. Whole-body protein utilization in humans. *Medicine and Science in Sports and Exercise.* 19:S157-S165, 1987.

4. Dangin, M., Y. Boirie, C. Garcia-Rodenas, P. Gachon, J. Fauquant, P. Callier, O. Ballevre, and B. Beaufrere. The digestion rate of protein is an independent regulating factor of postprandial protein retention. *American Journal of Physiology--Endocrinology and Metabolism.* 280:E340-348, 2001.

5. Food and Nutrition Board, Institute of Medicine. *Dietary Reference Intakes for Energy, Carbohydrate, Fiber, Fat, Fatty Acids, Cholesterol, Protein, and Amino Acids.* Washington D.C.: National Academy of Sciences, 2002.

6. Gausseres, N., I. Catala, S. Mahe, C. Luengo, F. Bornet, B. Guy-Grand, and D. Tome. Whole-body protein turnover in humans fed a soy protein-rich vegetable diet. *European Journal of Clinical Nutrition.* 51:308-311, 1997.

7. Gontzea, I., P. Sutzescu, and S. Dumitrache. The influence of adaptation of physical effort on nitrogen balance in man. *Nutrition Reports International.* 11:231-234, 1975.

8. Lemon, P. and J. Mullin. Effect of initial muscle glycogen levels on protein catabolism during exercise. *Journal of Applied Physiology.* 48:624-629, 1980.

9. Manore, M. and J. Thompson. *Sport Nutrition for Health and Performance.* Champaign, IL: Human Kinetics, 2000

10. Messina, V., A.R. Mangels, and M. Messina. *A Dietitian's Guide to Vegetarian Diets: Issues and Applications.* 2nd ed. Boston: Jones and Bartlett, 2004.

11. National Research Council. *Recommended Dietary Allowances.* Washington, DC: National Academy Press, 1989.

12. Nikawa, T., M. Ikemoto, T. Sakai, M. Kano, T. Kitano, T. Kawahara, S. Teshima, K. Rokutan, and K. Kishi. Effects of a soy protein diet on exercise-induced muscle protein catabolism in rats. *Nutrition.* 18:490-495, 2002.

13. Reddy, S.T., C.Y. Wang, K. Sakhaee, L. Brinkley, and C.Y. Pak. Effect of low-carbohydrate high-protein diets on acid-base balance, stone-forming propensity, and calcium metabolism. *American Journal of Kidney Diseases.* 40:265-274, 2002.

14. Simopoulos, A.P. Opening address. Nutrition and fitness from the first Olympiad in 776 BC to 393 AD and the concept of positive health. *American Journal of Clinical Nutrition.* 49:921-926, 1989.

15. Tarnopolsky, M. Protein requirements for endurance athletes. *Nutrition.* 20:662-668, 2004.

16. Tarnopolsky, M., S. Atkinson, J. MacDougall, A. Chesley, S. Phillips, and H. Schwarcz. Evaluation of protein requirements for trained strength athletes. *Journal of Applied Physiology.* 73:1986-1995, 1992.

17. American College of Sports Medicine, American Dietetic Association, and Dietitians of Canada. Nutrition and athletic performance. Joint position statement. *Medicine and Science in Sports and Exercise.* 32:2130-2145, 2000.

18. Young, V. Soy protein in relation to human protein and amino acid nutrition. *Journal of the American Dietetic Association.* 91:828-835, 1991.

19. Young, V. and P. Pellett. Plant proteins in relation to human protein and amino acid nutrition. *American Journal of Clinical Nutrition.* 59:1203S-1212S, 1994.

Chapter 6

1. American Dietetic Association and Dietitians of Canada. Position of the American Dietetic Association and Dietitians of Canada: Vegetarian diets. *Journal of the American Dietetic Association.* 103:748-765, 2003.

2. Barrett-Connor, E., J.C. Chang, and S.L. Edelstein. Coffee-associated osteoporosis offset by daily milk consumption: The Rancho Bernardo Study. *Journal of the American Medical Association.* 271:280-283, 1994.

3. Bauer, D.C., W.S. Browner, J.A. Cauley, E.S. Orwoll, J.C. Scott, D.M. Black, J.L. Tao, and S.R. Cummings. Factors associated with appendicular bone mass in older women: The Study of Osteoporotic Fractures Research Group. *Annals of Internal Medicine.* 118:657-665, 1993.

4. Cannell, J. Questions and answers. *Vitamin D Newsletter.* January, 2006. Retrieved June 30, 2006 from: www.vitamindcouncil.com/releases.shtml.

5. Centers for Disease Control and Prevention and National Center for Chronic Disease Prevention and Health Promotion. *National oral health surveillance system.* Retrieved January, 18, 2006, from: http://apps.nccd.cdc.gov/MWF/index.asp.

6. Chakkalakal, D.A. Alcohol-induced bone loss and deficient bone repair. *Alcoholism, Clinical and Experimental Research.* 29:2077-2090, 2005.

7. Chiu, J.F., S.J. Lan, C.Y. Yang, P.W. Wang, W.J. Yao, L.H. Su, and C. Hsieh. Long-term vegetarian diet and bone mineral density in postmenopausal Taiwanese women. *Calcified Tissue International.* 60:245-249, 1997.

8. Dawson-Hughes, B. Racial/ethnic considerations in making recommendations for vitamin D for adult and elderly men and women. *American Journal of Clinical Nutrition.* 80:1763S-1766S, 2004.

9. Feskanich, D., P. Weber, W.C. Willett, H. Rockett, S.L. Booth, and G.A. Colditz. Vitamin K intake and hip fractures in women: A prospective study. *American Journal of Clinical Nutrition.* 69:74-79, 1999.

10. Hallberg, L. Does calcium interfere with iron absorption? (Editorial). *American Journal of Clinical Nutrition.* 68:3-4, 1998.

11. Heaney, R., R. Recker, and P. Saville. Menopausal changes in calcium balance performance. *Journal of Laboratory and Clinical Medicine.* 92:953-962, 1978.

12. Heaney, R.P. Cofactors influencing the calcium requirement: Other nutrients. In *NIH Consensus Development Conference on Optimal Calcium Intakes.* Bethesda, Maryland, 1994.

13. Heaney, R.P. The Vitamin D requirement in health and disease. *Journal of Steroid Biochemistry and Molecular Biology.* 97:13-19, 2005.

14. Heaney, R.P., M.S. Dowell, K. Rafferty, and J. Bierman. Bioavailability of the calcium in fortified soy imitation milk, with some observations on method. *American Journal of Clinical Nutrition.* 71:1166-1169, 2000.

15. Heaney, R.P., K. Rafferty, M.S. Dowell, and J. Bierman. Calcium fortification systems differ in bioavailability. *Journal of the American Dietetic Association.* 105:807-809, 2005.

16. Holick, M.F. Environmental factors that influence the cutaneous production of vitamin D. *American Journal of Clinical Nutrition.* 61:638S-645S, 1995.

17. Holick, M.F. Evolution and function of vitamin D. *Recent Results in Cancer Research.* 164:3-28, 2003.

18. Jones, S., B.A. Burt, P.E. Petersen, and M.A. Lennon. The effective use of fluorides in public health. *Bulletin of the World Health Organization.* 83:670-676, 2005.

19. Kalkwarf, H.J., J.C. Khoury, and B.P. Lanphear. Milk intake during childhood and adolescence, adult bone density, and osteoporotic fractures in US women. *American Journal of Clinical Nutrition.* 77:257-265, 2003.

20. Kohlenberg-Mueller, K. and L. Raschka. Calcium balance in young adults on a vegan and lactovegetarian diet. *Journal of Bone and Mineral Metabolism.* 21:28-33, 2003.

21. Kok, D.J., J.A. Iestra, C.J. Doorenbos, and S.E. Papapoulos. The effects of dietary excesses in animal protein and in sodium on the composition and the crystallization kinetics of calcium oxalate monohydrate in urines of healthy men. *Journal of Clinical Endocrinology and Metabolism.* 71:861-867, 1990.

22. Manore, M.M. Nutritional needs of the female athlete. *Clinics in Sports Medicine.* 18:549-563, 1999.

23. Marsh, A.G., T.V. Sanchez, F.L. Chaffee, G.H. Mayor, and O. Mickelsen. Bone mineral mass in adult lacto-ovo-vegetarian and omnivorous males. *American Journal of Clinical Nutrition.* 37:453-456, 1983.

24. Marsh, A.G., T.V. Sanchez, O. Midkelsen, J. Keiser, and G. Mayor. Cortical bone density of adult lacto-ovo-vegetarian and omnivorous women. *Journal of the American Dietetic Association.* 76:148-151, 1980.

25. McArdle, W., F. Katch, and V. Katch. *Sports and Exercise Nutrition.* Baltimore: Lippincott Williams & Wilkins, 1999.

26. Messina, V., V. Melina, and A.R. Mangels. A new food guide for North American vegetarians. *Journal of the American Dietetic Association.* 103:771-775, 2003.

27. Minihane, A. and S. Fairweather-Tait. Effect of calcium supplementation on daily nonheme-iron absorption and long-term iron status. *American Journal of Clinical Nutrition.* 68:96-102, 1998.

28. Monsen, E.R. and J.L. Balintfy. Calculating dietary iron bioavailability: Refinement and computerization. *Journal of the American Dietetic Association.* 80:307-311, 1982.

29. Myburgh, K., J. Hutchins, A. Fataar, S. Hough, and T. Noakes. Low bone density is an etiologic factor for stress fractures in athletes. *Annals of Internal Medicine.* 113:754-759, 1990.

30. Pak, C.Y., K. Sakhaee, V. Piziak, R.D. Peterson, N.A. Breslau, P. Boyd, J.R. Poindexter, J. Herzog, A. Heard-Sakhaee, S. Haynes, B. Adams-Huet, and J.S. Reisch. Slow-release sodium fluoride in the management of postmenopausal osteoporosis: A randomized controlled trial. *Annals of Internal Medicine.* 120:625-632, 1994.

31. Palmer, C. and S.H. Wolfe. Position of the American Dietetic Association: The impact of fluoride on health. *Journal of the American Dietetic Association.* 105:1620-1628, 2005.

32. Peterson, B.A., R.C. Klesges, E.M. Kaufman, T.V. Cooper, and C M. Vukadinovich. The effects of an educational intervention on calcium intake and bone mineral content in young women with low calcium intake. *American Journal of Health Promotion.* 14:149-156, 2000.

33. Potter, S.M., J.A. Baum, H. Teng, R.J. Stillman, N.F. Shay, and J.W. Erdman, Jr. Soy protein and isoflavones: Their effects on blood lipids and bone density in postmenopausal women. *American Journal of Clinical Nutrition.* 68:1375S-1379S, 1998.

34. Raisz, L.G. Pathogenesis of osteoporosis: Concepts, conflicts, and prospects. *Journal of Clinical Investigation.* 115:3318-3325, 2005.

35. Ryder, K.M., R.I. Shorr, A.J. Bush, S.B. Kritchevsky, T. Harris, K. Stone, J. Cauley, and F. A. Tylavsky. Magnesium intake from food and supplements is associated with bone mineral density in healthy older white subjects. *Journal of the American Geriatrics Society.* 53:1875-1880, 2005.

36. Setchell, K.D. and E. Lydeking-Olsen. Dietary phytoestrogens and their effect on bone: Evidence from in vitro and in vivo, human observational, and dietary intervention studies. *American Journal of Clinical Nutrition.* 78:593S-609S, 2003.

37. Sogaard, C.H., L. Mosekilde, and A. Richards. Marked decrease in trabecular bone quality after five years of sodium fluoride therapy—assessed by biomechanical testing of iliac crest bone biopsies in osteoporotic patients. *Bone.* 15:393-399, 1994.

38. Teegarden, D., R.M. Lyle, W.R. Proulx, C.C. Johnston, and C.M. Weaver. Previous milk consumption is associated with greater bone density in young women. *American Journal of Clinical Nutrition.* 69:1014-1017, 1999.

39. The American College of Sports Medicine, the American Dietetic Association, and the Dietitians of Canada. Nutrition and athletic performance. Joint position statement. *Medicine and Science in Sports and Exercise.* 32:2130-2145, 2000.

40. Trang, H.M., D.E. Cole, L.A. Rubin, A. Pierratos, S. Siu, and R. Vieth. Evidence that vitamin D3 increases serum 25-hydroxyvitamin D more efficiently than does vitamin D2. *American Journal of Clinical Nutrition.* 68:854-858, 1998.

41. Tylavsky, F.A. and J.J. Anderson. Dietary factors in bone health of elderly lactoovovegetarian and omnivorous women. *American Journal of Clinical Nutrition.* 48:842-849, 1988.

42. Velazquez, E. and G. Bellabarba Arata. Testosterone replacement therapy. *Archives of Andrology.* 41:79-90, 1998.

43. Weaver, C. and K. Plawecki. Dietary calcium: Adequacy of a vegetarian diet. *American Journal of Clinical Nutrition.* 59:1238S-1241S, 1994.

44. Weaver, C.M., W.R. Proulx, and R. Heaney. Choices for achieving adequate dietary calcium with a vegetarian diet. *American Journal of Clinical Nutrition.* 70:543S-548S, 1999.

45. Wolman, R., P. Clark, E. McNally, M. Harries, and J. Reeve. Dietary calcium as a statistical determinant of trabecular bone density in amenorrhoeic and oestrogen-replete athletes. *Bone and Mineral.* 17:415-423, 1992.

46. Wyshak, G. Teenaged girls, carbonated beverage consumption, and bone fractures. *Archives of Pediatrics and Adolescent Medicine.* 154:610-613, 2000.

Chapter 7

1. American Dietetic Association and Dietitians of Canada. Position of the American Dietetic Association and Dietitians of Canada: Vegetarian diets. *Journal of the American Dietetic Association.* 103:748-765, 2003.

2. Ball, M.J. and M.A. Bartlett. Dietary intake and iron status of Australian vegetarian women. *American Journal of Clinical Nutrition.* 70:353-358, 1999.

3. Beard, J. and B. Tobin. Iron status and exercise. *American Journal of Clinical Nutrition.* 72:594S-597S, 2000.

4. Beard, J.L. Weekly iron intervention: The case for intermittent iron supplementation [see comments]. *American Journal of Clinical Nutrition.* 68:209-212, 1998.

5. Brownlie, T., V. Utermohlen, P.S. Hinton, and J.D. Haas. Tissue iron deficiency without anemia impairs adaptation in endurance capacity after aerobic training in previously untrained women. *American Journal of Clinical Nutrition.* 79:437-443, 2004.

6. Brutsaert, T.D., S. Hernandez-Cordero, J. Rivera, T. Viola, G. Hughes, and J.D. Haas. Iron supplementation improves progressive fatigue resistance during dynamic knee extensor exercise in iron-depleted, nonanemic women. *American Journal of Clinical Nutrition.* 77:441-448, 2003.

7. Davies, N.M. Toxicity of nonsteroidal anti-inflammatory drugs in the large intestine. *Diseases of the Colon and Rectum.* 38:1311-1321, 1995.

8. Eichner, E. Runner's macrocytosis: A clue to footstrike hemolysis. *American Journal of Medicine.* 78:321-325, 1985.

9. Food and Nutrition Board of the Institute of Medicine. *Dietary Reference Intakes for Vitamin A, Vitamin K, Arsenic, Boron, Chromium, Copper, Iodine, Iron, Manganese, Molybdenum, Nickel, Silicon, Vanadium, and Zinc.* Washington DC: National Academy Press, 2001.

10. Haddad, E.H., L.S. Berk, J.D. Kettering, R.W. Hubbard, and W.R. Peters. Dietary intake and biochemical, hematologic, and immune status of vegans compared with nonvegetarians. *American Journal of Clinical Nutrition.* 70:586S-593S, 1999.

11. Herbert, V. Everyone should be tested for iron disorders. *Journal of the American Dietetic Association.* 92:1502-1509, 1992.

12. Hinton, P.S., C. Giordano, T. Brownlie, and J.D. Haas. Iron supplementation improves endurance after training in iron-depleted, nonanemic women. *Journal of Applied Physiology.* 88:1103-1111, 2000.

13. Kandiah, J. Impact of tofu or tofu + orange juice on hematological indices of lacto-ovo vegetarian females. *Plant Foods for Human Nutrition.* 57:197-204, 2002.

14. Larson, D. and R. Fisher. Management of exercise-induced gastrointestinal problems. *Physician and Sportsmedicine.* 15:112-126, 1987.

15. Larsson, C.L. and G.K. Johansson. Dietary intake and nutritional status of young vegans and omnivores in Sweden. *American Journal of Clinical Nutrition.* 76:100-106, 2002.

16. Marx, J. Iron deficiency in developed countries: Prevalence, influence of lifestyle factors and hazards of prevention (Review). *European Journal of Clinical Nutrition.* 51:491-494, 1997.

17. Monsen, E.R. and J.L. Balintfy. Calculating dietary iron bioavailability: Refinement and computerization. *Journal of the American Dietetic Association.* 80:307-311, 1982.

18. Murray-Kolb, L.E., K.E. Whitfield, and J.E. Beard. Iron status alters cognitive functioning in women during reproductive years. Experimental Biology 2004 meeting. April 17-21. Washington, DC, Abstract #508. Retrieved July 6, 2006 from: http://select.biosis.org/faseb/eb2004_data/FASEB003128.html.

19. Nachtigall, D., P. Nielsen, R. Fischer, R. Engelhardt, and E.E. Gabbe. Iron deficiency in distance runners: A reinvestigation using Fe-labeling and non-invasive liver iron quantification. *International Journal of Sports Medicine.* 17:473-479, 1996.

20. Robertson, J., R. Maughan, and R. Davidson. Faecal blood loss in response to exercise. *British Medical Journal.* 295:303-305, 1987.

21. Rudzki, S.J., H. Hazard, and D. Collinson. Gastrointestinal blood loss in triathletes: Its etiology and relationship to sports anaemia. *Australian Journal of Science and Medicine in Sport.* 27:3-8, 1995.

22. Schumacher, Y.O., A. Schmid, D. Grathwohl, D. Bultermann, and A. Berg. Hematological indices and iron status in athletes of various sports and performances. *Medicine and Science in Sports and Exercise.* 34:869-875, 2002.

23. Sizer, F., and E. Whitney. *Nutrition Concepts and Controversies.* Belmont, CA: Thomson Learnine, 2000.

24. Snyder, A., L. Dvorak, and J. Roepke. Influence of dietary iron source on measures of iron status among female runners. *Medicine and Science in Sports and Exercise.* 21:7-10, 1989.

25. Telford, R.D., G.J. Sly, A.G. Hahn, R.B. Cunningham, C. Bryant, and J.A. Smith. Footstrike is the major cause of hemolysis during running. *Journal of Applied Physiology.* 94:38-42, 2003.

26. Waller, M. and E. Haymes. The effects of heat and exercise on sweat iron loss. *Medicine and Science in Sports and Exercise.* 28:197-203, 1996.

27. Weaver, C. and S. Rajaram. Exercise and iron status. *Journal of Nutrition.* 122:782-787, 1992.

28. Zoller, H. and W. Vogel. Iron supplementation in athletes: First do no harm. *Nutrition.* 20:615-619, 2004.

Chapter 8

1. American Dietetic Association and Dietitians of Canada. Position of the American Dietetic Association and Dietitians of Canada: Vegetarian diets. *Journal of the American Dietetic Association.* 103:748-765, 2003.

2. Barr, S.I. and C.A. Rideout. Nutritional considerations for vegetarian athletes. *Nutrition.* 20:696-703, 2004.

3. Belko, A. Vitamins and exercise: An update. *Medicine and Science in Sports and Exercise.* 19:S191-S196, 1987.

4. Block, G., B. Patterson, and A. Subar. Fruit, vegetables, and cancer prevention: A review of the epidemiological evidence. *Nutrition and Cancer.* 18:1-29, 1992.

5. Chasan-Taber, L., W.C. Willett, J.M. Seddon, M.J. Stampfer, B. Rosner, G.A. Colditz, F.E. Speizer, and S.E. Hankinson. A prospective study of carotenoid and vitamin A intakes and risk of cataract extraction in US women. *American Journal of Clinical Nutrition.* 70:509-516, 1999.

6. Clarkson, P. Antioxidants and physical performance. *Critical Reviews in Food Science and Nutrition.* 35:131-141, 1995.

7. Crohn, D. Perchlorate controversy calls for improving iodine nutrition. *Vegetarian Nutrition Update.* XIV:1,6-7, 2005.

8. De Luca, L.M. and S.A. Ross. Beta-carotene increases lung cancer incidence in cigarette smokers. *Nutrition Reviews.* 54:178-180, 1996.

9. Douglas, R.M., H. Hemila, R. D'Souza, E.B. Chalker, and B. Treacy. Vitamin C for preventing and treating the common cold. *Cochrane Database of Systematic Reviews.* CD000980, 2004.

10. Goldfarb, A.H. Antioxidants: Role of supplementation to prevent exercise-induced oxidative stress. *Medicine and Science in Sports and Exercise.* 25:232-236, 1993.

11. Goldfarb, A.H., S.W. Patrick, S. Bryer, and T. You. Vitamin C supplementation affects oxidative-stress blood markers in response to a 30-minute run at 75 percent $\dot{V}O_2$max. *International Journal of Sport Nutrition and Exercise Metabolism.* 15:279-290, 2005.

12. Grandjean, A. The vegetarian athlete. *Physician and Sportsmedicine.* 15:191-194, 1987.

13. Herrmann, W. and J. Geisel. Vegetarian lifestyle and monitoring of vitamin B-12 status. *Clinica Chimica Acta; International Journal of Clinical Chemistry.* 326:47-59, 2002.

14. Hickson, J.F., Jr., J. Schrader, and L.C. Trischler. Dietary intakes of female basketball and gymnastics athletes. *Journal of the American Dietetic Association.* 86:251-253, 1986.

15. Hunt, J., L. Matthys, and L. Johnson. Zinc absorption, mineral balance, and blood lipids in women consuming controlled lacto-ovo-vegetarian and omnivorous diets for 8 wk. *American Journal of Clinical Nutrition.* 67:421-430, 1998.

16. Hunt, J.R. Bioavailability of iron, zinc, and other trace minerals from vegetarian diets. *American Journal of Clinical Nutrition.* 78:633S-639S, 2003.

17. Kadrabova, J., A. Madaric, Z. Kovacikova, and E. Ginter. Selenium status, plasma zinc, copper, and magnesium in vegetarians. *Biological Trace Element Research.* 50:13-24, 1995.

18. Kanter, M. Free radicals and exercise: Effects of nutritional antioxidant supplementation. *Exercise and Sport Sciences Review.* 12:375-397, 1995.

19. Knekt, P., J. Ritz, M.A. Pereira, E.J. O'Reilly, K. Augustsson, G.E. Fraser, U. Goldbourt, B. L. Heitmann, G. Hallmans, S. Liu, P. Pietinen, D. Spiegelman, J. Stevens, J. Virtamo, W.C. Willett, E.B. Rimm, and A. Ascherio. Antioxidant vitamins and coronary heart disease risk: A pooled analysis of 9 cohorts. *American Journal of Clinical Nutrition.* 80:1508-1520, 2004.

20. Krajcovicova-Kudlackova, M., K. Buckova, I. Klimes, and E. Sebokova. Iodine deficiency in vegetarians and vegans. *Annals of Nutrition and Metabolism.* 47:183-185, 2003.

21. Krajcovicova-Kudlackova, M., M. Ursinyova, P. Blazicek, V. Spustova, E. Ginter, V. Hladikova, and J. Klvanova. Free radical disease prevention and nutrition. *Bratislavské Lekárske Listy.* 104:64-68, 2003.

22. Lange, H., H. Suryapranata, G. De Luca, C. Borner, J. Dille, K. Kallmayer, M.N. Pasalary, E. Scherer, and J.H. Dambrink. Folate therapy and in-stent restenosis after coronary stenting. *New England Journal of Medicine.* 350:2673-2681, 2004.

23. Law, M.R. and J.K. Morris. By how much does fruit and vegetable consumption reduce the risk of ischaemic heart disease? *European Journal of Clinical Nutrition.* 52:549-556, 1998.

24. Lightowler, H.J. and G.J. Davies. Iodine intake and iodine deficiency in vegans as assessed by the duplicate-portion technique and urinary iodine excretion. *British Journal of Nutrition.* 80:529-535, 1998.

25. Lodge, J.K. Vitamin E bioavailability in humans. *Journal of Plant Physiology.* 162:790-796, 2005.

26. Lukaski, H. Micronutrients (magnesium, zinc, and copper): Are mineral supplements needed for athletes? *International Journal of Sport Nutrition.* 5:S74-S73, 1995.

27. Lukaski, H.C. Low dietary zinc decreases erythrocyte carbonic anhydrase activities and impairs cardio-respiratory function in men during exercise. *American Journal of Clinical Nutrition.* 81:1045-1051, 2005.

28. Lukaski, H.C. Vitamin and mineral status: Effects on physical performance. *Nutrition.* 20:632-644, 2004.

29. Lukaski, H.C., W.W. Bolonchuk, L.M. Klevay, D.B. Milne, and H.H. Sandstead. Interactions among dietary fat, mineral status, and performance of endurance athletes: A case study. *International Journal of Sport Nutrition and Exercise Metabolism.* 11:186-198, 2001.

30. Manore, M., J. Helleksen, J. Merkel, and J. Skinner. Longitudinal changes in zinc status in untrained men: Effects of two different 12-week exercise training programs and zinc supplementation. *Journal of the American Dietetic Association.* 93:1165-1168, 1993.

31. Manore, M.M. Effect of physical activity on thiamine, riboflavin, and vitamin B-6 requirements. *American Journal of Clinical Nutrition.* 72:598S-606S, 2000.

32. Manore, M.M. Nutritional needs of the female athlete. *Clinics in Sports Medicine.* 18:549-563, 1999.

33. Messina, M. and V. Messina. *The Dietitian's Guide to Vegetarian Diets: Issues and Applications.* Gaithersburg, Maryland: Aspen, 1996.

34. Micheletti, A., R. Rossi, and S. Rufini. Zinc status in athletes: Relation to diet and exercise. *Sports Medicine.* 31:577-582, 2001.

35. Morillas-Ruiz, J.M., J.A. Villegas Garcia, F.J. Lopez, M.L. Vidal-Guevara, and P. Zafrilla. Effects of polyphenolic antioxidants on exercise-induced oxidative stress. *Clinical Nutrition.* 25:444-453, 2006. Retrieved January 19, 2006 from: www.ncbi.nlm.nih.gov/entrez/query.fcgi?cmd=Retrieve&db=PubMed&dopt=Citation&list_uids=16426710.

36. Morris, C.D. and S. Carson. Routine vitamin supplementation to prevent cardiovascular disease: A summary of the evidence for the U.S. Preventive Services Task Force. *Annals of Internal Medicine.* 139:56-70, 2003.

37. Omenn, G.S., G.E. Goodman, M.D. Thornquist, J. Balmes, M.R. Cullen, A. Glass, J.P. Keogh, F.L. Meyskens, B. Valanis, J.H. Williams, S. Barnhart, and S. Hammar. Effects of a combination of beta-carotene and vitamin A on lung cancer and cardiovascular disease. *New England Journal of Medicine.* 334:1150-1155, 1996.

38. Peters, E., J. Goetzsche, B. Grobbelaar, and T. Noakes. Vitamin C supplementation reduces the incidence of postrace symptoms of upper-respiratory-tract infection in ultramarathon runners. *American Journal of Clinical Nutrition.* 57:170-174, 1993.

39. Powers, S.K., K.C. DeRuisseau, J. Quindry, and K.L. Hamilton. Dietary antioxidants and exercise. *Journal of Sports Sciences.* 22:81-94, 2004.

40. Rauma, A., R. Torronen, O. Hanninen, and H. Mykkanen. Vitamin B-12 status of long-term adherents of a strict uncooked vegan diet ("living food diet") is compromised. *Journal of Nutrition.* 125:2511-2515, 1995.

41. Rauma, A.L. and H. Mykkanen. Antioxidant status in vegetarians versus omnivores. *Nutrition.* 16:111-119, 2000.

42. Remer, T., A. Neubert, and F. Manz. Increased risk of iodine deficiency with vegetarian nutrition. *British Journal of Nutrition.* 81:45-49, 1999.

43. Rousseau, A.S., S. Robin, A.M. Roussel, V. Ducros, and I. Margaritis. Plasma homocysteine is related to folate intake but not training status. *Nutrition, Metabolism, and Cardiovascular Diseases.* 15:125-133, 2005.

44. Singh, A., F. Moses, and P. Deuster. Chronic multivitamin-mineral supplementation does not enhance physical performance. *Medicine and Science in Sports and Exercise.* 24:726-732, 1992.

45. Soares, M., K. Satyanarayana, M. Bamji, C. Jacob, Y. Ramana, and S. Rao. The effect of exercise on the riboflavin status of adult men. *British Journal of Nutrition.* 69:541-551, 1993.

46. Steinmetz, K.A. and J.D. Potter. Vegetables, fruit, and cancer prevention: A review. *Journal of the American Dietetic Association.* 96:1027-1039, 1996.

47. Steinmetz, K.A. and J.D. Potter. Vegetables, fruit, and cancer. I. Epidemiology. *Cancer Causes and Control.* 2:325-357, 1991.

48. Than, T.-M., M.-W. May, K.-S. Aug, and M. Mya-Tu. The effect of vitamin B12 on physical performance capacity. *British Journal of Nutrition*. 40:269-273, 1978.

49. American College of Sports Medicine, American Dietetic Association, and Dietitians of Canada. Nutrition and athletic performance: Joint position statement. *Medicine and Science in Sports and Exercise*. 32:2130-2145, 2000.

50. Tucker, J.M. and D.M. Townsend. Alpha-tocopherol: Roles in prevention and therapy of human disease. *Biomedicine and Pharmacotherapy*. 59(7):380-387, 2005.

51. Urso, M.L. and P.M. Clarkson. Oxidative stress, exercise, and antioxidant supplementation. *Toxicology*. 189:41-54, 2003.

52. van Leeuwen, R., S. Boekhoorn, J.R. Vingerling, J.C. Witteman, C.C. Klaver, A. Hofman, and P.T. de Jong. Dietary intake of antioxidants and risk of age-related macular degeneration. *Journal of the American Medical Association*. 294:3101-3107, 2005.

53. Wapnir, R.A. Copper absorption and bioavailability. *American Journal of Clinical Nutrition*. 67:1054S-1060S, 1998.

Chapter 9

1. Almond, C.S., A.Y. Shin, E.B. Fortescue, R.C. Mannix, D. Wypij, B.A. Binstadt, C.N. Duncan, D.P. Olson, A.E. Salerno, J.W. Newburger, and D.S. Greenes. Hyponatremia among runners in the Boston Marathon. *New England Journal of Medicine*. 352:1550-1556, 2005.

2. American College of Sports Medicine. Position Stand: Exercise and fluid replacement. *Medicine and Science in Sports and Exercise*. 28:i-vi, 1996.

3. Balsom, P.D., K. Wood, P. Olsson, and B. Ekblom. Carbohydrate intake and multiple sprint sports: With special reference to football (soccer). *International Journal of Sports Medicine*. 20:48-52, 1999.

4. Below, P., R. Mora-Rodriguez, J. Gonzalez-Alonso, and E. Coyle. Fluid and carbohydrate ingestion independently improve performance during 1 h of intense exercise. *Medicine and Science in Sports and Exercise*. 27:200-210, 1995.

5. Broad, E.M., L.M. Burke, G.R. Cox, P. Heeley, and M. Riley. Body weight changes and voluntary fluid intakes during training and competition sessions in team sports. *International Journal of Sport Nutrition*. 6:307-320, 1996.

6. Chryssanthopoulos, C., C. Williams, A. Nowitz, C. Kotsiopoulou, and V. Vleck. The effect of a high carbohydrate meal on endurance running capacity. *International Journal of Sport Nutrition and Exercise Metabolism*. 12:157-171, 2002.

7. Fairchild, T.J., S. Fletcher, P. Steele, C. Goodman, B. Dawson, and P.A. Fournier. Rapid carbohydrate loading after a short bout of near maximal-intensity exercise. *Medicine and Science in Sports and Exercise*. 34:980-986, 2002.

8. Fallowfield, J.L., C. Williams, J. Booth, B.H. Choo, and S. Growns. Effect of water ingestion on endurance capacity during prolonged running. *Journal of Sports Sciences*. 14:497-502, 1996.

9. Gisolfi, C. and S. Duchman. Guidelines for optimal replacement beverages for different athletic events. *Medicine and Science in Sports and Exercise*. 24:679-687, 1992.

10. Goforth, H.W., Jr., D. Laurent, W.K. Prusaczyk, K.E. Schneider, K.F. Petersen, and G.I. Shulman. Effects of depletion exercise and light training on muscle glycogen supercompensation in men. *American Journal of Physiology--Endocrinology and Metabolism*. 285:E1304-1311, 2003.

11. Ivy, J.L., H.W. Goforth, Jr., B.M. Damon, T.R. McCauley, E.C. Parsons, and T.B. Price. Early postexercise muscle glycogen recovery is enhanced with a carbohydrate-protein supplement. *Journal of Applied Physiology*. 93:1337-1344, 2002.

12. Ivy, J.L., P.T. Res, R.C. Sprague, and M.O. Widzer. Effect of a carbohydrate-protein supplement on endurance performance during exercise of varying intensity. *International Journal of Sport Nutrition and Exercise Metabolism* 13:382-395, 2003.

13. Jentjens, R.L., C. Shaw, T. Birtles, R.H. Waring, L.K. Harding, and A.E. Jeukendrup. Oxidation of combined ingestion of glucose and sucrose during exercise. *Metabolism*. 54:610-618, 2005.

14. Kiens, B. Diet and training in the week before competition. *Canadian Journal of Applied Physiology.* 26 Suppl:S56-63, 2001.

15. Kirwan, J.P., D. Cyr-Campbell, W.W. Campbell, J. Scheiber, and W.J. Evans. Effects of moderate and high glycemic index meals on metabolism and exercise performance. *Metabolism.* 50:849-855, 2001.

16. Lancaster, S., R.B. Kreider, C. Rasmussen, C. Kerksick, M. Greenwood, P. Milnor, A.L. Almada, and C.P. Earnest. Effects of honey supplementation on glucose, insulin, and endurance cycling performance. *FASEB Journal.* 15:LB315, 2001.

17. Larson-Meyer, D.E., G.R. Hunter, and B.R. Newcomer. Influence of endurance running and recovery diet on intramyocellular lipid content in women: A ¹H-NMR study. *American Journal of Physiology.* 282:E95-E106, 2002.

18. Maffucci, D.M. and R.G. McMurray. Towards optimizing the timing of the pre-exercise meal. *International Journal of Sport Nutrition and Exercise Metabolism.* 10:103-113, 2000.

19. Robergs, R.A., S.B. McMinn, C. Mermier, G.R. Leadbetter, B. Ruby, and C. Quinn. Blood glucose and glucoregulatory hormone responses to solid and liquid carbohydrate ingestion during exercise. *International Journal of Sport Nutrition.* 8:70-83, 1998.

20. Saunders, M.J., M.D. Kane, and M.K. Todd. Effects of a carbohydrate-protein beverage on cycling endurance and muscle damage. *Med Sci Sports Exerc.* 36:1233-1238, 2004.

21. Schabort, E.J., A.N. Bosch, S.M. Weltan, and T.D. Noakes. The effect of a preexercise meal on time to fatigue during prolonged cycling exercise. *Medicine and Science in Sports and Exercise.* 31:464-471, 1999.

22. Seifert, J.G., J. Harmon, and P. DeClercq. Protein added to a sports drink improves fluid retention. *International Journal of Sports Nutrition and Exercise Metabolism*, (in press).

23. Sherman, W., G. Brodowicz, D. Wright, W. Allen, J. Somonsen, and A. Dernbach. Effects of 4 h pre-exercise carbohydrate feedings on cycling performance. *Medicine and Science in Sports and Exercise.* 21:598-604, 1989.

24. Siu, P.M. and S.H. Wong. Use of the glycemic index: Effects on feeding patterns and exercise performance. *Journal of Physiological Anthropology and Applied Human Science.* 23:1-6, 2004.

25. Speedy, D.B., J.M. Thompson, I. Rodgers, M. Collins, K. Sharwood, and T.D. Noakes. Oral salt supplementation during ultradistance exercise. *Clinical Journal of Sport Medicine.* 12:279-284, 2002.

26. American College of Sports Medicine, American Dietetic Association, and Dietitians of Canada. Nutrition and Athletic Performance: Joint Position Statement. *Medicine and Science in Sports and Exercise.* 32:2130-2145, 2000.

27. Thomas, D., J. Brotherhood, and J. Brand. Carbohydrate feeding before exercise: Effect of glycemic index. *International Journal of Sports Medicine.* 12:180-186, 1991.

28. Thomas, D., J. Brotherhood, and J. Miller. Plasma glucose levels after prolonged strenuous exercise correlate inversely with glycemic response to food consumed before exercise. *International Journal of Sport Nutrition.* 4:361-373, 1994.

29. Tokmakidis, S.P. and K.A. Volaklis. Pre-exercise glucose ingestion at different time periods and blood glucose concentration during exercise. *International Journal of Sports Medicine.* 21:453-457, 2000.

30. van der Brug, G.E., H.P. Peters, M.R. Hardeman, G. Schep, and W.L. Mosterd. Hemorheological response to prolonged exercise: No effects of different kinds of feedings. *International Journal of Sports Medicine.* 16:231-237, 1995.

31. Vergauwen, L., F. Brouns, and P. Hespel. Carbohydrate supplementation improves stroke performance in tennis. *Medicine and Science in Sports and Exercise.* 30:1289-1295, 1998.

32. Wallis, G.A., D.S. Rowlands, C. Shaw, R.L. Jentjens, and A.E. Jeukendrup. Oxidation of combined ingestion of maltodextrins and fructose during exercise. *Medicine and Science in Sports and Exercise.* 37:426-432, 2005.

33. Welsh, R.S., J.M. Davis, J.R. Burke, and H.G. Williams. Carbohydrates and physical/mental performance during intermittent exercise to fatigue. *Medicine and Science in Sports and Exercise.* 34:723-731, 2002.

34. Williams, C., J. Brewer, and M. Walker. The effect of a high carbohydrate diet on running performance during a 30-km treadmill time trial. *European Journal of Applied Physiology and Occupational Physiology.* 65:18-24, 1992.

35. Wright, D., W. Sherman, and A. Dernbach. Carbohydrate feedings before, during, or in combination improve cycling endurance performance. *Journal of Applied Physiology.* 71:1082-1088, 1991.

Chapter 10

1. Can you trust supplements? *Harvard Women's Health Watch.* November:4-5, 1998.

2. Online Resource for the National Collegiate Athletic Association. *Banned Drug List.* Retrieved January 20, 2006, from: www.ncaa.org.

3. Armstrong, L.E. Caffeine, body fluid-electrolyte balance, and exercise performance. *International Journal of Sport Nutrition and Exercise Metabolism.* 12:189-206, 2002.

4. Balsom, P., K. Soderlund, and B. Ekblom. Creatine in humans with special reference to creatine supplementation. *Sports Medicine.* 18:268-280, 1994.

5. Branch, J.D. Effect of creatine supplementation on body composition and performance: A meta-analysis. *International Journal of Sport Nutrition and Exercise Metabolism.* 13:198-226, 2003.

6. Burke, D.G., P.D. Chilibeck, G. Parise, D.G. Candow, D. Mahoney, and M. Tarnopolsky. Effect of creatine and weight training on muscle creatine and performance in vegetarians. *Medicine and Science in Sports and Exercise.* 35:1946-1955, 2003.

7. Clarys, P., E. Zinzen, and M. Hebbelinck. The effect of oral creatine supplementation on torque production in a vegetarian and non-vegetarian population: A double blind study. *Vegetarian Nutrition: An International Journal.* 1:100-105, 1997.

8. Cox, G.R., B. Desbrow, P.G. Montgomery, M.E. Anderson, C.R. Bruce, T.A. Macrides, D.T. Martin, A. Moquin, A. Roberts, J.A. Hawley, and L.M. Burke. Effect of different protocols of caffeine intake on metabolism and endurance performance. *Journal of Applied Physiology.* 93:990-999, 2002.

9. Davis, A.T., P.G. Davis, and S.D. Phinney. Plasma and urinary carnitine of obese subjects on very-low-calorie diets. *Journal of the American College of Nutrition.* 9:261-264, 1990.

10. Delanghe, J., J.-P. De Slypere, M. De Buyzere, J. Robbrecht, R. Wieme, and A. Vermeulen. Normal reference values for creatine, creatinine, and carnitine are lower in vegetarians. *Clinical Chemistry.* 35:1802-1803, 1989.

11. Graham, T.E. Caffeine and exercise: Metabolism, endurance, and performance. *Sports Medicine.* 31:785-807, 2001.

12. Green, A., E. Hultman, I. MacDonald, D. Sewell, and P. Greenhaff. Carbohydrate ingestion augments skeletal muscle creatine accumulation during creatine supplementation in humans. *American Journal of Physiology.* 271:E821-E826, 1996.

13. Harris, R.C., K. Soderlund, and E. Hultman. Elevation of creatine in resting and exercised muscle of normal subjects by creatine supplementation. *Clinical Science.* 83:367-374, 1992.

14. Juhn, M. Popular sports supplements and ergogenic aids. *Sports Medicine.* 33:921-939, 2003.

15. Juhn, M.S. and M. Tarnopolsky. Oral creatine supplementation and athletic performance: A critical review. *Clinical Journal of Sport Medicine.* 8:286-297, 1998.

16. Kreider, R.B., M. Ferreira, M. Wilson, and A.L. Almada. Effects of calcium beta-hydroxy-beta-methylbutyrate (HMB) supplementation during resistance-training on markers of catabolism, body composition and strength. *International Journal of Sports Medicine.* 20:503-509, 1999.

17. Kreider, R.B., M.P. Ferreira, M. Greenwood, M. Wilson, and A.L. Almada. Effects of conjugated linoleic acid supplementation during resistance training on body composition, bone density, strength, and selected hematological markers. *Journal of Strength and Conditioning Research.* 16:325-334, 2002.

18. Lukaszuk, J.M., R.J. Robertson, J.E. Arch, G.E. Moore, K.M. Yaw, D.E. Kelley, J.T. Rubin, and N.M. Moyna. Effect of creatine supplementation and a lacto-ovo-vegetarian diet on muscle creatine concentration. *International Journal of Sport Nutrition and Exercise Metabolism.* 12:336-348, 2002.

19. Nissen, S., R. Sharp, M. Ray, J.A. Rathmacher, D. Rice, J.C. Fuller, A.S. Connelly, and N. Arumrad. Effect of leucine metabolite B-hydroxy-B-methylbutyrate on muscle metabolism during resistance-exercise training. *Journal of Applied Physiology.* 81:2095-2103, 1996.

20. Nissen, S.L. and R.L. Sharp. Effect of dietary supplements on lean mass and strength gains with resistance exercise: A meta-analysis. *Journal of Applied Physiology.* 94:651-659, 2003.

21. Paluska, S.A. Caffeine and exercise. *Current Sports Medicine Reports.* 2:213-219, 2003.

22. Rainer, L. and C.J. Heiss. Conjugated linoleic acid: Health implications and effects on body composition. *Journal of the American Dietetic Association.* 104:963-968, quiz 1032, 2004.

23. Rebouche, C., and C. Chenard. Metabolic fate of dietary carnitine in human adults: Identification and quantification of urinary and fecal metabolites. *Journal of Nutrition.* 121:539-546, 1991.

24. Shomrat, A., Y. Weinstein, and A. Katz. Effect of creatine feeding on maximal exercise performance in vegetarians. *European Journal of Applied Physiology.* 82:321-325, 2000.

25. SupplementWatch. *Supplement decisions made easy.* Retrieved January 19, 2006 from: www.supplementwatch.com.

26. Terjung, R.L., P. Clarkson, E.R. Eichner, P.L. Greenhaff, P.J. Hespel, R.G. Israel, W.J. Kraemer, R.A. Meyer, L.L. Spriet, M.A. Tarnopolsky, A.J. Wagenmakers, and M.H. Williams. American College of Sports Medicine roundtable: The physiological and health effects of oral creatine supplementation. *Medicine and Science in Sports and Exercise.* 32:706-717, 2000.

27. Terpstra, A.H. Effect of conjugated linoleic acid on body composition and plasma lipids in humans: An overview of the literature. *American Journal of Clinical Nutrition.* 79:352-361, 2004.

28. Thom, E., J. Wadstein, and O. Gudmundsen. Conjugated linoleic acid reduces body fat in healthy exercising humans. *Journal of International Medical Research.* 29:392-396, 2001.

29. U.S. Food and Drug Administration. *Dietary Supplement Health and Education Act of 1994.* Retrieved January 18, 2006, from: www.fda.gov/opacom/laws/dshea.html.

Chapter 11

1. American Dietetic Association and Dietitians of Canada. Position of the American Dietetic Association and Dietitians of Canada: Vegetarian diets. *Journal of the American Dietetic Association.* 103:748-765, 2003.

2. Ahmed, S., J. Anuntiyo, C.J. Malemud, and T.M. Haqqi. Biological basis for the use of botanicals in osteoarthritis and rheumatoid arthritis: A review. *Evidence-Based Complementary and Alternative Medicine.* 2:301-308, 2005.

3. Ahmed, S., N. Wang, B.B. Hafeez, V.K. Cheruvu, and T.M. Haqqi. Punica granatum L. extract inhibits IL-1beta-induced expression of matrix metalloproteinases by inhibiting the activation of MAP kinases and NF-kappaB in human chondrocytes in vitro. *Journal of Nutrition.* 135:2096-2102, 2005.

4. Ariza-Ariza, R., M. Mestanza-Peralta, and M.H. Cardiel. Omega-3 fatty acids in rheumatoid arthritis: An overview. *Seminars in Arthritis and Rheumatism.* 27:366-370, 1998.

5. Beauchamp, G.K., R.S. Keast, D. Morel, J. Lin, J. Pika, Q. Han, C.H. Lee, A.B. Smith, and P.A. Breslin. Phytochemistry: Ibuprofen-like activity in extra-virgin olive oil. *Nature.* 437:45-46, 2005.

6. Bentley, S. Exercise-induced muscle cramp. Proposed mechanisms and management. *Sports Medicine.* 21:409-420, 1996.

7. Braham, R., B. Dawson, and C. Goodman. The effect of glucosamine supplementation on people experiencing regular knee pain. *British Journal of Sports Medicine.* 37:45-49; discussion 49, 2003.

8. Bye, A.M. and A.E. Kan. Cramps following exercise. *Australian Paediatric Journal.* 24:258-259, 1988.

9. Cannell, J. Questions and Answers. *Vitamin D Newsletter.* January, 2006.

10. Clark, N. *Nancy Clark's Sports Nutrition Guidebook.* 2nd ed. Champaign, IL: Human Kinetics, 1997.

11. Clarkson, P. and E. Haymes. Exercise and mineral status of athletes: Calcium, magnesium, phosphorus, and iron. *Medicine and Science in Sports and Exercise.* 27:831-843, 1995.

12. Clegg, D.O., D.J. Reda, C.L. Harris, M.A. Klein, J.R. O'Dell, M.M. Hooper, J.D. Bradley, C.O. Bingham, 3rd, M.H. Weisman, C.G. Jackson, N.E. Lane, J.J. Cush, L.W. Moreland, H.R. Schumacher, Jr., C.V. Oddis, F. Wolfe, J.A. Molitor, D.E. Yocum, T.J. Schnitzer, D.E. Furst, A.D. Sawitzke, H. Shi, K.D. Brandt, R.W. Moskowitz, and H J. Williams. Glucosamine, chondroitin sulfate, and the two in combination for painful knee osteoarthritis. *New England Journal of Medicine.* 354:795-808, 2006.

13. Firestein, G.S. and N.J. Zvaifler. Anticytokine therapy in rheumatoid arthritis. *New England Journal of Medicine.* 337:195-197, 1997.

14. Fredericson, M., B.J. Kim, and E.S. Date. Disabling foot cramping in a runner secondary to paramyotonia congenita: A case report. *Foot and Ankle International.* 25:510-512, 2004.

15. Grimble, R.F. and P.S. Tappia. Modulation of pro-inflammatory cytokine biology by unsaturated fatty acids. *Zeitschrift für Ernahrungswissenschaft.* 37Suppl 1:57-65, 1998.

16. Hansen, G., L. Nielsen, E. Kluger, M.H. Thysen, H. Emmertsen, K. Stengard-Pedersen, E.C. Lund, B. Unger, and P.W. Andersen. [Nutritional status of Danish patients with rheumatoid arthritis and effects of a diet adjusted in energy intake, fish content and antioxidants]. *Ugeskrift for Laeger.* 160:3074-3078, 1998.

17. Holick, M.F. Evolution and function of vitamin D. *Recent Results in Cancer Research.* 164:3-28, 2003.

18. Holick, M.F. Sunlight and vitamin D for bone health and prevention of autoimmune diseases, cancers, and cardiovascular disease. *American Journal of Clinical Nutrition.* 80:1678S-1688S, 2004.

19. Lawrence, R.C., C.G. Helmick, F.C. Arnett, R.A. Deyo, D.T. Felson, E.H. Giannini, S.P. Heyse, R. Hirsch, M.C. Hochberg, G.G. Hunder, M.H. Liang, S.R. Pillemer, V.D. Steen, and F. Wolfe. Estimates of the prevalence of arthritis and selected musculoskeletal disorders in the United States. *Arthritis and Rheumatism.* 41:778-799, 1998.

20. Litman, R.S. and H. Rosenberg. Malignant hyperthermia: Update on susceptibility testing. *Journal of the American Medical Association.* 293:2918-2924, 2005.

21. McAlindon, T.E., D.T. Felson, Y. Zhang, M.T. Hannan, P. Aliabadi, B. Weissman, D. Rush, P.W.F. Wilson, and P. Jacques. Relation of dietary intake and serum levels of Vitamin D to progression of osteoarthritis of the knee among participants in the Framingham study. *Annals of Internal Medicine.* 125:353-359, 1996.

22. McAlindon, T.E., P. Jacques, Y. Zhang, M.T. Hannan, P. Aliabadi, B. Weissman, D. Rush, D. Levy, and D.T. Felson. Do antioxidant micronutrients protect against the development and progression of knee osteoarthritis? *Arthritis and Rheumatism.* 39:648-656, 1996.

23. McAlindon, T.E., M.P. LaValley, J.P. Gulin, and D.T. Felson. Glucosamine and chondroitin for treatment of osteoarthritis: A systematic quality assessment and meta-analysis. *Journal of the American Medical Association.* 283:1469-1475, 2000.

24. Merlino, L.A., J. Curtis, T.R. Mikuls, J.R. Cerhan, L.A. Criswell, and K.G. Saag. Vitamin D intake is inversely associated with rheumatoid arthritis: Results from the Iowa Women's Health Study. *Arthritis and Rheumatism.* 50:72-77, 2004.

25. Moore, M.E., A. Piazza, Y. McCartney, and M.A. Lynch. Evidence that vitamin D3 reverses age-related inflammatory changes in the rat hippocampus. *Biochemical Society Transactions.* 33:573-577, 2005.

26. Riley, J.D. and S.J. Antony. Leg cramps: Differential diagnosis and management. *American Family Physician.* 52:1794-1798, 1995.

27. Riso, P., F. Visioli, S. Grande, S. Guarnieri, C. Gardana, P. Simonetti, and M. Porrini. Effect of a tomato-based drink on markers of inflammation, immunomodulation, and oxidative stress. *Journal of Agriculture and Food Chemistry.* 54:2563-2566, 2006.

28. Rosell, M.S., Z. Lloyd-Wright, P.N. Appleby, T.A. Sanders, N.E. Allen, and T.J. Key. Long-chain n-3 poly-unsaturated fatty acids in plasma in British meat-eating, vegetarian, and vegan men. *American Journal of Clinical Nutrition.* 82:327-334, 2005.

29. Schmid, B., R. Ludtke, H.K. Selbmann, I. Kotter, B. Tschirdewahn, W. Schaffner, and L. Heide. Efficacy and tolerability of a standardized willow bark extract in patients with osteoarthritis: Randomized placebo-controlled, double blind clinical trial. *Phytotherapy Research.* 15:344-350, 2001.

30. Schwellnus, M.P., E.W. Derman, and T.D. Noakes. Aetiology of skeletal muscle "cramps" during exercise: A novel hypothesis. *Journal of Sports Sciences.* 15:277-285, 1997.

31. Schwellnus, M.P., J. Nicol, R. Laubscher, and T.D. Noakes. Serum electrolyte concentrations and hydration status are not associated with exercise associated muscle cramping (EAMC) in distance runners. *British Journal of Sports Medicine.* 38:488-492, 2004.

32. Simopoulos, A.P., A. Leaf, and N. Salem, Jr. Workshop on the essentiality of and recommended dietary intakes for Omega-6 and Omega-3 fatty acids. *Journal of the American College of Nutrition.* 18:487-489, 1999.

33. Spector, T.D., P.A. Harris, D.J. Hart, F.M. Cicuttini, D. Nandra, J. Etherington, R.L. Wolman, and D.V. Doyle. Risk of osteoarthritis associated with long-term weight-bearing sports: A radiologic survey of the hips and knees in female ex-athletes and population controls. *Arthritis and Rheumatism.* 39:988-995, 1996.

34. Sulzer, N.U., M.P. Schwellnus, and T.D. Noakes. Serum electrolytes in Ironman triathletes with exercise-associated muscle cramping. *Medicine and Science in Sports and Exercise.* 37:1081-1085, 2005.

35. Torbergsen, T., A. Hodnebo, N.J. Brautaset, S. Loseth, and E. Stalberg. A rare form of painful non-dystrophic myotonia. *Clinical Neurophysiology.* 114:2347-2354, 2003.

36. Weller, E., P. Bachert, H.M. Meinck, B. Friedmann, P. Bartsch, and H. Mairbaurl. Lack of effect of oral Mg-supplementation on Mg in serum, blood cells, and calf muscle. *Medicine and Science in Sports and Exercise.* 30:1584-1591, 1998.

37. Williams, M.H. *Nutrition for Health, Fitness and Sport.* 5th ed. Boston: McGraw-Hill, 1999.

38. Williamson, S.I., R.W. Johnson, P.G. Hudkins, and S.M. Strate. Exertional cramps: A prospective study of biochemical and anthropometric variables in bicycle riders. *Cycling Science.* 15:20, 1993.

39. Young, G.L. and D. Jewell. Interventions for leg cramps in pregnancy. *Cochrane Database of Systematic Reviews.* CD000121, 2002.

40. Zittermann, A. Vitamin D in preventive medicine: Are we ignoring the evidence? *British Journal of Nutrition.* 89:552-572, 2003.

Chapter 12

1. Houtkooper, L. Food selection for endurance sports. *Medicine and Science in Sports and Exercise.* 24:S349-S359, 1992.

2. Messina, V., V. Melina, and A.R. Mangels. A new food guide for North American vegetarians. *Journal of the American Dietetic Association.* 103:771-775, 2003.

3. Welsh, S. A brief history of food guides in the United States. *Nutrition Today.* 27:6-11, 1992.

Chapter 13

1. Allen, N.E., P.N. Appleby, G.K. Davey, and T.J. Key. Hormones and diet: Low insulin-like growth factor-I but normal bioavailable androgens in vegan men. *British Journal of Cancer.* 83:95-97, 2000.

2. Burke, L.M., G.R. Collier, E.M. Broad, P.G. Davis, D.T. Martin, A.J. Sanigorski, and M. Hargreaves. Effect of alcohol intake on muscle glycogen storage after prolonged exercise. *Journal of Applied Physiology.* 95:983-990, 2003.

3. Butterfield, G., P. Lemon, S. Kleiner, and M. Stone. Roundtable: Methods of Weight Gain in Athletes. *Sports Science Exchange.* RT 21/Volume 5:1-4, 1995.

4. Crovetti, R., M. Porrini, A. Santangelo, and G. Testolin. The influence of thermic effect of food on satiety. *European Journal of Clinical Nutrition.* 52:482-488, 1998.

5. DellaValle, D.M., L.S. Roe, and B.J. Rolls. Does the consumption of caloric and non-caloric beverages with a meal affect energy intake? *Appetite.* 44:187-193, 2005.

6. Gunther, C.W., P.A. Legowski, R.M. Lyle, G.P. McCabe, M.S. Eagan, M. Peacock, and D. Teegarden. Dairy products do not lead to alterations in body weight or fat mass in young women in a 1-y intervention. *American Journal of Clinical Nutrition.* 81:751-756, 2005.

7. Han, L.K., T. Takaku, J. Li, Y. Kimura, and H. Okuda. Anti-obesity action of oolong tea. *International Journal of Obesity and Related Metabolic Disorders.* 23:98-105, 1999.

8. Hill, P., E. Wynder, L. Garbaczewski, H. Garnes, A.R. Walker, and P. Helman. Plasma hormones and lipids in men at different risk for coronary heart disease. *American Journal of Clinical Nutrition*. 33:1010-1018, 1980.

9. Hill, P.B. and E.L. Wynder. Effect of a vegetarian diet and dexamethasone on plasma prolactin, testosterone and dehydroepiandrosterone in men and women. *Cancer Letters*. 7:273-282, 1979.

10. Key, T.J., G.E. Fraser, M. Thorogood, P.N. Appleby, V. Beral, G. Reeves, M.L. Burr, J. Chang-Claude, R. Frentzel-Beyme, J.W. Kuzma, J. Mann, and K. McPherson. Mortality in vegetarians and nonvegetarians: Detailed findings from a collaborative analysis of 5 prospective studies. *American Journal of Clinical Nutrition*. 70:516S-524S, 1999.

11. Key, T.J., L. Roe, M. Thorogood, J.W. Moore, G.M. Clark, and D.Y. Wang. Testosterone, sex hormone-binding globulin, calculated free testosterone, and oestradiol in male vegans and omnivores. *British Journal of Nutrition*. 64:111-119, 1990.

12. Larson, D.E., R. Rising, R.T. Ferraro, and E. Ravussin. Spontaneous overfeeding with a "cafeteria diet" in men: Effects on 24-hour energy expenditure and substrate oxidation. *International Journal of Obesity*. 19:331-337, 1995.

13. Larson, D.E., P.A. Tataranni, R.T. Ferraro, and E. Ravussin. Ad libitum food intake on a "cafeteria diet" in Native American women: Relations with body composition and 24-hour energy expenditure. *American Journal of Clinical Nutrition*. 62:911-917, 1995.

14. Leeman, M., E. Ostman, and I. Bjorck. Vinegar dressing and cold storage of potatoes lowers postprandial glycaemic and insulinaemic responses in healthy subjects. *European Journal of Clinical Nutrition*. 59(11):1266-1271, 2005.

15. Lukaski, H.C. Body composition in exercise and sport. In: *Nutrition in Exercise and Sport*. I. Wolinsky (ed), pp. 621-657. New York: CRC Press, 1998.

16. Ostman, E., Y. Granfeldt, L. Persson, and I. Bjorck. Vinegar supplementation lowers glucose and insulin responses and increases satiety after a bread meal in healthy subjects. *European Journal of Clinical Nutrition*. 59:983-988, 2005.

17. Prentice, A.M. Manipulation of dietary fat and energy density and subsequent effects on substrate flux and food intake. *Journal of Clinical Nutrition*. 67:535S-541S, 1998.

18. Raben, A., B. Kiens, E.A. Richter, L.B. Rasmussen, B. Svenstrup, S. Micic, and P. Bennett. Serum sex hormones and endurance performance after a lacto-ovo vegetarian and a mixed diet. *Medicine and Science in Sports and Exercise*. 24:1290-1297, 1992.

19. Reed, M., R. Cheng, M. Simmonds, W. Richmond, and V. James. Dietary lipids: An additional regulator of plasma levels of sex hormone binding globulin. *Journal of Clinical Endocrinology and Metabolism*. 64:1083-1085, 1987.

20. Rolls, B.J. *The Volumetrics Eating Plan. Techniques and Recipes for Feeling Full on Fewer Calories*. New York: HarperCollins, 2005.

21. Suter, P., Y. Schutz, and E. Jequier. The effect of ethanol on fat storage in healthy subjects. *New England Journal of Medicine*. 326:983-987, 1992.

22. Tremblay, A. and S. St-Pierre. The hyperphagic effect of a high-fat diet and alcohol intake persists after control for energy density. *American Journal of Clinical Nutrition*. 63:479-482, 1996.

23. Westerterp-Plantenga, M.S., M.P. Lejeune, and E.M. Kovacs. Body weight loss and weight maintenance in relation to habitual caffeine intake and green tea supplementation. *Obesity Research*. 13:1195-1204, 2005.

24. Wyatt, H.R., G.K. Grunwald, C.L. Mosca, M.L. Klem, R.R. Wing, and J.O. Hill. Long-term weight loss and breakfast in subjects in the National Weight Control Registry. *Obesity Research*. 10:78-82, 2002.

25. Yajima, H., T. Noguchi, E. Ikeshima, M. Shiraki, T. Kanaya, N. Tsuboyama-Kasaoka, O. Ezaki, S. Oikawa, and K. Kondo. Prevention of diet-induced obesity by dietary isomerized hop extract containing isohumulones, in rodents. *International Journal of Obesity and Related Metabolic Disorders*. 29:991-997, 2005.

26. Young, L.R. and M. Nestle. Expanding portion sizes in the US marketplace: Implications for nutrition counseling. *Journal of the American Dietetic Association*. 103:231-234, 2003.

27. Zemel, M.B. Role of calcium and dairy products in energy partitioning and weight management. *American Journal of Clinical Nutrition*. 79:907S-912S, 2004.

Index

Note: The italicized *f* and *t* following page numbers refer to figures and tables, respectively.

A

adenosine triphosphate (ATP) 14
alcohol 77, 78*t,* 200
aldosterone 155, 158
alpha-linolenic acid (ALA) 48
amenorrhea 20
amino acids 56, 56*t,* 57
anabolism 203
anemia 84, 94
antidiuretic hormone (ADH) 155
antioxidants 98
antioxidants and anti-inflammatory agents
    herbs and plant products 168
    sources of 168
    studies 168, 169
arthritis 166
athletes
    carbohydrates 24-25
    fat 40-41, 42*f,* 42*t*
athletic anemia 94

B

B-complex vitamins
    description of 99
    other B vitamins 103-105, 104*t,* 105*t*
    riboflavin 101, 102*t*-103*t*
    role of 99
    sources of 100, 100*t,* 101
    vitamin B_{12} 101, 103
    and vitamin C for vegetarian athletes 100, 100*t*
beta-hydroxy-beta-methylbutyrate (HMB)
    benefits of 147
    dosage 147
bloating. *See* diarrhea, intestinal cramping, and bloating
Bonaly, Surya 2
bone health
    bone tissue 66-67
    bone turnover (remodeling) 66
    factors regulating 67-78
    importance of 66
    vegetarian diet and 78-80
bone health and hormones
    androgen deficiency 68
    estrogen 68
    parathyroid hormone (PTH) 67-68
    vitamin D and calcitonin 68
bone health and nutrition
    caffeine, alcohol, and soy isoflavones 77, 78*t*

    calcium 68-72, 70*t*-71*t,* 71*f*
    fluoride 75-76
    magnesium 73-75
    phosphorus 76
    vitamin D 72-73, 73*t*
    vitamins K, C, A 76-77
bone health and vegetarian diet
    optimal bone health 79-80
    poor bone health risks, research 78
Brown, Will 8

C

caffeine, alcohol, soy isoflavones and bone health 77, 78*t*
caffeine (theobromine)
    benefits 146
    central nervous system (CNS) stimulant 146
    habitual intake of 146, 147
    sources of 145-146, 146*t*
calcium
    calcium balance, factors 68-69
    muscle cramping 158-159
    requirements 69, 70*t*-71*t,* 71*f,* 72
    role of 68
    supplements 72
calories 14, 15
calories from plant sources, meeting
    250-calorie snacks 22
    daily energy requirements, estimating 21
    energy needs, estimating 18, 19*t,* 21, 22
    food choices 21, 22
    food supply, assessing 21
carbohydrate mix
    color and national nutrition campaigns 33, 33*t,* 34
    complex *vs.* simple carbohydrate 35, 36, 36*t*
    daily choices of foods 28*t,* 31
    getting right mix 36, 37*t,* 38
    grains *vs.* fruits *vs.* vegetables *vs.* dairy 31-32
    low glycemic *vs.* high glycemic index 36
    sport products and desserts 34-35
    whole *vs.* processed 34
carbohydrates
    bad training days 24
    carbohydrates as preferred fuel 24
    content of foods 28*t*-29*t*
    counting 27-30, 28*t*-29*t,* 30*t*
    counting log 28, 29, 30*t*
    fatigue and glycogen 24-25

carbohydrates *(continued)*
  intake, estimating 27-30
  loading (glycogen supercompensation)
    121-123
  needs, determining 26-27, 27*t*, 30*t*
  optimal intake, factors determining 26
  performance and 25-26
  right mix, getting 24
  training demands 26-27
  why athletes need 24-25
carbohydrates and performance
  high-carbohydrate diets, research 25
  magnetic resonance spectroscopy 26
  optimal bioenergetic state, study 26
carnitine
  role and sources of 145
  studies 145
carotenoids. *See* vitamin A and carotenoids
central nervous system (CNS) stimulant 146
Clark, Nancy 155, 159
conjugated linoleic acid (CLA)
  benefits of 148
  description of 147-148
  dosage 148
cookbooks 215, 226
copper 102*t*-103*t*, 112
cortical bone 67
creatine
  absorption and dosage 144-145
  long-term safety 144
  oral supplementation and vegetarian
    response 144
  studies 143-144
creatine phosphate (PCr) 14
creatine supplement study 135

D
daily energy expenditure (DEE) components
    16, 17
Devers, Gail 136
diarrhea, intestinal cramping, and bloating 118
diet and inflammation
  antioxidants and anti-inflammatory agents
    168-169
  nutrition tips for reducing 164
  omega-3 fatty acids 164-165
  vitamin D 165-167
diet and muscle cramping
  calcium 158-159
  carbohydrate 159, 160
  cramps caused by mineral deficiency 162
  fluid imbalances and dehydration 155
  improvements in 162
  magnesium 70*t*, 159, 160*t*
  malignant hyperthermia (MH) 162
  nutritional causes, ruling out (box 11.2) 161
  potassium 157, 157*t*, 158
  sodium 155-156
  sweat 156
dietary fat. *See* fat
Dietary Guidelines for Americans 184
dietary reference intakes for vitamins and
    minerals 233-235
dietary supplement 137. *See also* supplement(s)

dilutional anemia 94
disordered eating 20
docosahexaenoic acid (DHA) 48
doubly labeled water technique 15, 16

E
eicosanoids 51, 164
eicosapentaenoic acid (EPA) 48
endurance and ultraendurance events 128,
    129, 130-131
endurance performance and fat, research
    42-43
energy costs of physical activity 227-229
energy expenditure during nontraining
    activities (NTEE) 16, 17
energy expenditure during training (TEE) 16,
    17
energy intake, dangers of inadequate
  female-athlete triad 20
  neutral energy balance 18
  sufficient energy consumption 18, 20
energy needs
  activity level 17
  calories and joules 14, 15
  daily energy requirements, components
    16-17
  doubly labeled water 15, 16
  energy, description of 14
  estimating, methods of 15-18, 19*t*
  estimating DEE from its components 17, 19*t*
  kilocalorie 15
  meeting 14
  resting energy expenditure (REE), studies
    15
  of vegetarian athletes, studies 14, 15
ergocalciferol (vegetarian vitamin D) 73
ergogenic aid 137
ergonomics in kitchen 210-211
essential amino acids 56, 56*t*, 57
excess postexercise oxygen consumption
    (EPOC) 16-17

F
fat
  benefits of 39-40
  dietary fat and body fat, studies 46-47
  dietary fats 48
  diets low in fat 45-46
  droplets 41*f*
  eating too much or too little,
    recommendations 45, 45*t*
  energy source 40
  good fat and bad fat 47-51
  intake as percentage of daily energy 44, 45,
    45*t*
  monounsaturated fat and omega-3s 48-51,
    50*t*, 52*f*, 53*t*
  muscle fat as fuel 41, 42*f*
  need for 39
  needs, determining 44-46, 45*t*
  performance and 42-43
  smart fat 51-54
  stored in adipose tissue 40, 41, 42*f*, 42*t*
  used to fuel exercising muscle 40, 41*f*
ferritin 82

fluid and carbohydrate guidelines 128, 129, 130-131
fluid imbalances and dehydration 155
fluids and nutrition during exercise
    carbohydrate supplementation 123
    dehydration and overhydration 124
    fluid intake 123-124, 126
    hyponatremia (water intoxication) 124, 125
    protein, carbohydrates, and fluids, study 125
    sweat rate and fluid requirements during exercise 125
fluoride
    function of 75
    public water supply 75-76
    sources of 75
folate 103-104, 104*t*
folic acid 103
food guidance systems 230-231
food labels
    description of 186
    ingredient list 186, 187-188, 187*t*, 188*f*
food *vs.* supplements 114
formation 66
free radicals 98
fruit juices 128, 130

G
gluconeogenesis 24, 56
glycemic index of common foods 232
grab-and-go breakfasts 220, 221
grills 224
grocery store tour 212, 212*t*, 213-214
Guide to Food Ingredients 187

H
heartburn 117
hematuria 83
hemoglobin 82
hemolysis 83
hemosiderin 82
herbs and spices 212
hormones and bone health
    androgen deficiency 68
    estrogen 68
    parathyroid hormone (PTH) 67-68
    vitamin D and calcitonin 68
Howard, Desmond 2
hunger 117
hydrogenated fats and trans fats 49
hydroxyapatite 66
hyperkalemia 158
hypokalemia 158
hyponatremia (water intoxication) 124, 125

I
inflammation and diet
    antioxidants and anti-inflammatory agents 168-169
    nutrition tips for reducing 164
    omega-3 fatty acids 164-165
    vitamin D 165-167
inflammation and injury
    diet 163-169
    role of inflammation 162
    tissue damage 1, 162-163, 163*f*

inflammation and muscle cramps
    causes of 152, 153
    diet 154-160
    dietary factors and inflammation 152
    fatigue 153
    occurrences of 151, 152
    passive stretching 153
    research 152
    treatment for 153
injury. *See* inflammation and injury
intestinal cramping. *See* diarrhea, intestinal cramping, and bloating
iodine
    iodized salt 111
    role and status 111
iron
    daily iron requirements 83
    excessive 93
    function of 82
    hematuria 83
    hemolysis 83
    importance of 82
    losing through GI bleeding 83
    nonheme and heme 87, 89
    requirements for athletes 83-84
    supplements 92-93, 94
iron deficiency
    absorption from plant sources 89, 90*t*
    anemia 84
    cognitive function 84, 85
    food sources of 87, 88*t*-89*t*
    intake and absorption, boosting 92
    iron skillet or iron egg 87
    performance impairment 85-86
    plant sources inhibiting absorption 89, 90*t*, 91*t*, 92
    prevalence of 86
    research 86
    results of 84-86
    risk factors for 86-92
    stages of 85
    sufficient iron intake and absorption 87-92
    vitamin C foods with iron 89, 91*t*

J
joules 14, 15
Jurek, Scott 2

K
King, Billie Jean 2

L
limiting amino acids or acids 57
low bone density and osteoporosis 20

M
magnesium
    deficiencies in 74, 75
    food sources of 75
    importance of 73-74
magnetic resonance spectroscopy 26
malignant hyperthermia (MH) 162
Manetti, Bill 2
meal plan
    adding or subtracting servings 184, 185
    3,000-calorie vegan meal plan 178, 179, 180*t*

meal plan *(continued)*
 3,000-calorie vegetarian meal plan 178, 179, 179*t*
 checklist approach 181, 182*f*
 coffee, tea and alcohol 184
 customizing 176-185
 eating intuitively, learning 185-186
 evaluating 181
 food combinations 180-181
 food combinations with 250 additional calories 178, 178*t*
 food groups, reasons for 172-173, 174*t*, 176*f*
 food guidance systems 172
 food labels, using 186-188
 key nutrients in food guidance systems 174*t*
 models for vegetarian athletes 175-176, 176*f*
 personal nutritional goals 181, 183
 rest day 185
 USDA or other nutrient databases 188
 using USDA Food Guide Pyramid or Vegetarian Food Guide Pyramid 176, 177*t*
 variety, importance of 173, 175
meals, postexercise
 carbohydrate consumption 132-133
 factors influencing 132
 importance of 132
 mixed meal 133, 134
 recommendations 132, 133, 133*t*
meals and snacks
 basics, keeping 215-224
 cookbooks 215
 difference taste preferences 210
 ergonomics 210-211
 getting started 210-215, 212*t*
 grab-and-go breakfasts 220, 221
 grocery store tour 211, 211*t*, 213-214
 healthy smoothies 222*t*
 healthy snacks 221
 herbs and spices 211
 keeping it exciting 224-226
 menu plan 215-216, 217*t*
 pantry, organizing 210
 planned-overs 216
 portable lunches 220, 221, 222-223
 quick and simple plans 216, 218, 218*t*, 219
 salad 218, 220
 storage containers 211
 store list 223-224
meat eating, history of 55-56
medium-chain triglycerides (MCTs) 49
metric conversions for common measures 236
minerals
 copper 112
 iodine 111
 trace minerals 112, 113*t*
 zinc 109-111
monosaturated fats 48
monounsaturated fat and omega-3s
 benefits of 48-49 50, 51
 recommendations 50*t*, 51, 52*f*, 53*t*
multivitamins
 better food choices 97-99

 B vitamins 99-105
 free radicals and antioxidants 98
 fruits and vegetables *vs.* supplements 99
 with less reliance on supplements 99-109
 macronutrients and micronutrients 96
 retaining nutrients in food 99
 taking, considerations 112, 113-114
 vegetarians deficiencies, claims 95-96
 vitamin A and carotenoids 106-107, 107*t*
 vitamin C 105-106
 vitamin E 108, 108*t*, 109
 vitamins *vs.* minerals 97
muscle cramping and diet
 calcium 158-159
 carbohydrate 159, 160
 cramps caused by mineral deficiency 162
 fluid imbalances and dehydration 155
 improvements in 162
 magnesium 70*t*, 159, 160*t*
 malignant hyperthermia (MH) 162
 nutritional causes, ruling out (box 11.2) 161
 potassium 157, 157*t*, 158
 sodium 155-156
 sweat 156
muscle cramps and inflammation
 causes of 152, 153
 diet 154-160
 dietary factors and inflammation 152
 fatigue 153
 occurrences of 151, 152
 passive stretching 153
 research 152
 treatment for 153
muscle-electrolyte concentrations 153
myoglobin 82
MyPyramid 172, 176

N

nausea 117
Navratilova, Martina 2
neutral energy balance 18
nonessential amino acids 56, 56*t*
nutrition, preevent
 carbohydrate loading and nutrition 121-123
 concerns for preevent meals 116, 117-118
 fasting and early-morning workouts 121
 improved performance and 116, 118
 preevent meals, importance of 116
 when and what to eat 117-118, 119-121, 119*t*, 120*t*
nutrition and bone health
 caffeine, alcohol, and soy isoflavones 77, 78*t*
 calcium 68-72, 70*t*-71*t*, 71*f*
 fluoride 75-76
 magnesium 73-75
 phosphorus 76
 vitamin D 72-73, 73*t*
 vitamins K, C, A 76-77, 91*t*, 107*t*
nutrition and fluids during exercise
 carbohydrate supplementation 123
 dehydration and overhydration 124
 fluid intake 123-124, 126
 hyponatremia (water intoxication) 124, 125
 protein, carbohydrates, and fluids, study 125

sweat rate and fluid requirements during exercise 125
nutrition during training and competition
  dehydration and sweat rate 125, 126
  fluid and carbohydrate intake 119t, 126
  higher carbohydrate intakes 126, 127f
  personal fluid intake plan 127-128

O

omega-3 fatty acids
  description of 48
  eicosanoids 164
  inflammatory response 164-165
  nagging athletic injuries, studies 165, 166
  role of 164
  sources of 165, 167t
omega-6 fatty acids 48
omega-3 fatty acids and monounsaturated fat
  benefits of 48-4950, 51
  recommendations 50t, 51, 52f, 53t
osteoarthritis 166
osteoblasts 66
osteoclasts 66
osteoporosis and low bone density 20
overreaching 30

P

pantry, organizing 210, 212t
Parish, Robert 2
Parrish, Louis 210
passive stretching 153
pedometer 201
performance
  fat's influence on 42-43
performance and carbohydrates
  high-carbohydrate diets, research 25
  magnetic resonance spectroscopy 26
  optimal bioenergetic state, study 26
performance benefits
  early feats of vegetarian athletes 8, 8t
  endurance performance 8, 9
  short-term intervention studies 9
  studies 7-9
phosphorus 76
phytochemicals 97-98
polyunsaturated fats 48
portable lunches 220, 221, 222-223
potassium 157, 157t, 158
pressure cookers 224
protein
  essential and nonessential amino acids 56, 56t, 57
  excess 62-63
  importance of 56
  isolated protein 63-64
  supplements 63-64
protein needs
  athletes vs. general population 59, 59t
  determining 57-59
  energy and carbohydrate intake 57, 58
  food combinations with all essential amino acids 60, 60t
  meeting 59-62
  protein intake, counting 60, 61t, 62, 62t
  training program considerations 57

vegetarian athletes in intense training 60
vegetarian diet 59-60
vegetarians 58
Prudhomme, Paul 39

R

Ramaala, Hendrick 136
rebound hypoglycemia 117
recovery benefits
  antioxidants (or phytochemicals), studies 9
  free radicals, studies 9-10
research and vegetarian advantage
  data from Adventist Health Study 6, 7t
  health benefits 5-6, 7t
  lifestyle factors 6
  meat intake and health risks, studies 5-6
  performance benefits 7-9, 8t
  plant foods, benefits 6
  recovery benefits 9-10
resting energy expenditure (REE) 15, 16, 17
rheumatoid arthritis 166
riboflavin 101, 102t-103t
rice cookers 224
Rolls, Barbara 200
Runner's World 151

S

saturated fats and trans fats
  assessing diet 49-50, 50t
  dietary fats 48
  high-density lipoprotein (HDL) cholesterol 49
  recommendations 47, 49
  saturated fats, description of 48
  sources of 47
  unnatural trans fats 49
Scott, Dave 2
selenium 112, 113t
serum ferritin 82
slow cookers 224
smart fat
  benefits of 51, 53t, 54
  choosing 52f, 54
snacks, healthy 221
sodium 155-156
soy isoflavones 77, 78t
sport drinks and gels 128, 129
sports anemia 94
storage containers 211
store list 223-224
supplement evaluation
  keeping watchful eye 140, 141
  product and claims 141
  regular use, questions before taking 138, 140
  research regarding claims 141-142
  risks and costs 142-143
  safe, vegetarian, and legal 139t, 142
  SupplementWatch 139t, 141
supplement(s)
  appeal of 136-137
  FDA safeguards 138
  Germany's Commission E 138
  glucosamine and chondroitin 169
  primer 136-137

supplement(s) *(continued)*
  regulation of 137-138
  sources for information about 138, 139*t*
supplements of interest to vegetarians
  beta-hydroxy-beta-methylbutyrate (HMB)
    147
  caffeine 145-147, 146*t*
  carnitine 145
  conjugated linoleic acid (CLA) 147-148
  creatine 143-145
  herbals and other supplements 139*t*, 148,
    149*t*
  questions before taking 140
sweat, diet and muscle cramping 156
sweat rate and fluid requirements during
    exercise 125

T

team sports, carbohydrates and fluids 131
Tergat, Paul 136
testosterone myth 205
thermic effect of food (TEF) 16, 17
trabecular bone 67
trans fats and hydrogenated fats 49
trans fats and saturated fats
  assessing diet 49-50, 50*t*
  dietary fats 48
  high-density lipoprotein (HDL) cholesterol
    49
  recommendations 47, 49
  saturated fats, description of 48
  sources of 47
  unnatural trans fats 49
transferrin 82
triglycerides 48

U

USDA National Database for Standard
    Reference 188
USDA pyramid 172

V

vegetarian athletes
  percentage of 2
  types of 2-4
vegetarian diet and bone health
  optimal bone health 79-80
  poor bone health risks, research 78
vegetarian diets
  athletes of ancient Olympics 4
  categorizing vegetarians 3
  Daniel (Bible) 4
  historical advantages of 4
  including fish and poultry, study 3, 4
  interest in 2
  purists *vs.* eating dairy or animal foods 10,
    12
  reasons for following 2
  research supporting 5-10
  scientific evidence 5-10
  vegetarian diet, transitioning to 11-12
  vs. omnivorous diets 1
Vegetarian Food Guide Pyramid 176, 176*f*

vinegar 200-201
vitamin A and carotenoids 106-107, 107*t*
vitamin B₆ 104, 105, 105*t*
vitamin C
  benefits of 106
  recovery from intense training 106
  roles of 105
  sources of 106
vitamin D
  deficiency in 72, 73
  dosage 167
  food sources of 72, 73*t*
  recommended amounts of 73
  role of 165, 166
  studies 167
  sunlight exposure 72, 73
vitamin E 108, 108*t* 109
vitamins K, C, and A 76-77, 91*t*, 107*t*

W

water intoxication 124, 125
weight management and meal plan
  customizing plan 197, 198, 199*t*
  gaining weight 204
  low testosterone myth 205
  overweight issues 191
  physics of 190-191
  promoting weight gain 204, 206, 207
  tricks or maintenance 197, 199-203
  vegetarian athletes 189-190
  weight gain, physics of 203
  weight-loss plan, considerations 192
  weight-reduction plan 192-197
weight-reduction plan
  alcohol 200
  breakfast, don't skip 199
  calcium 201-202
  carbohydrates 193-194
  D word and aids in weight loss 202-203
  fat 195
  fluids and cutting back on supplements
    195-196
  food records 201
  fruits, vegetables, vitamins, minerals, and
    energy-dense foods 195
  losing slowly 196-197
  low-calorie, high-volume appetizer 200
  pedometer 201
  portion sizes 196
  protein 194-195
  restricting calories 192-193
  vinegar 200-201
woks 224

Z

Zemel, Michael 201
zinc
  absorption rate 109-110
  role of 109
  sources of 102*t*-103*t*, 110
  vegetarian diet and 109-110
  zinc status 110, 111

About the Author

D. Enette Larson-Meyer, PhD, RD, FACSM, is an assistant professor of Human Nutrition at the University of Wyoming, where she also serves as director of the nutrition and exercise laboratory. She is a registered dietitian with training in exercise physiology and has experience working with vegetarian (and nonvegetarian) athletes. Her research focuses on how nutrition and metabolism influence the health and performance of active people.

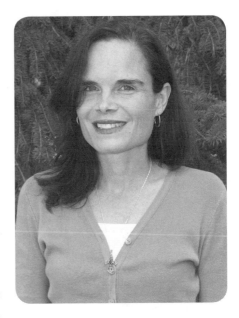

Dr. Larson-Meyer served as the sports nutritionist for the University of Alabama at Birmingham Athletic Department from 1995 to 2000, and she has consulted with numerous athletes throughout her career. She is a fellow of the American College of Sports Medicine and is past chair of the Vegetarian Nutrition Dietetic Practice Group. Dr. Larson-Meyer has published numerous scientific and consumer articles, has been featured in publications like *Vegetarian Journal*, and has served as a chapter contributor to publications including the American Dietetic Association's *Sports Nutrition: A Guide for the Professional Working with Active People* and the International Olympic Committee Medical Commission's *Volleyball (Handbook of Sports Medicine and Science)*. She completed her dietetic internship at Massachusetts General Hospital in 1988 and also completed an internship at the Olympic Training Center in Colorado Springs during her undergraduate training. Larson-Meyer received her PhD in Nutrition Sciences from the University of Alabama in 1998.

A serious recreational athlete for close to 20 years, Larson-Meyer enjoys running distance events, cycling, and dancing in her spare time. She lives in Laramie, Wyoming with her husband and three children.

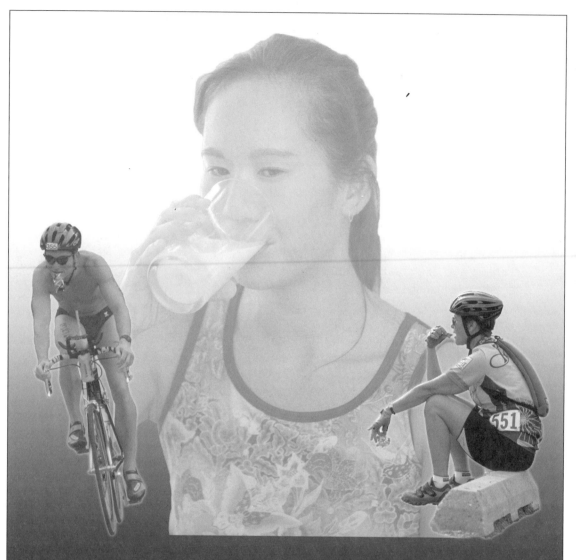